Biochemistry of Schizophrenia and Addiction

Biochemistry of Schizophrenia and Addiction

In Search of a Common Factor

Edited by

Gwynneth Hemmings
Honorary Secretary,
The Schizophrenia Association of Great Britain

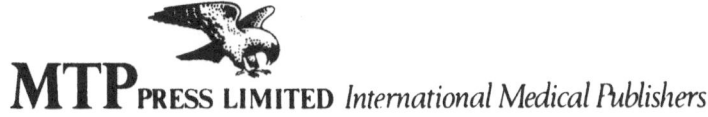

MTPPRESS LIMITED *International Medical Publishers*

Published by
MTP Press Limited
Falcon House
Lancaster, England

Copyright © 1980 MTP Press Limited
Softcover reprint of the hardcover 1st edition 1980

British Library Cataloguing in Publication Data

Biochemistry of Schizophrenia and Addiction
  1. Schizophrenia – Congresses
  2. Drug abuse – Congresses
  I. Hemmings, Gwynneth II. Schizophrenia
Association of Great Britain
616.8'982   RC514

ISBN-13: 978-94-009-8708-1   e-ISBN-13: 978-94-009-8706-7
DOI: 10.1007/978-94-009-8706-7

Contents

SECTION 3: ADDICTION

SECTION 4: PUERPERAL PSYCHOSES

SECTION 5: ENZYMOLOGY

SECTION 6: PHYSIOLOGY

SECTION 7: MORBIDITY AND MORTALITY

SECTION 8: DRUG TREATMENTS

List of Contributors

C. W. ABELL
Department of Human Biological
  Chemistry and Genetics
Division of Biochemistry
The University of Texas Medical Branch
Galveston, Texas 77550, USA

A. ASHKENAZI
Department of Pediatrics A
  and Pediatric Research Laboratory
Kaplan Hospital
Rehovot, Israel

J. A. BALDWIN
Unit of Clinical Epidemiology
University of Oxford
Oxford, United Kingdom

J. F. BRIDGES
Department of Gastroenterology
University of Manchester
Manchester, United Kingdom

I. F. BROCKINGTON
Department of Psychiatry
University Hospital of South Manchester
Manchester, United Kingdom

B. COSTALL
Postgraduate School of Studies in
  Pharmacology
University of Bradford
Bradford, United Kingdom

T. J. CROW
Division of Psychiatry
Clinical Research Centre
Harrow HA1 3UJ, United Kingdom

S. C. CUNNANE
P.O. Box 10
Nun's Island, Montreal H3E 1J8
Canada

J. F. W. DEAKIN
Departments of Neurophysiology
  and Neuropharmacology
National Institute for Medical Research
Mill Hill, London, United Kingdom

A. DELL
Department of Biochemistry
Imperial College
London SW7, United Kingdom

A. M. DENMAN
Division of Immunology
Clinical Research Centre and
  Northwick Park Hospital
Harrow HA1 3UJ, United Kingdom

M. DONNER
Research Unit of Experimental
  Cancerology and Radiobiology (U.95)
I.N.S.E.R.M.
Plateau de Brabois
54500 Vandoeuvre-lès-Nancy, France

A. T. ETIENNE
Department of Biochemistry
Imperial College
London SW7, United Kingdom

W. P. FAULK
Blond McIndoe Centre for Transplantation
  Biology
Queen Victoria Hospital
East Grinstead, United Kingdom

L. FAULKNER
Department of Biological Sciences
University of Keele
Keele, United Kingdom

T. FORSYTH
Department of Biological Sciences
University of Keele
Keele, United Kingdom

D. L. FRANCIS
Research Department
Miles Laboratories Ltd.
Stoke Poges, Slough SL2 4LY
    United Kingdom

D. L. FREED
Departments of Bacteriology and Virology
University of Manchester Medical School
Manchester, United Kingdom

A. C. GIBSON
Department of Psychiatry
St Ann's Hospital
Canford Cliffs, Poole, United Kingdom

Y. GINAT
Department of Psychiatry H
Talbieh Psychiatric Hospital
Jerusalem, Israel

K. GREGORY
Department of Psychiatry
University Hospital of South Manchester
Manchester, United Kingdom

G. H. HALL
Department of Pharmacology
School of Pharmacy
Sunderland Polytechnic
Sunderland SR1 3SD, United Kingdom

B. HALPERIN
Department of Psychiatry D
Talbieh Psychiatric Hospital
Jerusalem, Israel

W. Th. J. M. HEKKENS
Department of Gastroenterology
University Hospital
Leiden, The Netherlands

S. M. HILTON
Department of Physiology
The Medical School
University of Birmingham
Birmingham, United Kingdom

D. F. HORROBIN
P.O. Box 10
Nun's Island, Montreal H3E 1J8
    Canada

D. IDAR
Pediatric Research Laboratory
Kaplan Hospital
Rehovot, Israel

M. KALIAN
Department of Psychiatry D
Talbieh Psychiatric Hospital
Jerusalem, Israel

W. A. KLEE
Laboratory of General and Comparative
    Biochemistry
National Institute of Mental Health
Bethesda, Maryland 20014, USA

D. KRASILOWSKY
Talbieh Psychiatric Hospital
Jerusalem, Israel

S. LEVIN
Department of Pediatrics A and Pediatric
    Research Laboratory
Kaplan Hospital
Rehovot, Israel

J. M. LITTLETON
Department of Pharmacology
King's College
London, United Kingdom

J. LUCY
Department of Biological Sciences
University of Keele
Keele, United Kingdom

J. A. MCINTYRE
Blond McIndoe Centre for Transplantation
    Biology
Queen Victoria Hospital
East Grinstead, United Kingdom

A. MAKIN
Department of Biological Sciences
University of Keele
Keele, United Kingdom

M. S. MANKU
P.O. Box 10
Nun's Island, Montreal H3E 1J8
    Canada

D. L. MARGULES
Department of Psychology
Temple University
Philadelphia, Pennsylvania 19122, USA

J. N. MEHRISHI
Department of Medicine
University of Cambridge
Addenbrooke's Hospital
Cambridge CB2 2QQ, United Kingdom

H. R. MORRIS
Department of Biochemistry
Imperial College
London SW7, United Kingdom

R. J. NAYLOR
Postgraduate School of Studies in
    Pharmacology
University of Bradford
Bradford, United Kingdom

M. OKA
P.O. Box 10
Nun's Island, Montreal H3E 1J8
    Canada

A. OR
Pediatric Research Laboratory
Kaplan Hospital
Rehovot, Israel

E. PULKKINEN
Kellokoski Hospital
04500 Kellokoski, Finland

A. J. M. SCHIPPERIJN
Department of Internal Medicine
Psychiatric Clinic "Sancta Maria"
Noordwijkerhout, The Netherlands

E. SCHOFIELD
Department of Psychiatry
University Hospital of South Manchester
Manchester, United Kingdom

E. E. STERCHI
Abteilung für Gastroenterologie
Universitäts-Kinderklinik
Bern, Switzerland

J. F. WOODLEY
Department of Biological Sciences
University of Keele
Keele, United Kingdom

C. ZIOUDROU
Department of Biology
Nuclear Research Center "Democritos"
Aghia Paraskevi, Attiki, Greece

Preface

The main theme of this book concerns the relationship, if any, between schizophrenia and addiction. Are they linked biochemically? Is there a common factor for all addictions? We need to know whether the chemistry of addiction can help clarify the biochemistry of schizophrenia and vice versa. There is much anecdotal evidence that many sufferers from schizophrenia *are* addicted to smoking, *are* adversely affected by even small amounts of alcohol and do have their schizophrenic illness worsened by street drugs. We would urge our readers to try to find correlations between some of the findings described here on the biology of schizophrenia and what they read in the up-to-date chapters on addictions.

We would like to thank all the authors for the excellence of their work and for their cooperation and understanding of our needs and also, for the second time this year, to thank MTP Press for their willingness to publish a perhaps somewhat provocative book. We thank them for their humanity.

Gwynneth Hemmings
Tyr Twr
Llanfair Hall
Caernarvon
Gwynedd
Wales

Foreword

The Schizophrenia Association is committed to the belief that schizophrenia is a biochemical disorder affecting the brain and also influencing many other systems of the body. The Association has been strongly criticized for this belief which many think is based on inadequate evidence. However the history of science and medicine demonstrates conclusively that most major advances have been achieved by those who began to believe in a concept long before the evidence was fully convincing. It is this type of faith which has so often provided the driving force enabling people to carry on when faced with enormous difficulties and great scepticism. When the faith proves justified, the outcome is triumph; when the critics are right there is tragedy.

Is the final outcome of the efforts of the Schizophrenia Association and its friends to be tragedy or triumph? It now seems to me that the hypothetical impartial observer must be convinced that triumph is a more likely result. The evidence that schizophrenics are physically and chemically different from others, that schizophrenia is a disease of the body which particularly affects the brain, is increasingly persuasive. This book gathers together much of that evidence in a most valuable way. This evidence comes from many different fields of study and the overall impression is that while much remains to be done, the outcome is now almost certain. Within the next twenty years schizophrenia will be shown to be a disease – or more probably several diseases – in which biochemical disarray leads to brain malfunction.

Turning from the general question of schizophrenia I should like to use this foreword to pay a particular tribute to the efforts of Mrs Gwynneth Hemmings and her family and friends who have overcome formidable obstacles in order to keep the Association going and to organize a series of conferences of which this is the latest. Only great enthusiasm and great determination could have achieved what they have done and it seems to me that the worlds of schizophrenics and of researchers on schizophrenia owe them a great debt. Such a debt can, of course, never be repaid, but I know that the Hemmings family will be more than satisfied if as now seems likely their efforts have contributed in a real way to the control of this most difficult disease.

David F. Horrobin

List of Abbreviations

AA	arachidonic acid
ACh	acetylcholine
ACTH	adrenocorticotrophic hormone
ADA	adenosine deaminase
ADH	antidiuretic hormone
ADP	adenosine diphosphate
AFC	antibody forming cells
BGG	bovine gammaglobulin
BLM	bucco-linguo-masticatory
cAMP / cyclic AMP	cyclic 3′,5′-adenosine monophosphate
CDR	calcium dependent regulator
cGMP / cyclic GMP	cyclic 3′,5′-guanosine monophosphate
CK	cholecystokinin
cLA	*cis*-linoleic acid
CMI	cell mediated immunity
CPZ	chlorpromazine
DA	dopamine
DGLA	dihomogammalinolenic acid
DNLCA	3′,4′-deoxynorlaudanosolinecarboxylic acid
DOPS	dihydroxyphenylserine
DPA	n-dipropylacetate
EB	Epstein–Barr (virus infections)
EFA	essential fatty acids
EPM	electrophoretic mobility
Flu	fluphenazine
FSH	follicle stimulating hormone
GABA	gamma amino butyric acid
GLA	gamma linolenic acid

GTP	guanosine triphosphate
HC	hydrocortisone
HCG	human chorionic gonadotropin
HLA	human leukocyte antigens
HPLC	high pressure liquid chromatography
HRBC	horse erythrocytes
HRP	horse-radish peroxidase
5HT	5-hydroxytryptamine
HVA	homovanillic acid
IBMX	3-isobutyl-1-methylxanthine
IMPS	inpatient multidimensional psychiatric scale
KLH	keyhole limpet haemocyanin
LH	luteinizing hormone
LHRH	luteinizing hormone releasing factor
LIF	leukocyte migration inhibition factor
MAF	macrophage activating factor
MAO	monoamine oxidase
MHC	major histocompatibility complex
MIF	macrophage inhibition factor
MLC	mixed lymphocyte culture
MNLCA	3'-O-methylnorlaudanosolinecarboxylic acid
MPS	methylprednisolone
MSH	melanocyte stimulating hormone
NA	noradrenaline
αNOAA	α-naphthyloxyacetic acid
PAAS	premorbid asocial adjustment scale
PAG	periaqueductal grey
PAL	phenylalanine ammonia-lyase
PBL	peripheral blood lymphocytes
PCPA	parachlorophenylalanine
PDE	phosphodiesterase
PG	prostaglandin
PHA	phytohaemagglutinin
PMN	polymorphonuclear
PWM	pokeweed mitogen
QMWS	quasi morphine withdrawal syndrome
REM	rapid eye movements
RIA	radioimmunoassay

SCID   Swiss type combined immunodeficiency disease
SKSD   streptokinase-streptodornase
SLE   systemic lupus erythematosus
SRBC   sheep erythrocytes
SSS   pneumococcal polysaccharides
STH   somatotropin

TD   tardive dyskinesia
Thio   thioridazine
TRH   thyrotropin releasing hormone
TSH   thyroid stimulating hormone

VIP   vasoactive intestinal polypeptides

WBI   word behaviour inventory

Section 1:
PATHOGENESIS

1
The role of a prostaglandin E_1 deficiency in schizophrenia: interactions with dopamine and opiates

D. F. HORROBIN, M. S. MANKU, M. OKA and S. C. CUNNANE

INTRODUCTION

There is evidence for a prostaglandin (PG) E_1 deficiency in schizophrenia. Dopamine is able to antagonize some of the effects of PGE_1 on excitable tissues and the fundamental problem may therefore be an elevated dopamine: PGE_1 ratio. Schizophrenia should therefore be made worse by factors which raise this ratio and alleviated by factors which lower it. Opiates and various dietary deficiencies may lower PGE_1 formation whereas prolactin and melatonin may enhance it. Most of the existing antischizophrenic drugs may function because they have three separate actions which will tend to lower the effective dopamine/PGE_1 ratio. They block dopamine receptors, they enhance prolactin secretion and they enhance melatonin secretion. This concept leads to new therapeutic strategies which seem worthy of trial.

The idea that schizophrenia may be related to a defect in the formation of prostaglandins (PGs) of the 1 series, probably accompanied by normal or even excess production of PGs of the 2 series has been discussed in detail previously (Horrobin, 1977a and b; Horrobin *et al.*, 1978; Horrobin, 1979). The main pieces of evidence are as follows:

(1) Schizophrenics are resistant to such conditions as rheumatoid arthritis and pain in which increased PG synthesis may play a part.

3

(2) Schizophrenic states may temporarily remit during fever and after epileptiform convulsions, situations in which brain PG synthesis is enhanced.

(3) Most effective antischizophrenic drugs enhance the secretion of prolactin, a hormone which increases the production of PGE_1 (Manku *et al.*, 1979a).

(4) Platelet preparations from schizophrenics when subjected to a complex preparative procedure fail to form PGE_1 in the usual way when exposed to ADP (Abdulla and Hamadah, 1975). In preliminary studies using the much simpler procedure of simply incubating the radioactive precursor of PGE_1 (dihomogammalinolenic acid, DGLA) with whole platelets, we have been able to confirm that platelets from schizophrenics seem to form much less PGE_1 than those from normals.

(5) Platelets from schizophrenics fail to form normal amounts of cAMP when exposed to PGE_1 (Rotrosen *et al.*, 1978). A similar defect has been described in platelets from severely essential fatty acid deficient animals in which endogenous PGE_1 production is defective (Vincent *et al.*, 1974).

(6) Clozapine, the only effective antischizophrenic agent whose potency is much greater than expected on the basis of its weak prolactin-stimulating action, has actions similar to PGE_1 in a rat vascular preparation and has a structure which is related to known PG agonists/antagonists (Manku and Horrobin, unpublished results). In animal behavioural studies, clozapine and PGs have similar effects (Bloss and Singer, 1978). It therefore seems possible that clozapine is able to activate PGE_1 receptors directly.

DOPAMINE AND PGE_1

In one or other of its various forms the 'dopamine concept' is perhaps the dominant one in schizophrenia at the moment. Although direct evidence has proved difficult to obtain, the indirect evidence is strong and has often been reviewed (Crow *et al.*, 1977; Iversen, 1977; Gruen, 1978). The consistent ability of most antischizophrenic drugs to block dopamine receptors, the similarity between amphetamine psychosis (believed to be due to enhanced dopamine release) and schizophrenia, and the apparently increased dopamine receptor levels in some areas of schizophrenic brains (Lee *et al.*, 1978; Owen *et al.*, 1978) are the most striking points.

The strength of the evidence that in some way the biological activity of dopamine is enhanced in schizophrenics led us to investigate the interactions between dopamine and PGE_1, in an isolated excitable tissue preparation, the mesenteric vascular muscle of the rat. In this preparation PGE_1 has biphasic actions (Manku et al., 1979a). At low to moderate concentrations it enhances calcium release in response to activating agents but at high concentrations it inhibits such release. In isolated nerve preparations, at the same concentrations at which PGE_1 enhances calcium release, it increases action potential amplitude and conduction velocity (Horrobin et al., 1977). At the concentrations at which PGE_1 inhibits calcium release, it also reduces action potential amplitude and slows conduction velocity. These effects occur at strictly physiological concentrations and if they take place in the brain as well can be expected to modify brain function profoundly.

Our studies on PGE_1 and dopamine in the mesenteric muscle have revealed a series of complex, concentration-dependent interactions (Oka, Manchu and Horrobin, in preparation). In essence we can say that dopamine interferes with the effects of PGE_1 in enhancing calcium release, without blocking those effects which inhibit calcium release. Therefore in order to have normal calcium release in an excitable tissue, the ratio between dopamine and PGE_1 effects must be correct. Similar problems will be caused both by very low and very high PGE_1 : dopamine ratios. Dopamine antagonism of PGE_1 stimulation of cAMP formation in a cultured nerve cell line has also been reported (Myers et al., 1978). In schizophrenia, because of the evidence for low PGE_1 levels and excess dopamine activity, we propose that the ratio of PGE_1 activity to dopamine activity is low and that measures which restore this ratio to the normal range will be therapeutically effective.

Opiates, opioids and PGE_1

Recently considerable interest has been generated by the possible involvement of the endogenous opiate compounds, the opioids, or endorphins and enkephalins in schizophrenia. On injection into animals these agents can produce a catatonic state (Bloom et al., 1976). The opioid antagonist, naloxone, can relieve hallucinations in some patients, and although there have been several negative reports it seems possible that these studies have used inadequate doses (Gunne et al., 1977; Watson et al., 1978). Much more naloxone may be required to reverse the effects of an endogenous opioid than of exogenous morphine. Increased amounts of endorphin have been found in cerebrospinal fluid (CSF) from schizophrenics, particularly in the acute phase (Terenius et al., 1976; Domschke et al., 1979) and an apparently abnormal leu-endorphin has been found in dialysis fluid from schizophrenics (Palmour and Ervin, 1977).

The opioid concept has recently unexpectedly linked with another idea, that schizophrenia is related to increased consumption of wheat, rye and other cereals and that in those with abnormal gastrointestinal permeability certain peptide products of digestion of these cereals may enter the body and disturb brain function. The idea was first proposed by Dohan, who has recently reviewed the concept (Dohan, 1979). A dietary study under controlled conditions demonstrated that withdrawal of wheat and other cereals may improve schizophrenics (Singh and Kay, 1976). However the approach generated relatively little interest until Zioudrou et al. (1979) demonstrated that a number of proteins, including some from cereals and α-casein from milk, were able to generate in the gut substances which behaved as opioids and which have been termed exorphins. Hemmings (1978) has shown that surprisingly large peptides may pass the gut wall and reach the brain. It therefore seems possible that both endogenous opioids and exogenous opioids generated by food may modify brain function.

We have demonstrated that β-endorphin has actions consistent with inhibition of PGE_1 formation in the rat mesentery (Manku et al., 1978). We have recently explored this opiate/PG interaction in human platelets incubated with either DGLA, the precursor of PGE_1, or with arachidonic acid, the precursor of 2 series PGs. Using l- and d-levorphanol, the former having opiate activity, and the latter not, we have been able to demonstrate the following (Manku, Oka and Horrobin, in preparation).

(1) l-levorphanol modulates the formation of PGE_1 from DGLA but the d-isomer has no effect.

(2) l-levorphanol has no significant effects on the formation of 2 series PGs from arachidonic acid.

(3) l-levorphanol has biphasic effects, enhancing PGE_1 formation at low concentrations and blocking PGE_1 formation at high concentrations. Both these effects are prevented by the opiate antagonist, naloxone.

It is currently believed that many biphasic effects in pharmacology are dependent on the activation of two types of receptor (Horrobin, 1977a). We therefore suggest that in human platelets there may be two types of receptor for opiates, one of which activates PGE_1 formation and the other of which blocks it. An alternative explanation is that there is one receptor which is activated by low concentrations and blocked by higher concentrations. Either way we predict that by further analysis of this effect some opiate/opioid compounds will be identified which will act selectively on one or other function, i.e. some will be relatively pure stimulators of PGE_1 formation while others will be relatively pure inhibitors. Other relevant effects of opiates include their ability to inhibit cAMP formation in response to PGE_1 (Collier and Roy, 1974) and to lead to dopamine super-sensitivity (Lal, 1975) both observations being consistent with the concepts outlined in this paper.

Other factors which may influence PGE_1 formation

We have recently been exploring the possible factors which may regulate the formation of PGE_1. They may be divided into two groups; those which seem to be specific for 1 series PGs, and those which are likely to involve both the 1 series and the 2 series. Figure 1 outlines the pathways of biosynthesis.

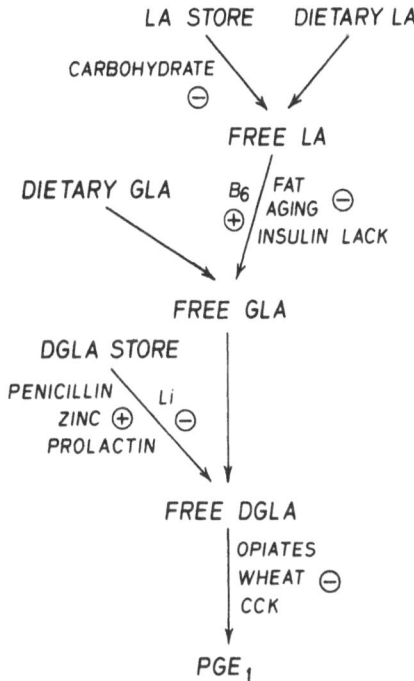

Figure 1 An outline of the pathway of prostaglandin E_1 biosynthesis. LA, linoleic acid; GLA, gammalinolenic acid; DGLA, dihomogammalinolenic acid; B6, pyridoxine; CCK, cholecystokinin. A plus sign indicates activation and a minus sign inhibition. The site of pyridoxine action is not yet clear and could be at the GLA–DGLA step. Niacin may be necessary for the conversion of DGLA to PGE_1, as may vitamin C

FACTORS AFFECTING BOTH 1 AND 2 SERIES

The 1 series PGs are derived immediately from DGLA while the 2 series are formed from arachidonic acid (AA). Neither can be synthesized by the body from simple precursors and the two compounds are essential fatty acids (EFAs) which are sometimes known as vitamin F. There are moderate amounts of AA in meat and dairy products but only very small amounts of DGLA in most foods. DGLA is in large part derived from dietary cis-linoleic acid (cLA), a major constituent of some vegetable oils such as corn, sunflower and safflower but not of others such as olive, peanut and coconut. Trans-linoleic acid (tLA) cannot act as a precursor for DGLA, which is important since hydrogenation of vegetable oils converts much of the cLA to the trans form.

cLA may be oxidized like any other fat, may be esterified and stored, or may be converted to gammalinolenic acid (GLA) the first step in conversion to DGLA and AA. In between meals and during starvation cLA stores become important. The mobilization of cLA is blocked in humans by high blood glucose levels, possibly acting via insulin (Wene et al., 1975). In animals the conversion of cLA to GLA has been shown to be blocked by a high fat intake, by ageing and by insulin deficiency (Brenner, 1974) and the conversion of dietary cLA to GLA therefore seems to be a very vulnerable process, particularly in those on Western style diets.

Pyridoxine (vitamin B6) deficiency leads to symptoms very similar to those of EFA deficiency. Pyridoxine enhances conversion of cLA to AA, although the step at which it acts is uncertain (Witten and Holman, 1952). The most likely candidates are the conversion of cLA to GLA, or of GLA to DGLA, or both.

Finally tryptophan seems to be a necessary co-factor for PG synthesis (Ho et al., 1976) although its relative effects on the 1 and 2 series have not been studied. Niacin may well have a tryptophan-like effect since the vascular flush which follows high dose administration can be blocked by inhibitors of PG synthesis (Kunin, 1976).

Therefore deficiencies in intake of EFAs, of pyridoxine and of tryptophan/niacin are likely to lead to defects in formation of both 1 and 2 series PGs.

Factors specific to the 1 series

There are two rate-limiting steps specific to formation of 1 series PGs. The first is the mobilization of free DGLA from the DGLA stores in the body and the second is the conversion of the free DGLA to the 1 series PGs.

We have explored the first of these steps in the mesenteric bed of the rat. By the following criteria we have come to the conclusion that prolactin, zinc ions, penicillin and penicillamine are able to enhance specifically the mobilization of DGLA without affecting AA mobilization.

(1) These agents have biological effects which are accompanied by the

outflow of PG-like material as indicated by rat stomach bioassay. This is a non-specific assay sensitive to both 1 and 2 series PGs.

(2) The biological effects of these agents can be blocked by aspirin, indomethacin and mefenamic acid which inhibit conversion of both DGLA and AA to their respective prostaglandins.

(3) The biological effects can be imitated by DGLA or PGE_1, but not by AA or any 2 series product.

(4) The biological effects can be blocked by lithium and/or cortisol which do not interfere with the effects of DGLA itself. This indicates that the agents modify the formation of free DGLA but not its conversion to PGE_1.

The arguments for prolactin and zinc have recently been summarized (Manku et al., 1979a). The pineal product, melatonin, does not by itself enhance PGE_1 output in this preparation but it does dramatically increase the effects of the other agents, particularly zinc (Cunnane et al., 1979).

On the basis of these observations we would therefore predict that PGE_1 formation is likely to be defective in those deficient in zinc or melatonin or in those exposed to excess cortisol or lithium. Cortisol is equally effective in blocking AA and DGLA mobilization and will therefore have similar effects on 1 and 2 series PGs, whereas at the concentrations relevant to human use (up to 2 mmol/l), lithium has a relatively selective effect on DGLA alone. Our work on zinc and melatonin is of interest because defects in both zinc metabolism and in pineal function have been postulated in schizophrenics.

Zinc intake is below the daily requirement in many parts of North America and probably in other parts of the world (National Research Council, 1978; Klevay et al., 1979). Acrodermatitis enteropathica, a zinc absorption defect, is associated with schizoid states (Horrobin et al., 1978) and abnormal globulins which have been reported to occur in schizophrenic plasma can bind zinc (Frohman, 1973). Skin striae, similar to those observed in zinc deficiency states, can develop in schizophrenics, and some schizophrenics seem to respond to zinc therapy (Pfeiffer and Cott, 1974). Defects in pineal function have been postulated on two main grounds: (i) a defect in melatonin biosynthesis could lead to formation of harmaline-like hallucinogens (McIsaac, 1961); and (ii) the disorders of pigment deposition in schizophrenic tissues could be explained by melatonin deficiency (Nicolson et al., 1966).

More recently it has been shown that untreated schizophrenics have very low circulating melatonin levels and that phenothiazines may stimulate melatonin production (Ozaki et al., 1976; Smith, 1978). The excess of schizophrenic births in late winter/early spring could be related to changes in melatonin/PGE_1 interactions at this time. We have shown that at the latitude of Montreal the ability of zinc to enhance PGE_1 formation falls precipitously in March/April, that a similar effect follows pinealectomy in mid-winter and that the effect can be reversed by melatonin *in vitro* (Cunnane *et al.*, 1979). There is preliminary evidence that blindness may protect against schizophrenia (Horrobin, 1979). This must be checked by careful epidemiological studies, but if true would be interesting because of the elevated melatonin levels which have been reported in blind people.

Having looked at the mobilization of DGLA we turned to investigate the conversion of AA and DGLA to their respective products by human platelets. We did this without any great optimism because the current dogma is that the first cyclo-oxygenase step in conversion of DGLA and AA is the same for both compounds, and therefore that factors which will affect one or other selectively are unlikely to exist. To our surprise we found that several agents could modify the DGLA conversion without affecting AA and the work on opiates has already been described.

Two other compounds of relevance to psychiatry which had this selective effect were ascorbic acid and ethanol. Over the range 10 μg/ml to 1 mg/ml ascorbic acid caused a dose-dependent increase in PGE_1 formation with little effect on AA metabolism.

Ethanol had a generally similar effect, the threshold in this case being about 30 mg/100 ml exactly the concentration at which the first intoxicating effects in humans begin to be apparent (Manku *et al.*, 1979b, 1979c). The ethanol action is likely to prove of particular importance in psychiatry (Horrobin and Manku, 1979). It suggests that alcoholic intoxication is associated with increased formation of PGE_1. Increased formation of PGE_1 has been described in mania, a condition which is in many ways similar to alcoholic intoxication (Abdulla and Hamadah, 1975); these authors also reported that, in depression, platelet PGE_1 production was lower than normal, though not as low as in schizophrenia. Since body stores of DGLA are limited, excess formation of PGE_1 is likely to be followed by depletion of DGLA, reduced PGE_1 formation and depression. This concept, which is at this stage clearly only speculative, offers an attractive explanation for the mood swings in alcoholism and in manic-depressive psychosis and for the reported therapeutic effects of lithium in both bipolar affective disorders and alcoholism (Kline *et al.*, 1974). Lithium, which inhibits mobilization of DGLA stores, would be expected to limit the level of intoxication and/or mania and would, by conserving DGLA, limit the subsequent fall in PGE_1 production and depression. These concepts have been fully explored elsewhere (Horrobin and Manku, 1979).

The platelet studies therefore suggest that PGE_1 formation may be enhanced selectively by ascorbic acid and by alcohol. Different opioids and opiates may either enhance or inhibit depending on structure and concentration. The effect of opiate antagonists will obviously depend on the background opiate situation. It must be emphasized that the overall effects on the body of these various agents will be quite different, depending on the distribution patterns and on the pattern of opiate receptors. Alcohol and ascorbic acid have quite different distributions among different cells.

CONCEPTS OF SCHIZOPHRENIA

The idea developed in this paper is that schizophrenia-like states will occur when the PGE_1:dopamine ratio is too low. By this ratio we mean the ratio of biological activities of the two compounds, factors which will depend both on rates of formation and release, and on receptor numbers and sensitivity. Since the effects of low and very high PGE_1 levels are similar, a state with schizoid features could occur with a very high PGE_1/dopamine ratio but in our view this is likely to be much less common.

A low PGE_1:dopamine ratio could occur as a result of excess dopamine formation or release, or of supersensitivity of dopamine receptors, or of activation of dopamine receptors by dopamine agonists. The psychoses associated with amphetamine, with L-dopa and with bromocriptine may be of this form. On the other hand the primary abnormality could be on the PGE_1 side. Defective intakes of essential fatty acids, of pyridoxine, of niacin/tryptophan, of zinc and of vitamin C would all affect PGE_1 formation at different sites. A defect in pineal function, excess formation or abnormal formation or defective excretion and degradation of endorphins or enkephalins, and production of exorphins in the gut would also all lead to defective PGE_1 production and a low PGE_1:dopamine ratio.

It is our suspicion that in the end the schizophrenia syndrome will be found to have one or two major causes which will be involved in 90–95% of patients and a whole variety of much rarer causes. Our current guess is that opioid excess and pineal deficiency are the most likely candidates for major causes. It is possible that these are related since opioids may well modify pineal function and vice versa.

In terms of therapy it is already possible to make tentative recommendations starting from the firm base of the known antischizophrenic effects of existing neuroleptics. There is an excellent correlation between the ability of these drugs to block dopamine receptors concerned in the inhibition of prolactin secretion and their therapeutic effects (Meltzer and Gang, 1976; Gruen, 1978). However, maximal effects on prolactin secretion are achieved at drug levels which are therapeutically suboptimal and it is quite clear that all their therapeutic effect cannot be attributed to stimulation of prolactin and therefore of PGE_1 production. But it seems a mistake to swing to the opposite extreme and to state that *none* of the effect can be attributed to prolactin. The other possible effect, the stimulation of melatonin production, has to date been inadequately explored. It is our view, that in the end all three factors, blockade of dopamine receptors and enhancement of prolactin, melatonin and therefore PGE_1 formation, will be found to contribute to the therapeutic action.

While it seems probable that some of the therapeutic actions of these drugs can be attributed to dopamine blockade, it is certain that many of the undesirable side effects, notably the extra-pyramidal problems and the tardive dyskinesias are also caused by dopamine block. Since these side effects are dose dependent, it seems appropriate to enhance the PGE_1 stimulating effects of the drugs so that lower doses may achieve the same change in PGE_1 : dopamine ratio. In principle there are three main ways of influencing PGE_1 formation.

(1) By ensuring that the formation of DGLA in the body is adequate. In order to achieve this there must be sufficient intake of both EFAs and pyridoxine. Because the cLA to GLA step is so susceptible to inhibition, there is potential value in Evening Primrose oil as an EFA source. This contains about 70% cLA but is unique in containing about 10% of GLA (Vaddadi, 1979).

(2) By ensuring that mobilization of DGLA from body stores is adequate. Zinc may be a necessary co-factor and in occasional individuals zinc deficiency may be a cause of a schizophrenic state. Possibly much more important is the idea that, even if not a primary cause, zinc deficiency will limit the biological effectiveness of prolactin and melatonin and will therefore limit the possible therapeutic response. The effects of penicillamine (Nicolson et al., 1966) and penicillin (Chouinard et al., 1978; Vaddadi, 1979) in producing some improvement in some schizophrenics may relate to their mobilization of DGLA.

(3) By ensuring that conversion of DGLA to PGE_1 is adequate. Tryptophan/niacin and ascorbic acid both may be necessary co-factors here. Again deficiencies of these nutrients may be rare causes of the schizophrenia syndrome by themselves but are likely to be more important as factors limiting therapeutic effects. It is our current belief that a major cause of schizophrenia is likely to be inhibition of this reaction by endogenous and/or exogenous opioids. It is possible that the exogenous opioids are important mainly in those who already have an endogenous defect and who may be susceptible to being 'pushed over the edge' by an exogenous source. The encouraging preliminary results with naloxone deserve following up with attention to two concepts which have not been adequately considered so far. Doses of naloxone have been such as would inhibit the actions of exogenous opiate drugs. It is possible that the relevant endogenous opioid has a much higher affinity for the receptors and

therefore that much higher antagonist concentrations will be required to displace it. Secondly it has been assumed that the effects of the opioids are rapid membrane effects and will therefore be very rapidly reversed: trial periods have therefore been extremely short. There is no doubt that these rapid effects do occur, but if part of the action is related to regulation of PGE_1 synthesis, much longer time periods than the usual hour or two will be required to explore the action of naloxone. Furthermore, if naloxone does reverse an inhibitory effect on PGE_1 synthesis, PGE_1 levels will rise only if there are adequate amounts of DGLA precursor available.

CONCLUSIONS

We suggest that the time has come for a different approach to concepts of schizophrenia and to clinical trials in the disease. Much effort has been expended in trying to prove that a particular approach is 'right' or 'wrong'. We suggest that as with the blind men and the elephant (Horrobin, 1978) none of the current approaches is right and perhaps even none is wrong. They are all different aspects of the same fundamental problem which we suggest is a low ratio of PGE_1 to dopamine activity.

The converse of this approach is that none of the current therapeutic concepts is right and that therapeutic attempts to correct a single defect will at best be only partially effective. In particular, if agents are found which have some therapeutic action, the best approach may not be to increase the dose to the limit since at that stage other side effects will inevitably appear. It may be more sensible to combine different approaches in order to achieve the optimum effect. The strategies we would suggest are as follows:

(1) Elimination of possible dietary deficiencies. These, if they exist, will limit the effectiveness of all other therapies. The particular problem areas in Western diets would appear to be essential fatty acids, pyridoxine, tryptophan/niacin, zinc and vitamin C. We are not proposing the use of very large doses of any of these but only that doses should be more than adequate, which probably means several times higher than the minimal recommended daily allowances. 4–6 ml of Evening Primrose oil, 100–200 mg of pyridoxine, 20–40 mg of zinc, 1–2 g of vitamin C and 100–200 mg of niacin per day should be adequate to ensure that no deficiencies are present.

(2) Blockade of dopamine receptors. The existing neuroleptics are effective and most of the sedative and motor problems occur with high doses. If one is trying to restore a normal dopamine : PGE_1 ratio only by dopamine blockade, such high doses may be necessary. On the other hand if dopamine blockade is combined with enhanced PGE_1

formation, the desired ratio may be reached at a level of dopamine blockade which does not produce intolerable side effects.

(3) Enhancement of mobilization of DGLA stores. This may be achieved by either penicillin or penicillamine. Penicillamine is likely to prove extremely difficult to use because it chelates zinc which will tend to inhibit DGLA mobilization. It may therefore be almost impossible to find the right dose.

(4) Enhanced conversion of DGLA to PGE_1. If opioids are a factor in blocking this, then an opioid antagonist should be used. Such an antagonist will have little effect if adequate amounts of DGLA are not available. Conversely, provision of large quantities of free DGLA will be useless if their conversion to PGE_1 is blocked by an opioid. It should be noted that our human platelet work suggests that opiates and opioids will be found which will *enhance* PGE_1 formation. Apart from antagonizing opioid effects, their removal by haemodialysis or avoidance by dietary manipulation may be important. Seeley (1979) has recently pointed out that sweating may achieve the same results as haemodialysis in a much simpler though slower manner. Given the number of patients likely to be involved this may turn out to be a more practical approach.

(5) Use of agents which enhance PGE_1 formation indirectly. Melatonin seems to be in this class since it has little effect itself but greatly enhances the action of zinc; colchicine competes for melatonin binding sites and has a similar effect, so that it might be worthy of trial.

In summary we suggest that careful attention to diet plus the combined administration of drugs which will block dopamine receptors, will mobilize DGLA and will enhance DGLA conversion to PGE_1, may allow successful treatment of schizophrenia without intolerable side effects. This multiple therapy is not an indiscriminate shotgun approach but is the logical consequence of an understanding of dopamine/PGE_1 interactions and of the regulation of PGE_1 biosynthesis. The relevance of the PGE_1 concept for the understanding of the immunological problems in schizophrenia is explored in Chapter 13.

References

Abdulla, Y. H. and Hamadah, K. (1975). Effect of ADP on PGE formation in blood platelets from patients with depression, mania and schizophrenia. *Br. J. Psychiatry*, **127**, 591

Bloom, F., Segal, D. and Ling, N. (1976). Endorphins: profound behavioral effects in rats suggest new etiological factors in mental illness. *Science*, **194**, 630

Bloss, J. L. and Singer, G. H. (1978). Neuropharmacological and behavioral evaluation of prostaglandin E2 and 11-thiol-11-deoxy prostaglandin E2 in the mouse and rat. *Psychopharmacology*, **57**, 295

Brenner, R. R. (1974). The oxidative desaturation of unsaturated fatty acids in animals. *Mol. Cell. Biochem.*, **3**, 41

Chouinard, G., Horrobin, D. F. and Annable, L. (1978). An antipsychotic action of penicillin in schizophrenia. *IRCS J. Med. Sci.*, **6**, 187

Collier, H. O. J. and Roy, A. C. (1974). Morphine-like drugs inhibit the stimulation by E prostaglandins of cyclic AMP formation by rat brain homogenates. *Nature*, **248**, 24

Crow, T. J., Johnstone, E. C., Longden, A., Owen, F. and Riley, G. (1977). The role of dopamine in the antipsychotic effect and the pathogenesis of schizophrenia. *Proc. R. Soc. Med.*, **70** (Suppl.), 15

Cunnane, S. C., Horrobin, D. F., Manku, M. S., Oka, M. and Ally, A. I. (1979). The vascular response to zinc varies seasonally: effect of pinealectomy and melatonin. (Submitted for publication.)

Dohan, F. C. (1979). Schizophrenia and neuroactive peptides from food. *Lancet*, **1**, 1031

Domschke, W., Dickschas, A. and Mitznegg, P. (1979). CSF beta-endorphin in schizophrenia. *Lancet*, **1**, 1024

Frohman, C. E. (1973). Plasma proteins and schizophrenia. In Mendels, J. (ed.) *Biological Psychiatry*, p. 131. (New York: John Wiley)

Gruen, P. H. (1978). The prolactin response in clinical psychiatry. *Med. Clin. N. Am.*, **62**, 409

Gunne, L. M., Lindstrom, L. and Terenius, L. (1977). Naloxone-induced reversal of schizophrenia hallucinations. *J. Neurol. Transm.*, **40**, 13

Hemmings, W. A. (1978). The absorption of large breakdown products of dietary proteins into the body tissues, including brain. In Hemmings, G. and Hemmings, W. A. (eds.) *The Biological Basis of Schizophrenia*, pp. 239–257. (Lancaster: MTP Press)

Ho, P. P. K., Walters, P. and Sullivan, H. R. (1976). Biosynthesis of thromboxane B2: assay, isolation and properties of the enzyme in human platelets. *Prostaglandins*, **12**, 951

Horrobin, D. F. (1977a). Interactions between prostaglandins and calcium: the importance of bell-shaped dose response curves. *Prostaglandins*, **14**, 667

Horrobin, D. F. (1977b). Schizophrenia as a prostaglandin deficiency disease. *Lancet*, **1**, 936

Horrobin, D. F. (1978). Dopamine supersensitivity, endorphin excess and prostaglandin E1 deficiency: three aspects of the same schizophrenic elephant. *Schizophrenia Bull.*, **4**, 487

Horrobin, D. F. (1979). Schizophrenia: reconciliation of the dopamine, prostaglandin and opioid concepts and the role of the pineal. *Lancet*, **1**, 529

Horrobin, D. F., Ally, A. I., Karmali, R. A., Karmazyn, M., Manku, M. S. and Morgan, R. O. (1978). Prostaglandins and schizophrenia. Further discussion of the evidence. *Psychol. Med.*, **8**, 43

Horrobin, D. F., Durand, L. G. and Manku, M. S. (1977). Prostaglandin E1 modifies nerve conduction and interferes with local anaesthetic action. *Prostaglandins*, **14**, 103

Horrobin, D. F. and Manku, M. S. (1979). The possible role of prostaglandin E1 in the affective disorders and in alcoholism. *Br. Med. J.* (In press)

Iversen, L. L. (1977). Dopaminergic mechanisms in schizophrenia *Proc. R. Soc. Med.*, **70** (Suppl.), 1

Klevay, L. M., Reck, S. J. and Barcome, D. F. (1979). Evidence of dietary copper and zinc deficiencies. *J. Am. Med. Assoc.*, **241**, 1916

Kline, N. S., Wnen, J. C., Cooper, T. B., Varga, E. and Canal, O. (1974). Evaluation of lithium therapy in chronic and periodic alcoholism. *Am. J. Med. Sci.*, **268**, 15

Kunin, R. A. (1976). The action of aspirin in preventing the niacin flush and its relevance to the anti-schizophrenic action of megadose niacin. *J. Orthomol. Psychiatry*, **5**, 89

Lal, H. (1975). Narcotic dependence, narcotic action and dopamine receptors. *Life Sci.*, **17**, 483

Lee, T., Seeman, P., Tourtelotte, W. W., Farley, I. J. and Hornykiewicz, O. (1978). Binding of ^{3}H-neuroleptics and ^{3}H-apomorphine in schizophrenic brains. *Nature (London)*, **274**, 897

McIsaac, W. M. (1961). A biochemical concept of mental disease. *Postgrad. Med. J.*, **30**, 111

Manku, M. S., Horrobin, D. F., Seidah, N. and Chrétien, M. (1978). Beta-endorphin at physiological concentrations blocks prolactin and zinc-induced synthesis of a prostaglandin E1-like substance. Presented at the *Conference on Central Nervous System, Effects of Hypothalamic Hormones and Other Peptides*, May 2, Montreal

Manku, M. S., Horrobin, D. F., Karmazyn, M., Cunnane, S. C. (1979a). Prolactin and zinc effects on rat vascular reactivity: possible relationship to dihomo-gammalinolenic acid and to prostaglandin synthesis. *Endocrinology*, **104**, 774

Manku, M. S., Oka, M. and Horrobin, D. F. (1979b). Differential regulation of the formation of prostaglandins and related substances from arachidonic acid and from dihomo-gammalinolenic acid. I. Effects of ethyl alcohol. *Prostaglandins Med.*, **3**, 129

Manku, M. S., Oka, M. and Horrobin, D. F. (1979c). Differential regulation of the formation of prostaglandins and related substances from arachidonic acid. II. Effects of vitamin C. *Prostaglandins Med.*, **3**, 138

Meltzer, H. Y. and Gang, V. S. (1976). The effect of neuroleptics on serum prolactin in schizophrenic patients. *Arch. Gen. Psychiat.*, **33**, 279

Myers, P. R., Blosser, J. and Shaw, W. (1978). Neurotransmitter modulation of prostaglandin E1 stimulated increases in cyclic AMP. *Biochem. Pharmacol.*, **27**, 1173

National Research Council (Subcommittee on Zinc). (1978). *Zinc*. (Baltimore: University Park Press)

Nicolson, G. A., Greiner, A. C., McFarlane, W. J. G. and Baker, R. A. (1966). Effect of penicillamine on schizophrenic patients. *Lancet*, **1**, 344

Owen, F., Crow, T. J., Poulter, M., Cross, A. J., Longden, A. and Riley, G. J. (1978). Increased dopamine receptor sensitivity in schizophrenia. *Lancet*, **2**, 223

Ozaki, Y., Lynch, H. J. and Wurtman, R. J. (1976). Melatonin in rat pineal, plasma and urine: 24 hour rhythmicity and effect of chlorpromazine. *Endocrinology*, **98**, 1418

Palmour, R. M. and Ervin, F. R. (1977). Characteristics of a peptide derived from the serum of psychiatric patients. Presented at the *Annual Meeting of the Society for Neuroscience*, Anaheim, California

Pfeiffer, C. C. and Cott, A. (1974). A study of zinc and manganese dietary supplements in the copper-loaded schizophrenic. In Pories, W. J., Strain, W. H., Hsu, J. M. and Woosley, R. L. (eds.) *Clinical Applications of Zinc Metabolism*, pp. 260–278. (Springfield, Illinois: C. C. Thomas)

Rotrosen, J., Miller, A. D., Mandio, D., Traficante, L. J. and Gershon, S. (1978). Reduced PGE1-stimulated cAMP accumulation in platelets from schizophrenics. *Life Sci.*, **23**, 1989

Seeley, S. (1979). The therapeutic effect of hemodialysis on schizophrenia: comments and further possibilities. *Med. Hypotheses*, **5**, 303

Singh, M. M. and Kay, S. R. (1976). Wheat gluten as a pathogenic factor in schizophrenia. *Science*, **191**, 401

Smith, J. A. (1978). The pineal gland: its possible significance in schizophrenia. In Hemmings, G. and Hemmings, W. A. (eds.) *The Biological Basis of Schizophrenia*, pp. 105–110. (Lancaster: MTP Press)

Terenius, L., Wahlstrom, A., Lindstrom, L. and Widerlov, E. (1976). Increased CSF levels of endorphines in chronic psychoses. *Neurosci. Lett.*, **3**, 157

Vaddadi, K. S. (1979). Treatment of schizophrenia with penicillin and essential fatty acids. *Prostaglandins Med.*, **2**, 77

Vincent, J. E., Melai, A. and Bonta, I. L. (1974). Comparison of the effects of prostaglandin E1 on platelet aggregation in normal and essential fatty acid deficient rats. *Prostaglandins*, **5**, 369

Watson, S. J., Berger, P. A., Akil, H., Mills, M. J. and Barchas, J. D. (1978). Effects of naloxone in schizophrenia: reduction in hallucinations in a sub-population of subjects. *Science*, **201**, 73

Wene, J. D., Connor, W. E. and DenBesten, L. (1975). The development of essential fatty acid deficiency in healthy men fed fat-free diets intravenously and orally. *J. Clin. Invest.*,

56, 127

Witten, P. W. and Holman, R. T. (1952). Effect of pyridoxine on essential fatty acid conversions. *Arch. Biochem. Biophys.*, **41**, 266

Zioudrou, C., Streaty, R. A. and Klee, W. A. (1979). Opioid peptides derived from food proteins: the exorphins. *J. Biol. Chem.*, **254**, 2446

2
The pathogenesis of schizophrenia

T. J. CROW

Schizophrenia remains an elusive concept. Opinions on causation are heavily determined by views on the nature of the disease. Yet some assumptions of historical importance in the development of the concept are thrown into a new light by recent observations; other assumptions appear questionable. Thus Bonhoeffer (1909) held that the psychoses provoked by drugs and other toxins (the 'exogenous psychoses') had in common that consciousness was disturbed, and in this respect could be distinguished from schizophrenia. Yet descriptions of the amphetamine psychosis (Connell, 1958; Ellinwood, 1967) make it apparent that there is at least one exogenous psychosis in which disturbance of consciousness is not prominent, and the features of this psychosis resemble closely those of acute paranoid schizophrenia. Again Bleuler, and to a lesser extent Kraepelin, maintained that schizophrenic illnesses were characterized by an absence of true intellectual impairment, and that even in the chronic states orientation was undisturbed. Recent observations establish that there are some chronic patients who, by the criteria of these authors, would be considered to suffer from schizophrenia who do have intellectual impairment, and some are disorientated for time. There is evidence that some of these patients also have structural changes in the brain.

Thus, the borderline between the organic and functional psychoses is less distinct than is conventionally believed. Some exogenous toxins are sufficiently selective in their effects on the nervous system that they induce only those changes which are characteristic of acute paranoid schizophrenia. By contrast some chronic schizophrenic states have features which are often associated with the organic dementias. Both these observations may be relevant to an understanding of the nature of schizophrenia; together they suggest that more than one pathological process may be involved.

THE MECHANISM OF THE ANTIPSYCHOTIC EFFECT

Some schizophrenic illnesses are ameliorated by neuroleptic drugs. This suggests that in these cases there is a reversible element and that this component has a chemical basis. The mechanism of the antipsychotic effect has been the focus of much recent work.

One of the most striking properties of the neuroleptics is their ability to induce extrapyramidal symptoms resembling those of Parkinson's disease. Flügel (1953) and Deniker (1960) suggested this was related to the therapeutic effect, but this view was discounted largely because some drugs (e.g. thioridazine) have fewer extrapyramidal effects than the prototype chlorpromazine but yet are equally effective as antipsychotics. However, with the introduction of new groups of compounds such as the butyrophenones and thiaxanthenes, extrapyramidal effects have remained and, following the work of Ehringer and Hornykiewicz (1960) and Carlsson and Lindqvist (1963) have been attributed to blockade of dopamine receptors. Thus the original hypothesis that extrapyramidal and antipsychotic effects are related can be restated in the form that both are due to dopamine receptor blockade.

The relationship between dopamine antagonism and antipsychotic potency has been examined in two *in vitro* assays of the dopamine receptor – in the dopamine-sensitive adenylate cyclase system and with the butyrophenone binding, both of which can be assessed in corpus striatum. With the adenylate cyclase system the correlation is good for phenothiazines and thiaxanthenes, but the butyrophenones are less effective than would be expected from their clinical potency (Miller, Horn and Iversen, 1974). In the inhibition of butyrophenone binding assay the correlation is also good and in this system the effectiveness of the butyrophenones is in line with their clinical effects (Burt, Creese and Snyder, 1976; Seeman, Lee, Chau-Wong and Wong, 1976).

Some stereoisomeric effects have been discovered for dopamine antagonist activity. The thiaxanthene compounds exist in two isomeric forms and only the α- (cis-) isomers have been found to have significant dopamine receptor blocking activity (Miller *et al.*, 1974). In a clinical trial (Johnstone *et al.*, 1978) it was demonstrated that only the α- (cis-) isomer of the thiaxanthene flupenthixol has antipsychotic activity, the β- (trans-) isomer being no more effective than placebo. This result is consistent with the hypothesis that dopamine blockade is the mechanism of the antipsychotic effect and rules out a number of alternative theories.

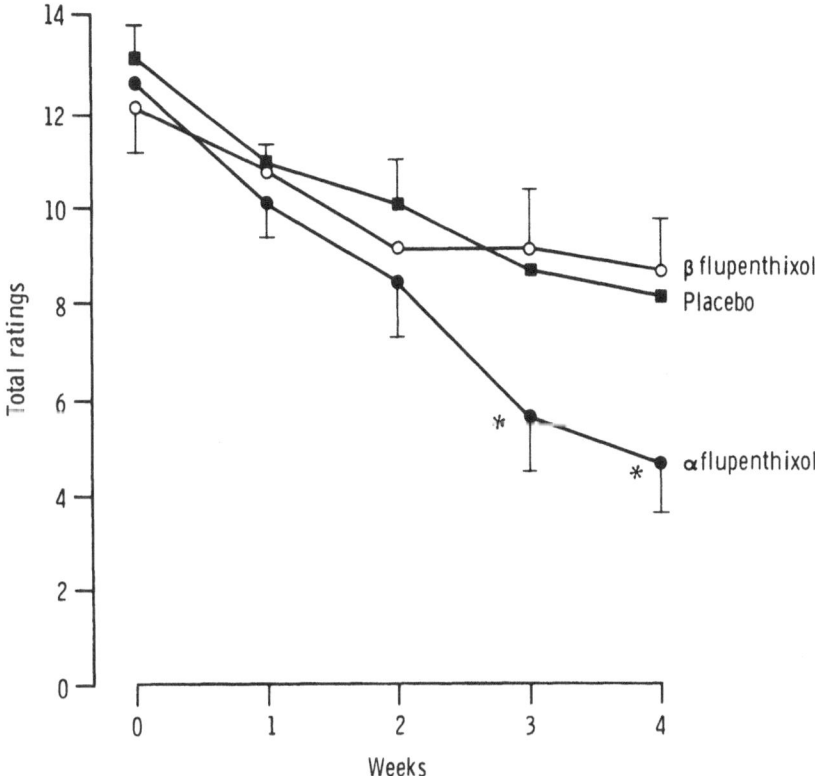

Figure 1 The relative effectiveness of the α- (*cis*-) and β- (*trans*-) isomers of flupenthixol and placebo in the treatment of acute schizophrenia (from Johnstone *et al.*, 1978a) $p < 0.05$ versus β-Flupenthixol or placebo

It remains to be explained why, if both are due to the same mechanism, extrapyramidal and therapeutic effects are not more closely related. One possibility is that some drugs (e.g. thioridazine) have relatively high anti-cholinergic potency (Miller and Hiley, 1974) and thus have 'in-built' anti-Parkinsonian activity.

THE SITE OF THE ANTIPSYCHOTIC EFFECT

It is possible that extrapyramidal and antipsychotic effects occur at different sites in the brain. The motor effects presumably occur by dopamine antagonism in the corpus striatum. Andén (1972) first suggested that the antipsychotic effect might take place within the 'mesolimbic' dopamine system, for example in the nucleus accumbens. The corpus striatum receives its dopaminergic innervation from the pars compacta of the substantia nigra (the A_9 area) and the mesolimbic system receives terminals from cell bodies located (in the A_{10} area) more medially in the ventral mid-brain and situated directly above the interpeduncular nucleus. Whereas the corpus striatum receives non-dopaminergic afferents from the neocortex the nucleus accumbens receives similar afferents from the hippocampus and other limbic lobe structures. Thus it appears that the striatum integrates information from the cortex with ascending messages in dopaminergic pathways while the nucleus accumbens may perform a similar function with respect to the hippocampus. Although there are similarities of organization in the two pathways there are indications that the dopaminergic-cholinergic interaction which takes place in the striatum is absent in the mesolimbic system (Andén 1972).

When three neuroleptic drugs (chlorpromazine, fluphenazine, and thioridazine) with a differing incidence of extrapyramidal effects were compared the effects of equipotent therapeutic doses on dopamine turnover (assessed as accumulation of the metabolite homovanillic acid) in the nucleus accumbens correlated well with the antipsychotic potency while effects in the corpus striatum were better related to extrapyramidal effects (Crow, Deakin and Longden, 1977; Figure 2). These findings are consistent with the view that the antipsychotic action is due to dopamine

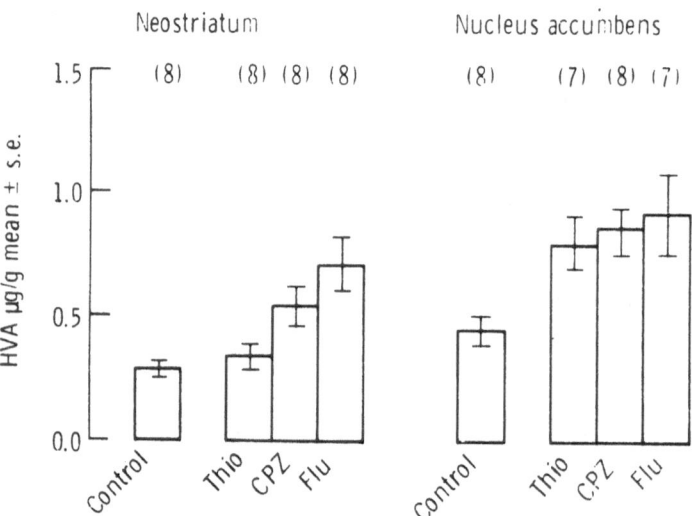

Figure 2 The effects of therapeutically equipotent doses of thioridazine (Thio), chlorpromazine (CPZ), and fluphenazine (Flu) on dopamine turnover, assessed as the concentrations of the metabolite homovanillic acid (HVA) in corpus striatum and nucleus accumbens in rat brain. Effects in the striatum are related to extrapyramidal actions but in the nucleus accumbens are more closely related to the antipsychotic effect. Figures in brackets indicate numbers of animals (from Crow, Deakin and Longden, 1977)

blockade within the nucleus accumbens, but it is possible that actions elsewhere in the mesolimbic system (e.g. in that area of the frontal cortex which receives a dopaminergic innervation) are important.

THE TIME COURSE OF THE ANTIPSYCHOTIC EFFECT

An unexplained aspect of the action of neuroleptic drugs is the time course of the therapeutic effect. It has long been recognized (for references see Klein and Davis, 1969) that drug–placebo differences in clinical trials develop rather slowly and may be increasing even after 4 or more weeks of drug treatment. This time course can be contrasted with that of dopamine receptor blockade as reflected in the increase in patients on active medication in prolactin secretion, presumed to be due to blockade of dopamine receptors in the pituitary which inhibit prolactin release, (Figure 3). There is a discrepancy of at least two weeks between the therapeutic effect attributable to drugs (calculated as difference in ratings in patients on active and inactive medication) and dopamine blockade assessed by increased prolactin secretion. This suggests that dopamine receptor blockade may be necessary for some other change with a slow time course to take place before there is a change in clinical state (Cotes *et al.*, 1978).

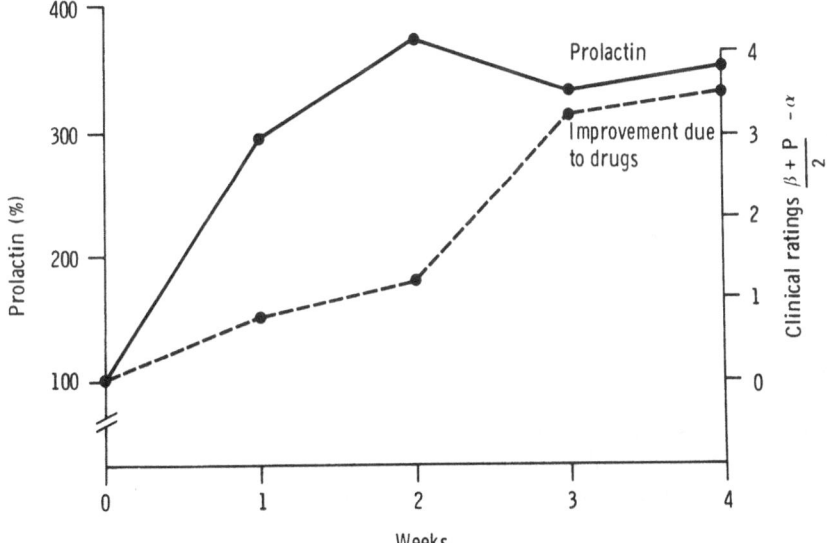

Figure 3 The time course of the antipsychotic effect (calculated as the difference in scores between patients on active and inactive medication) compared with the time course of the rise in prolactin observed in patients on active medication (from Cotes *et al.*, 1978)

DOPAMINERGIC MECHANISMS IN SCHIZOPHRENIA

The features of the amphetamine psychosis resemble those of acute para-noid schizophrenia and many of the behavioural effects of the ampheta-mines have been shown in animal experiments to be due to central dopamine release (Randrup and Munkvad, 1966; Creese and Iversen, 1975). Both the symptoms of the amphetamine psychosis and the amphetamine-induced behavioural changes in animals are reversed by neuroleptic drugs. For these reasons as well as because dopamine recep-tor blockade appears to be of value in treatment it is of interest to know whether there is any abnormality of dopaminergic transmission in schizophrenia.

The first approach to this question was by assessment of dopamine metabolites in cerebrospinal fluid after administration of probenecid, which blocks the egress of the acid metabolites of monoamines. These studies yielded no evidence of increased dopamine turnover (Bowers, 1974; Post et al., 1975). Indeed increasing severity of symptoms (Post et al., 1975) and poor prognosis (Bowers, 1974) were correlated with decreased dopamine turnover.

These findings have been substantiated in post-mortem studies. Con-centrations of homovanillic acid or dihydroxyphenylacetic acid were not increased in areas of corpus striatum or nucleus accumbens in patients with schizophrenia by comparison with patients dying from a variety of physical illnesses (Owen et al., 1978). The findings are particularly sur-prising in view of the fact that many of these patients had been on neurol-eptic medication which by itself might have been expected to increase dopamine turnover. Presumably, as demonstrated in animal experi-ments, tolerance to this action of neuroleptic drugs develops with contin-ued administration. However this may be, the findings give no support to the hypothesis that dopamine neurones are overactive in schizophre-nia.

An alternative hypothesis (Bowers, 1974; Crow et al., 1976) is that the abnormality lies not in the presynaptic neurone but in the post-synaptic receptor. Using isotopically-labelled butyrophenones as ligands for the dopamine receptor it has now been demonstrated that the numbers of dopamine receptors are increased both in corpus striatum and nucleus accumbens in schizophrenic brain (Figure 4).

The above findings with spiroperidol (Owen et al., 1978) are in agree-ment with those of a study using haloperidol as ligand (Lee et al., 1978). The best estimate of the numbers of receptors is given by maximum spiro-peridol binding (an index which is uninfluenced by residual neuroleptic in the brain after death), and this index gives a mean increase of 100% in

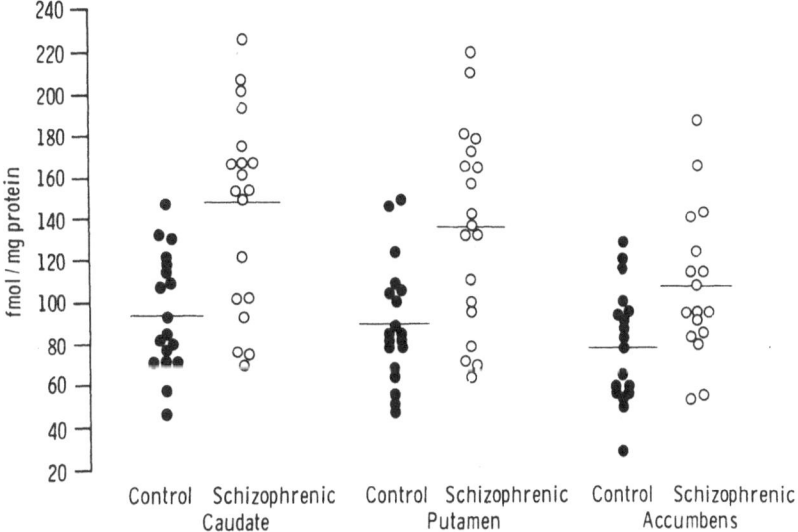

Figure 4 Dopamine receptors assessed with 0.8 nm [³H]spiroperidol in the brains of patients with schizophrenia and controls (from Owen *et al.*, 1978)

schizophrenics by comparison with controls (Figure 5).

The values for approximately two-thirds of patients lie outside the normal range although it is clear there are some patients whose values are not abnormal. A possible explanation for the increase is that it is a consequence of neuroleptic drug administration since increased numbers of receptors have been observed following chronic drug administration in animal experiments. However this seems unlikely for the following two reasons – (i) A significant increase is observed in some patients who apparently had been free of medication for at least a year before death (Owen et al., 1978). (ii) There is no increase in binding of the dopamine agonist ADTN in schizophrenic brain (Owen *et al.*, 1980). The binding of agonists may well occur to sites other than those binding antagonists (i.e. there may be more than one type of dopamine receptor), and since both agonist and antagonist binding is known to increase following neuroleptic administration it seems that these findings indicate that the increase in dopamine receptors in schizophrenic brain may be selective to one type of receptor and is not due to neuroleptic administration.

Other receptors, e.g. for GABA, 5-hydroxytryptamine and acetylcholine have been examined in schizophrenic brain and have been found not to be abnormal (Owen *et al.*, 1980).

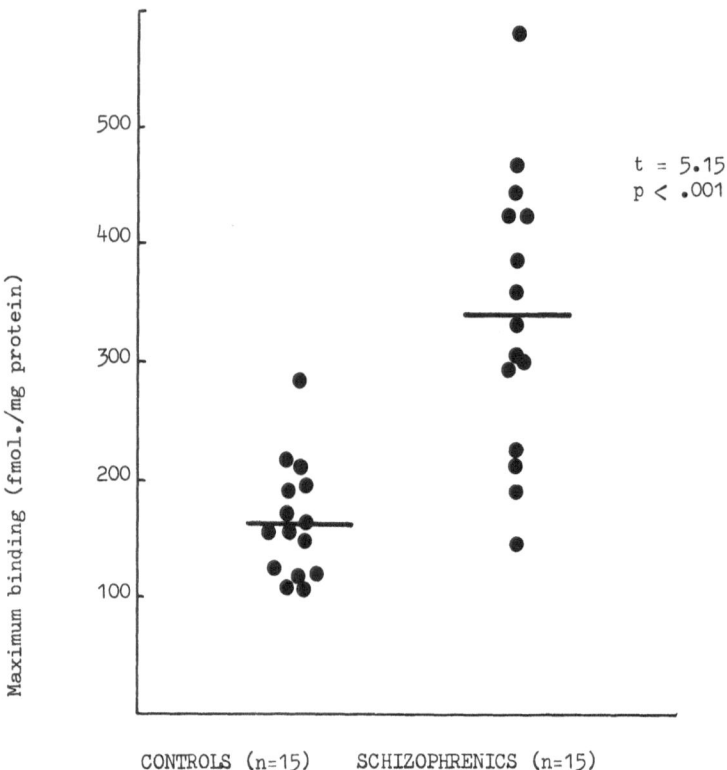

Figure 5   Maximum spiroperidol binding (assessed from a saturation analysis) in caudate nucleus in the brains of patients with schizophrenia and controls (from Owen *et al.*, 1978)

OTHER MONOAMINE HYPOTHESES

Other hypotheses of the primary disturbance in schizophrenia have been tested in post-mortem brain. Thus it has been found that monoamine oxidase activity in platelets is reduced in schizophrenics by comparison with controls (Murphy and Wyatt, 1972). This has not been a consistent finding (Owen *et al.*, 1976) but raised the possibility that there might be some abnormality of the enzyme in brain. This was tested with four substrates in fourteen different brain areas (Crow *et al.*, 1979) but no differences in enzyme activity between schizophrenics and controls were found.

The hypothesis that the primary defect is a degeneration of central noradrenergic reward pathways (Stein and Wise, 1971) has been assessed by measurements of the enzyme dopamine-β-hydroxylase. (Cross *et al.*, 1978). Again no consistent differences in enzyme activity between patients and controls were detected. Finally the hypothesis of Gaddum (1954), based on the psychotomimetic properties of LSD, that serotonergic transmission is diminished, has been evaluated by assessing various aspects of serotonergic function. Although serotonin concentrations were modestly increased the concentrations of tryptophan, of its metabolite kynurenin, and of the serotonin metabolite 5-hydroxyindoleacetic acid were within the normal range. Moreover serotonin receptors assessed either with 5-HT or LSD as ligands were unchanged (Owen *et al.*, 1980).

Thus from these post-mortem studies there is no support for the hypotheses that a deficiency of monoamine oxidase, degeneration of central noradrenaline neurones or failure of serotonergic transmission is a general finding in schizophrenia. It is of course possible that such defects may occur in a proportion or a sub-group of patients but to detect such sub-groups will require more extensive post-mortem studies than have so far been conducted.

ACUTE AND CHRONIC SCHIZOPHRENIA

Some pharmacological findings are consistent with the view that there are substantial differences in the mechanisms underlying different groups of symptoms. Thus while amphetamine-like substances exacerbate symptoms in acute schizophrenia there is evidence (Kornetsky, 1976) that patients with chronic schizophrenia are resistant to the amphetamines. The effects of neuroleptic drugs may also be selective to certain symptoms. Thus while positive symptoms (delusions, hallucinations and thought disorder) which are characteristic of acute episodes do respond to medication, negative symptoms (flattening of affect, poverty of speech) which are much more frequently observed in chronic schizophrenia are resistant (Figure 6).

There is also evidence (Letemendia and Harris, 1967) that chronic schizophrenic patients are relatively resistant to therapeutic improvement by neuroleptics.

THE NATURE OF CHRONIC SCHIZOPHRENIA

The possibility that the defect in chronic schizophrenia may be more akin to that in the organic psychoses (i.e. the dementias) than has previously been thought is suggested by some recent observations. Thus it has been found (Crow and Mitchell, 1975; Stevens *et al.*, 1978) that approximately 25% of chronic institutionalized patients show severe defects of temporal orientation. It seems that acquisition of new information is severely impaired. For many of these patients 'time stands still', and the nature of the impairment is such as might be expected in organic brain disease

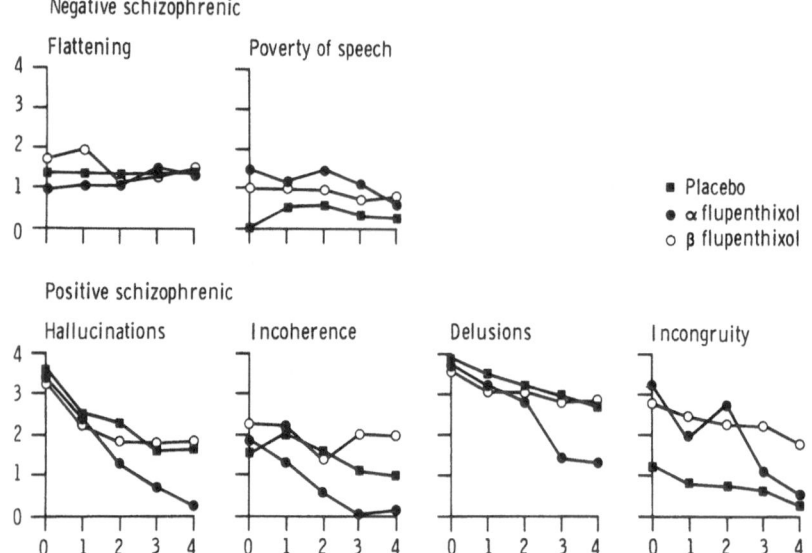

Figure 6   The selectivity of the antipsychotic effect with respect to the symptoms of schizo-phrenia. Positive symptoms (delusions, hallucinations, thought disorder and incongruity of affect) improve faster in patients on α-flupenthixol, than on β-flupenthixol or placebo. Negative symptoms (flattening of affect and poverty of speech) show little change over the four weeks of the trial and are not differentially affected by active medication (from John-stone *et al.*, 1978a)

(Crow and Stevens, 1978).

There is also evidence of structural changes in the brain. Thus Haug (1962) and Asano (1967) found in pneumoencephalographic studies that patients with evidence of clinical deterioration, or with more typically 'nuclear' illnesses, respectively, were more likely to show abnormalities of ventricular shape or size (Table 1).

In a recent study with the computerized axial tomography (Johnstone *et al.*, 1976; Johnstone *et al.*, 1978), a group of chronic schizophrenics were found to have larger ventricles than an age-matched control group, and within the schizophrenic group increased ventricular size was correlated with evidence of intellectual impairment and presence of negative symptoms.

MORE THAN ONE PROCESS IN SCHIZOPHRENIA?

It seems possible that two syndromes can be distinguished in schizophrenia and that each may have a specific underlying pathology. The first syndrome (labelled type I in Table 2) is manifest as positive symptoms

Table 1 Controlled studies of ventricular size in chronic schizophrenia

Authors	Technique	Type of patient and comparison	Result
Haug (1962)	pneumoencephalography	278 psychiatric patients divided into 3 groups (i) non-organic (ii) schizophrenic (iii) organic (schizophrenic patients were selected to exclude those over 60 years and those with evidence of complicating disorders)	schizophrenic patients have larger ventricles than those with non-organic disorders ($p < 0.05$); within the schizophrenic group there is a correlation ($p < 0.001$) between clinically assessed deterioration and ventricular size
Storey (1966)	pneumoencephalography	18 schizophrenic patients compared with patients investigated for neurological disease but reported as normal	no significant differences
Asano (1967)	pneumoencephalography	53 schizophrenics (mean age 28.9 years) divided into nuclear and peripheral subtypes	ventricular enlargement in 94% of nuclear and 43% of peripheral schizophrenic patients
Johnstone et al. (1978)	computer-assisted tomography	17 chronic schizophrenic patients compared with controls matched for age, sex and premorbid occupation	ventricular size larger in patients than controls ($p < 0.01$)
Weinberger et al. (1979 a,b)	computer-assisted tomography	58 chronic schizophrenic patients compared with 56 asymptomatic volunteers (mostly relatives of patients with Huntington's chorea) – all subjects aged less than 50 years	Ventricular size larger in schizophrenic patients ($p < 0.0001$): the difference is unexplained by age or duration of illness or hospitalization; schizophrenic patients also have more cortical abnormalities and these may be independent of ventricular change

(delusions, hallucinations and thought disorder) and is characteristic of acute schizophrenic episodes. These symptoms are exacerbated by the amphetamines and ameliorated by neuroleptic drugs. Presumably dopaminergic processes are particularly relevant to this type of disturbance although it remains to be demonstrated that the changes in the dopamine receptor are specifically associated with the type I syndrome.

The second (type II in Table 2) syndrome is equivalent to the defect state and is characterized by the negative symptoms of flattening of affect, poverty of speech and loss of drive. It seems likely that this syndrome is unresponsive to neuroleptic drugs and for this reason is probably unrelated to changes in dopaminergic transmission. The presence of these symptoms may constitute the irreversible component in schizophrenia and may contribute substantially to the poor long-term outlook. It seems that this syndrome at least sometimes has features which resemble those of the organic states, although the question of whether the defect state is always associated with intellectual deterioration and structural changes in the brain, and if so the location and nature of these changes, remains to be decided.

Table 2 Two syndromes of schizophrenia

	Type I		*Type II*	
Symptoms	hallucinations delusions thought disorder }	positive symptoms	affective flattening poverty of speech }	negative symptoms
Response to neuroleptics	present		absent	
Course	reversible		irreversible	
Intellectual impairment	absent		present	
Underlying pathology	increased dopamine receptors		structural changes in the brain	

Types I and II schizophrenia are clearly not independent diseases but the relationship between the two syndromes is variable. Episodes of the type I syndrome are often followed by development of type II symptoms. Type I illnesses may also occur without progression to the type II syndrome (this phenomenon representing a type of 'good prognosis' schizophrenia). Less commonly the type II syndrome develops without any type I features. Such an illness may be described as 'simple' or 'pseudoneurotic' schizophrenia. Since negative symptoms are less readily defined than those of the type I syndrome, diagnosis in this case is more difficult to establish.

CAUSATION OF SCHIZOPHRENIA

The one accepted fact about the causation of schizophrenia is that genetic factors make a contribution. However, from the fact that concordance in monozygotic twins (between 50 and 60% at the highest) falls short of 100% and because schizophrenia is an illness which often has an onset at a definable point in adult life, other factors must also be relevant. One possibility is that genes predispose to certain pathogenic life stresses. Another is that they predispose (as in the case of poliomyelitis and tuberculosis) to an infectious agent.

The possibility that schizophrenia might be caused by a virus was considered by those who observed the psychiatric sequelae of the influenza epidemic of 1918 (Menninger, 1926) and of the epidemic of encephalitis lethargica that occurred not long after (Jelliffe, 1927; Hendrick, 1928). Schizophrenia-like psychoses occurred in close relation to both of these illnesses. Both the type of influenza virus responsible for the epidemic of 1918 and the virus presumed responsible for encephalitis lethargica have disappeared, but sporadic cases of encephalitis-like illnesses with schizophrenic symptoms have been reported (for review see Crow, 1978). However the viruses responsible are seldom identified and the criteria by which such illnesses are to be distinguished from schizophrenia are unclear. Organic-type psychological changes may be absent in such cases (Misra and Hay, 1971), and as noted above are sometimes present in apparently typical cases of schizophrenia. CSF changes are seldom looked for in schizophrenia but when they are sought they are found to be present in a number of cases (Hunter, Jones and Malleson, 1969). Such considerations suggest that the borderline between encephalitis-like illnesses caused by an unidentified virus and schizophrenia is not easily defined. Investigation of the possible role of viruses in schizophrenia is required.

In a recent study (Tyrrell et al., 1979; Crow et al., 1979b) tissue culture techniques were used to investigate possible viral infection in a series of recently-admitted schizophrenic patients. Viruses were detected in specimens taken by throat swab in a number of cases but these were such (e.g. adenoviruses, poliovirus III and herpes simplex) as might be detected in a sample of the general population. No viruses were detected in samples of cerebrospinal fluid but it became clear that cerebrospinal fluid from a proportion (between one and two-thirds, probably depending on the precise details of the tissue culture technique) of schizophrenic patients induced a cytopathic effect in cell cultures which resembled that induced by some rhinoviruses. This effect was seen best in MRC5 fibro-blasts maintained in stationary culture. Only with difficulty could the effect be passaged and then only on one or two occasions. Therefore although the cytopathic effect resembles that induced by certain viruses the agent cannot be identified as a virus by the test of replication. None-theless general properties of the agent have been established by pretreat-ing the CSF before it is added to cell culture (Table 3).

Table 3 Characteristics of virus-like agent detected in CSF from some patients with schizo-phrenia and other neurological disorders (e.g. Huntington's chorea)

Size: 50–100 nm
Resistant to heat at 56 °C for 1 hour
  and to chloroform
Not inhibited by bromodeoxyuridine
  (a DNA synthesis inhibitor)

Thus the agent does pass a filter of 100 nm but not one of 50 nm pore size. It is therefore presumably a particle of less than 100 nm diameter. It is resistant to treatment with chloroform and therefore does not have a lipid envelope. It is relatively resistant to heat and also to the DNA syn-thesis inhibitor bromodeoxyuridine. Thus the findings are consistent with the possibility that the agent is an RNA-containing virus without a lipid envelope and of less than 100 nm in diameter (Tyrrell et al., 1979).

The agent was found to be present in the cerebrospinal fluid of 18 of 47 patients with schizophrenia (Crow et al., 1979a). Of these, 10 patients had nuclear (Schniederian first rank) symptoms. The remaining patients received a diagnosis either of delusional psychosis, on the basis of their current mental state, or were diagnosed as suffering from definite schizo-phrenia by application of the Feighner criteria which take into account the course of the illness over time. A comparison of the symptoms, mode of onset, number of previous episodes of illness, family history and other characteristics of the patients in whose CSF a virus-like agent was and was not detected revealed no significant differences although, a follow-up of between 3 and 18 months suggested that patients in whom the virus-like agent was detected had higher scores for persisting positive symptoms and evidence of the defect state.

Detection of a virus-like agent with these characteristics in cerebrospin-al fluid is not limited to schizophrenia. Similar effects have been seen with CSF from some patients with Huntington's chorea and multiple sclerosis, and are also seen in some patients with obscure neurological syndromes in whom a definite diagnosis has been difficult to reach (Tyr-rell et al., 1979; Crow et al., 1979a). More recently a similar agent has also been detected in some patients with affective disorders, but cytopathic effects are seen only occasionally in patients without serious psychiatric and neurological disease.

Three interpretations of these findings have to be considered:

(i) That the presence of the virus-like agent (or agents, since it is possible that a number of different agents are detected with these techniques but cannot yet be distinguished) is a secondary consequence of CNS disease. Thus cell dysfunction or death might allow the growth or replication of an infectious agent not otherwise found in the nervous system.

(ii) That the presence of the virus-like agent is a consequence of another factor, e.g. drug treatment, associated with psychiatric or neurological disease.

(iii) That the virus-like agent is causally-related to one or more of the diseases in which it has been found.

At the present time none of these explanations can be ruled out although the possibility that the presence of the virus-like agent is a secondary consequence of drug treatment seems unlikely since in schizophrenic patients at least the agent has been detected in patients who have not recently received neuroleptic drugs and in a few patients who have never received these drugs (Crow et al., 1979b). The simplest version of interpretation (i), that the presence of the agent is secondary to neural damage or disturbance of any kind is called into question by the fact that the agent has not been detected in CSF taken from a number of cases of meningitis and febrile fits. More complex interpretations of the relationship (e.g. that the agent is able to replicate only where the cellular disturbance is long-standing) cannot be excluded.

Two causal relationships are possible between the virus-like agent(s) and schizophrenia and other neurological diseases, (i) that a single agent is responsible for different disease syndromes and that the particular disease process is determined by genetic predisposition, and (ii) that there are a number of different agents at present indistinguishable and that each is responsible for a different disease process. In the second case genetic factors, particularly in Huntington's chorea, would also play a critical role in predisposition. Genetic factors are known to predispose to a number of viruses, including those such as polio which have a predilection for the CNS and some slow viruses (e.g. scrapie) which cause CNS disease in animals (Dickinson, 1975).

Slow virus diseases in general appear to have a predilection for the nervous system (ter Meulen and Katz, 1977), and this raises the possibility that the defence mechanisms of this compartment may be at a disadvantage in dealing with such agents. In those conditions which are well studied immune responses are variable.

In Creuzfeldt–Jacob disease and scrapie no antibody response has been identified perhaps because the agent is too small to elicit one. In subacute sclerosing panencephalitis the agent persists in spite of a pronounced response (ter Meulen *et al.*, 1969). The case of visna in sheep is of potential interest in the present context. Here the virus has conventional characteristics, can be isolated from CSF and can be grown in cell culture. There is an antibody response which apparently is evaded by rapid spontaneous mutations in the organism (Narayan, Griffin and Clements, 1978). The pathological changes in the brain are predominantly periventricular (Sigurdsson, Palsson and van Bogaert, 1962). Thus, visna is a slow infection by a conventional virus which affects particularly those structures which are in contact with cerebrospinal fluid. It may be a model for those chronic schizophrenic illnesses with evidence of changes in ventricular structure and chronic deterioration.

Some neurotropic viruses have a well-marked selectivity for particular neural systems. Thus polio virus affects anterior horn cells, herpes simplex and zoster viruses have an affinity for sensory ganglia, and rabies virus for certain hypothalamic nuclei. If encephalitis lethargica and idiopathic Parkinson's disease are viral illnesses these agents must also have a high degree of selectivity for particular neurons. This selectivity presumably depends upon an affinity for particular receptors on the cell surface, and it seems entirely possible that these are the neurotransmitter receptors. Thus it will be of particular interest to determine whether the virus-like agent detected in some patients with schizophrenia has any affinity for the dopamine receptor, or a structure related to this receptor.

Such speculations may have some relevance to possible drug therapy. The characteristics of pharmacological agents which interact with the dopamine receptor are fairly well known. Thus if agents with antiviral activity can be found it should be possible to direct them to this particular site. Amantadine has actions on dopaminergic transmission and also has antiviral activity, inhibiting replication of some strains of influenza virus. Unfortunately it does not seem to be effective in inhibiting the virus-like agent detected in CSF from patients with schizophrenia (unpublished observations). However the possibility of synthesizing agents which combine neurochemical specificity with antiviral activity is one which should be pursued.

CONCLUSIONS

Recent evidence is consistent with the view that dopamine receptor blockade is the mechanism of the antipsychotic effect although the time course of clinical change suggests that other changes, taking place over 2–3 weeks, are also necessary. Post-mortem studies have shown dopamine turnover not to be increased in schizophrenia but increased numbers of dopamine receptors (assessed by binding of butyrophenones but not of dopamine agonists) have been found in two-thirds of patients. These changes may be related to the disease process, since they have been found in some patients who apparently were untreated with neuroleptic drugs for at least a year before death.

The apparent selectivity of the effects of neuroleptic drugs and the nature of the psychological disorder in some chronic patients suggests that two constellations of symptoms can be distinguished and that these may be associated with separate pathological processes. Positive symptoms (delusions, hallucinations and thought disorder) are characteristic of acute schizophrenic episodes and often respond to medication. A disorder of dopaminergic transmission (e.g. at the receptor) might well be involved in this (labelled as the type I) syndrome. Negative symptoms (the type II syndrome) respond less well, if at all, to neuroleptics and may be associated with intellectual impairment and structural changes in the brain.

The fact that concordance for schizophrenia in monozygotic twins falls well short of 100% and the onset of the disease is often in adult life suggest that environmental factors must be relevant to causation. A viral aetiology of schizophrenia seems entirely possible and a virus-like agent has recently been detected in cerebro-spinal fluid from some patients with schizophrenia and some other neurological and psychiatric diseases (e.g. multiple sclerosis and Huntington's chorea). This agent is probably between 50 and 100 nm in size, is resistant to heat and chloroform, and to a DNA synthesis inhibitor. It has yet to be demonstrated that this agent is causally related to the disease process or processes underlying schizophrenia but if this is the case it is clear that either one agent is related to more than one disease, or that several agents causing similar cytopathic effects cannot be distinguished with current techniques. In either case it is apparent that in these diseases of the nervous system, as with other viral infections, genetic factors influence susceptibility.

References

Asano, N. (1967). Pneumoencephalographic study of schizophrenia. In Mitsuda, H. (ed.) *Clinical Genetics in Psychiatry*, (Tokyo: Igaku-Shoin)

Andén, N. E. (1972). Dopamine turnover in the corpus striatum and the limbic system after treatment with neuroleptic and anti-acetylcholine drugs. *J. Pharm. Pharmacol.*, **24**, 905

Bonhoeffer, K. (1909). 'Zur Frage der exogenen Psychosen'. *Zentlbl. Nervenheilk*, **32**, 499. Translated and reprinted in *Themes and Variations in European Psychiatry*, S. Hirsch & M. Shepherd (eds.), John Wright, Bristol, 1974

Bowers, M. B. (1974). Central dopamine turnover in schizophrenic syndromes. *Arch. Gen. Psychiatry*, **31**, 50

Carlsson, A. and Lindqvist, M. (1963). Effect of chlorpromazine and haloperidol on formation of 3-methoxy-tyramine and normetanephrine in mouse brain. *Acta Pharm. Toxicol.*,
20, 140

Cotes, P. M., Crow, T. J., Johnstone, E. C., Bartlett, W. and Bourne, R. C. (1978). Neuroendocrine changes in acute schizophrenia as a function of clinical state and neuroleptic
medication. *Psychol. Med.*, **8**, 657

Connell, P. H. (1958). *Amphetamine Psychosis.* (London: Oxford University Press)

Creese, I., Burt, D. R. and Snyder, S. H. (1976). Dopamine receptor binding predicts clinical and pharmacological potencies of anti-schizophrenic drugs. *Science*, **192**, 481

Creese, I. and Iversen, S. D. (1975). The pharmacological and anatomical substrates of the
amphetamine response in the rat. *Brain Res.*, **83**, 419

Crow, T. J. (1978). Viral causes of psychiatric disease. *Postgrad. Med. J.*, **54**, 763

Crow, T. J., Baker, H. F., Cross, A. J., Joseph, M. H., Lofthouse, R., Longden, A.,
Owen, F., Riley, G. J., Glover, M. and Killpack, W. S. (1979a). Monoamine mechanisms in
chronic schizophrenia: post-mortem findings. *Br. J. Psychiatry*, **134**, 249

Crow, T. J., Deakin, J. F. W., Johnstone, E. C. and Longden, A. (1976). Dopamine and
schizophrenia. *Lancet*, **2**, 563

Crow, T. J., Deakin, J. F. W. and Longden, A. (1977). The nucleus accumbens – possible
site of antipsychotic action of neuroleptic drugs? *Psychol. Med.*, **7**, 213

Crow, T. J., Ferrier, I. N., Johnstone, E. C., Macmillan, J. F., Owens, D. G. C.,
Parry, R. P. and Tyrrell, D. A. J. (1979b). Characteristics of patients with schizophrenia or
neurological disorder and virus-like agent in cerebrospinal fluid. *Lancet*, **1**, 842

Crow, T. J. and Mitchell, W. S. (1975). Subjective age in chronic schizophrenia: evidence
for a sub-group of patients with defective learning capacity? *Br. J. Psychiatry*, **126**, 360

Crow, T. J. and Stevens, M. (1978). Age disorientation in chronic schizophrenia: the nature
of the cognitive deficit. *Br. J. Psychiatry*, **133**, 137

Crow, T. J., Tyrrell, D. A. J., Ferrier, I. N., Johnstone, E. C., Macmillan, J. F.,
Owens, D. G. C. and Parry, R. P. (1979). Virus-like particles in csf in schizophrenia.
Lancet, **2**, 35

Deniker, P. (1960). Experimental neurological syndromes and the new drug therapies in
psychiatry. *Comprehensive Psychiat.*, **1**, 92

Dickinson, A. G. (1975). Host-pathogen interactions in scrapie. *Genetics*, **79**, (Suppl.), 387

Ehringer, H. and Hornykiewicz, O. (1960). Verteilung von Noradrenalin und Dopamin (3-
Hydroxytyramin) im Gehirn des Menschen und ihr Verhalten bei Erkrankungen des
Extrapyramidalen-Systems. *Klin. Wochenschr.*, **38**, 1236

Ellinwood, E. H. (1967). Amphetamine psychosis: I. Description of the individuals and process. *J. Nerv. Ment. Dis.*, **144**, 274

Flügel, F. (1953). Thérapeutique par medication neuroleptique obtenue en réalisant syste-
matiquement des états Parkinsoniformes. *L'Encephale*, **45**, 1090

Gaddum, J. H. (1954). Drugs antagonistic to 5-hydroxytryptamine. In: Wolstenholme, G. W., *Ciba Foundation Symposium on Hypertension*, pp. 75–77, (Boston: Little,
Brown)

Haug, J. O. (1962). Pneumoencephalographic studies in mental disease. *Acta Psychiatr. Scand.*, **38**, Suppl. 165

Hendricks, I. (1927). Encephalitis lethargica and the interpretation of mental disease.
Am. J. Psychiatry, **7**, 989

Hunter, R., Jones, M. and Malleson, A. (1969). Abnormal cerebrospinal fluid total protein
and gamma-globulin levels in 256 patients admitted to a psychiatric unit. *J. Neurol. Sci.*, **9**,
11

Jelliffe, S. E. (1927). The mental pictures in schizophrenia and epidemic encephalitis. *Am. J.
Psychiatry*, **6**, 413

Johnstone, E. C., Crow, T. J., Frith, C. D., Husband, J. and Kreel, L. (1976). Cerebral ventricular size and cognitive impairment in chronic schizophrenia. *Lancet*, **2**, 924

Johnstone, E. C., Crow, T. J., Frith, C. D., Carney, M. W. P. and Price, J. S. (1978a). Mechanism of the antipsychotic effect in the treatment of acute schizophrenia. *Lancet*, **1**, 848

Johnstone, E. C., Crow, T. J., Frith, C. D., Stevens, M., Kreel, L. and Husband, J. (1978b). The dementia of dementia praecox. *Acta Psychiatr. Scand.*, **57**, 305

Klein, D. F. and Davis, J. M. (1969). *Diagnosis and Drug Treatment of Psychiatric Disorder.* (Baltimore: Williams & Wilkins)

Kornetsky, C. (1976). Hyporesponsivity of chronic schizophrenic patients to dexamphetamine. *Arch. Gen. Psychiatry*, **33**, 1425

Lee, T., Seeman, P., Tourlelotte, W. W., Farley, I. J. and Hornykiewicz, O. (1978). Binding of ³H-neuroleptics and ³H-apomorphine in schizophrenic brains. *Nature (London)*, **274**, 897

Letemendia, F. J. J. and Harris, A. D. (1967). Chlorpromazine and the untreated chronic schizophrenic: a long-term trial. *Br. J. Psychiatry*, **113**, 950

Menninger, K. A. (1926). Influenza and schizophrenia. An analysis of post-influenzal 'dementia praecox' as of 1918, and five years later. *Am. J. Psychiatry*, **5**, 469

ter Meulen, V. and Katz, M. (eds.) (1977). *Slow Virus Infections of the Central Nervous System.* (New York: Springer-Verlag)

ter, Meulen, V., Enders-Ruckle, G., Müller, D. and Joppich, G. (1969). Immunobiological and microscopic studies on encephalitis. III. Subacute progressive panencephalitis, virology and immunohistology. *Acta Neuropathologica, (Berlin)*, **12**, 244

Miller, R. J. and Hiley, C. R. (1974). Antimuscarinic properties of neuroleptics and drug-induced Parkinsonism. *Nature (London)*, **248**, 596

Miller, R. J., Horn, A. S. and Iversen, L. L. (1974). The action of neuroleptic drugs on dopamine-stimulated adenosine cyclic 3', 5'-monophosphate production in neostriatum and limbic forebrain. *Molec. Pharmacol.*, **10**, 759

Misra, P. C. and Hay, G. G. (1971). Encephalitis presenting as acute schizophrenia. *Br. Med. J.*, **1**, 532

Murphy, D. L. and Wyatt, R. J. (1972). Reduced MAO activity in blood platelets from schizophrenic patients. *Nature (London)*, **238**, 225

Narayan, O., Griffin, D. E. and Clements, J. E. (1978). Virus mutation during slow infection: temporal development and characterisation of mutants of visna virus recovered from sheep. *J. Gen. Virol.*, **41**, 343

Owen, F., Bourne, R. C., Crow, T. J., Johnstone, E. C., Bailey, A. R. and Hershon, H. I. (1976). Platelet monoamine oxidase in schizophrenia: an investigation in drug-free chronic hospitalised patients. *Arch. Gen. Psychiat.*, **33**, 1370

Owen, F., Cross, A. J., Crow, T. J., Lofthouse, R. and Poulter, M. (1980). Neurotransmitter receptors in brain in schizophrenia. *Acta Psychiat. Scand.*, Suppl. (In press)

Owen, F., Cross, A. J., Crow, T. J., Longden, A., Poulter, M. and Riley, G. J. (1978). Increased dopamine receptor sensitivity in schizophrenia. *Lancet*, **2**, 223

Post, R. M., Fink, E., Carpenter, W. T. and Goodwin, F. K. (1975). Cerebrospinal fluid amine metabolites in acute schizophrenia. *Arch. Gen. Psychiat.*, **32**, 1013

Randrup, A. and Munkvad, I. (1966). On the role of catecholamines in the amphetamine excitatory response. *Nature (London)*, **211**, 540

Seeman, P., Lee, T., Chau-Wong, M. and Wong, K. (1976). Antipsychotic drug doses and neuroleptic/dopamine receptors. *Nature (London)*, **261**, 717

Sigurdsson, B., Palsson, P. A. and Bogaert, L. van, (1962). Pathology of visna. *Acta Neuropathol.*, **1**, 343

Stein, L. and Wise, C. D. (1971). Possible etiology of schizophrenia: progressive damage to the noradrenergic reward system by 6-hydroxydopamine. *Science*, **171**, 1032

Stevens, M., Crow, T. J., Bowman, M. and Coles, E. C. (1977). Age disorientation in chronic schizophrenia: a constant prevalence of 25% in a mental hospital population? *Br. J. Psychiatry*, **133**, 130

Storey, P. B. (1966). Lumbar air encephalography in chronic schizophrenia: a controlled experiment. *Br. J. Psychiatry*, **112**, 135

Tyrrell, D. A. J., Crow, T. J., Parry, R. P., Johnstone, E. C. and Ferrier, I. N. (1979). Possible virus in schizophrenia and some neurological disorders. *Lancet*, **1**, 839

Weinberger, D. R., Torrey, E. F., Neophytides, A. N. and Wyatt, R. T. (1979a). Lateral cerebral ventricular enlargement in chronic schizophrenia. *Arch. Gen. Psychiatry*, **36**, 735

Weinberger, D. R., Torrey, E. F., Neophytides, A. N. and Wyatt, R. J. (1979b). Structural abnormalities in the cerebral cortex of chronic schizophrenic patients. *Arch. Gen. Psychiatry*, **36**, 935

3
Opiates, opioid peptides and their possible relevance to schizophrenia

J. F. W. DEAKIN

HISTORICAL OVERVIEW

The poppy plant *Papaver somniferum* has been known to man for many thousands of years. Cuneiform inscriptions on clay tablets excavated from the library of Ashurbanipal in Nineveh describe how the women-folk tended the poppy fields of ancient Mesopotamia, and earlier Sumerian writings are referred to, which describe the medicinal use of opium some 4000 years ago. It was not until 1805, however, that the active ingredient of opium was isolated by the German pharmacist Serturner (1783–1841). He named it 'morpheum' after the Greek god of dreams, Morpheus, and its structure is shown in Figure 1.

OPIATE RECEPTORS

In the 1940s it was recognized that certain substitutions of opiate molecules conferred antagonistic properties. For example *N*-allyl substitution of morphine produced nalorphine, a substance with opiate actions when administered alone, but with the ability to antagonize the effects of large doses of morphine. More strikingly, naloxone (Figure 1), another *N*-allyl substituted opiate derivative, has no opiate actions when administered alone yet very small doses will completely reverse the effects of a severe overdose of morphine. The development of these 'competitive' antagonists gave rise to the concept that the brain contains a set of receptors into which opiate molecules fit, resulting in their various pharmacological effects, and from which they can be displaced by antagonists. This

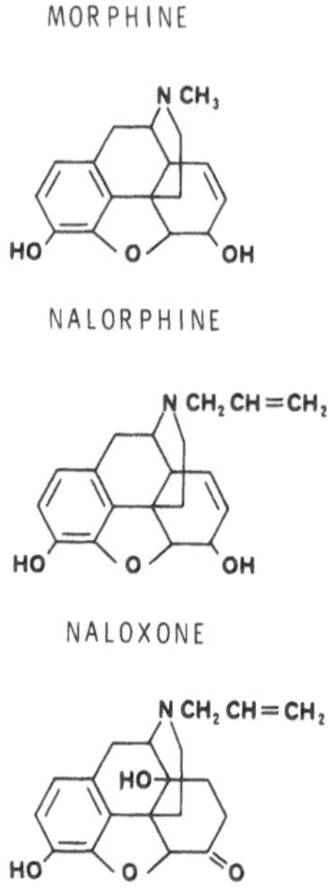

MORPHINE

NALORPHINE

NALOXONE

Figure 1   Structure of morphine and antagonists

receptor concept may be likened to a lock and key mechanism where the keyhole represents the receptor and keys which fit the keyhole and turn the lock represent opiate molecules. Opiate antagonists might be represented by keys which fit the keyhole, thus preventing access of opiate keys, but which are incapable of turning the lock.

OPIOID PEPTIDES

The development of the opiate receptor concept begged the teleological question of the reason the brain contains a set of receptors for substances derived from plants. One answer was that the brain might contain its own morphine-like compounds which interact with the opiate receptor. The search for the endogenous ligand of the opiate receptor culminated in the announcement by Hughes (1975) of the isolation of a substance from pig brain which behaved like morphine in standard pharmacological opiate bioassays. The substance was named 'Enkephalin' but was later found to consist of two pentapeptides of identical structure except that the C-terminal amino acid was leucine in the case of leu-enkephalin and methionine in met-enkephalin (Figure 2) (Hughes *et al.*, 1975). Enkephalin was found to have a number of opiate actions *in vitro* and *in vivo*

although in many cases they were short lasting due to the high susceptibility of the pentapeptides to enzymic degradation (Hambrook *et al.*,
1976).

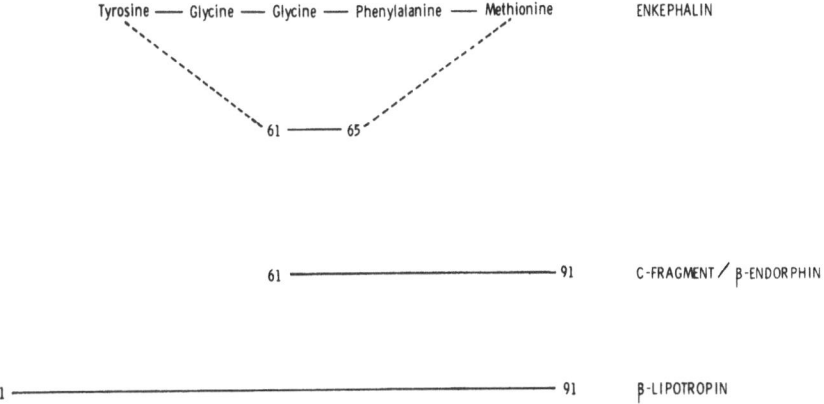

Figure 2 Structure of enkephalin, β-endorphin and β-lipotropin: β-Lipotropin is cleaved
between its 60th and 61st amino acids to produce β-endorphin (C-fragment), the first 5
amino acids of which correspond to the enkephalin sequence

Prior to the discovery of enkephalin, Smyth and colleagues had
demonstrated that the pituitary gland contained two fragments of the 91
amino acid hormone β-lipotrophin, the C-fragment comprising amino
acids 61-91 of the lipotrophin sequence and C^1-fragment comprising
β LPH 61–87 (Figure 2) (Bradbury *et al.*, 1975). Morris, who with co-
workers had recently determined the sequence of enkephalin (Hughes *et
al.*, 1975), noticed that the first five N-terminal amino acids of these fragments corresponded exactly to methionine enkephalin and this seemed
too much to expect of chance. Therefore the fragments were tested for
opiate activity and it was demonstrated that C-fragment (now more commonly known as β-endorphin) had high affinity for the opiate receptor
(Bradbury *et al.*, 1976) and caused potent and prolonged analgesia in contrast to the fleeting analgesic effects of even large doses of enkephalin
(Feldberg and Smyth, 1976; Bradbury *et al.*, 1977). The contrasting effects
of β-endorphin and enkephalin are due to the extra amino acids of
β-endorphin which protect the enkephalin part of the molecule from
enzymic degradation. In addition the four N-terminal amino acids of
β-endorphin at the opposite end of the molecule to the N-terminal enkephalin sequence increase its morphine-like potency several hundred fold
(Geisow *et al.*, 1977).

A number of peptides intermediate in length to β-endorphin and enkephalin have since been described. It remains to be established whether

these are specific cleavage products of β-endorphin, perhaps with distinct functions, or whether they represent steps on a degradative pathway. It is clear, however, as will be seen below, that the distribution of β-endorphin and enkephalins in the brain is quite different. This makes it unlikely that met-enkephalin is formed from β-endorphin and a separate precursor for enkephalin may be found.

DISTRIBUTION OF OPIOID PEPTIDES

β-Endorphin cell bodies are located in a circumscribed region of the basolateral part of the hypothalamus and their fibres have a distribution confined to periventricular areas of the brain (Bloom *et al.*, 1978). In contrast enkephalins are very widely distributed from the spinal cord to the forebrain (Elde *et al.*, 1976). A striking feature of this distribution is that it overlaps to a considerable extent the distribution of monoamine-containing neuronal systems. Of particular relevance to the present topic is the finding that enkephalin is present in high concentration around dopamine-containing cell bodies of the substantia nigra and ventral tegmental area and in the corpus striatum and nucleus accumbens which receive a prominent dopaminergic innervation. Furthermore, there is evidence that opiate and enkephalin receptors are located on presynaptic dopaminergic nerve terminals (Pollard *et al.*, 1977). This anatomical association of enkephalins and dopaminergic systems is of considerable significance in view of the evidence summarized in Table 1 implicating an overactivity of dopaminergic mechanisms in the aetiology of schizophrenia.

Table 1   Evidence for schizophrenia as a dopaminergic disease*

---

(1) Amphetamines release dopamine and cause a paranoid psychosis in abusers and normal subjects clinically indistinguishable from acute paranoid schizophrenia. (Connell, 1958)
(2) Antischizophrenic drugs (neuroleptics) block dopamine receptors *in vitro* and *in vivo* in proportion to their clinical potency. (Creese, Burt and Snyder, 1976)
(3) Dopamine receptors are increased in number in postmortem brains of schizophrenic subjects. (Owen *et al.*, 1978)

---

* See e.g. Crow, Deakin, Johnstone and Longden (1976)

ARE ENDOGENOUS OPIOID PEPTIDES ENDOGENOUS NEUROLEPTICS?

The central administration of low doses of β-endorphin in rats results in profound catalepsy, characterized by rigidity, immobility and the prolonged maintenance of abnormal postures (Jaquet and Marks, 1976). Catalepsy is produced by most antischizophrenic (neuroleptic) drugs; this has given rise to suggestions that opioid peptides may be endogenous neuroleptics. Opiates, opioid peptides and neuroleptics have a number of other properties in common summarized in Table 2. While some differences between the actions of the two classes of compounds are well established (see Table 2), their similarities raise the possibility that deficiency in opioid peptide function might predispose to the development of schizophrenia and that opiates and opioid peptides may have some potential as antischizophrenic agents.

Table 2 Neuroleptic-like properties of opiates

---

(1) Catalepsy* (Jaquet and Marks, 1976)
(2) Blockade dopamine sensitive adenylate cyclase. (Minneman and Iversen, 1977)
(3) Increased dopamine synthesis and neuronal firing.* (Fukui and Takagi, 1972)
(4) Prolactin release.* (Rivier et al., 1977)
(5) Chronic treatment leads to behavioural supersensitivity to dopamine agonists. (Halliwell and Kumar, 1977).

BUT

(1) Opiates do not directly interact with the dopamine receptor.* (Enna et al., 1976)
(2) Opiate catalepsy is hypertonic* and not modified by anticholinergics. (Segal et al., 1977).
(3) Opiates do not produce Parkinsonism.

---

* True of β-endorphin

Opium was not uncommonly used as a means of sedation in British psychiatric institutions of the 18th and 19th centuries, yet its use fell into disfavour despite its protagonists. No doubt problems of tolerance and dependence were partly responsible for the decline in opium treatment. Nevertheless it is difficult to believe this would have occurred in the face of significant antipsychotic activity. With the discovery of opioid peptides, interest in this approach to treatment has been renewed although adequate controlled trials have yet to be carried out. Kline et al. (1977) investigated the effects of intravenous injections of synthetic β-endorphin in several psychiatric patients including three schizophrenic subjects. No clear antipsychotic effect was observed in this non-placebo controlled, non-'blind' study. More recently, Jorgensen et al. (1979) have claimed an antipsychotic effect of a synthetic pentapeptide resistant to enzymic degradation (Tyr-D-Ala-Gly-MePhe-Met-ol) administered daily for three days by intramuscular injection to nine chronic psychotic patients. Unfortunately this study was neither placebo controlled nor 'blind' and the criteria used in selecting the patients are unclear; the results are therefore inconclusive.

De Weid et al. (1978) reported that γ-endorphin (βLPH 61–77) showed neuroleptic-like activity in delaying extinction of active and passive shock avoidance tasks, and that removal of the first tyrosine residue producing (des-tyr-γ-endorphin; βLPH 62–77) increased neuroleptic-like activity while destroying its opioid actions (Van Ree et al., 1978a). Des-tyr-γ-endorphin has been investigated for antischizophrenic activity and encouraging results have been reported in a pilot study in six chronic schizophrenic subjects, later extended in a double blind crossover study of a further six patients (Van Ree et al., 1978b). However, these reports are very brief, the number of patients small and their means of selection unstated. If this peptide proves to have clear cut antipsychotic effects on more extensive testing, this will not be due to actions on opiate receptors since the compound has no in vitro or in vivo opiate receptor activity.

ARE ENDOGENOUS OPIOID PEPTIDES SCHIZOPHRENOGENIC?

The neuroleptic-like actions of opiates and opioid peptides have been discussed above. However these compounds also have paradoxical amphetamine-like actions apparently mimicking the effects of increased dopaminergic neurotransmission (see Table 3).

Table 3   Amphetamine-like actions of opiates and opioid peptides

---

(1) Opiate receptor stimulation in mice and cats produces almost exclusively hyperactivity and stereotypy and this behaviour follows the cataleptic phase in rats (Babbini and Davis, 1972). These effects are antagonized by neuroleptics (Kuschinsky, 1976).

(2) In rats with unilateral lesions of the nigrostriatal tract, opiates, β-endorphin and amphetamines cause turning towards the lesioned side (Pert et al., 1979).

(3) Amphetamine and opiate abuse can result in addiction. Their rewarding effects in animals can be blocked by neuroleptics. (Schwartz and Marchok, 1974).

These amphetamine-like actions of opiate receptor stimulation generate an opposite set of predictions to their neuroleptic-like actions. Opiates should precipitate rather than alleviate psychosis; increased rather than diminished activity in opioid peptide pathways might be associated with the development of schizophrenia and this might be reversible by opiate antagonists such as naloxone.

Psychotic effects of opiate administration to normal subjects have not been reported; more commonly dysphoric effects are experienced (Smith and Beecher, 1961). Furthermore there is no evidence that prolonged abuse of opiates in addicted subjects is associated with the development of psychosis although this question has not been systematically investigated. However, there is good evidence that the atypical narcotics, cyclazosine and pentazocine, and the mixed agonist–antagonist, nalorphine, can induce LSD-like responses in questionnaire studies of these drugs in postaddicted subjects (Jasinski *et al.*, 1967) and delusions and hallucinations have been associated with their clinical use (Jaffe and Martin, 1975). Further evaluation of these states as model psychoses would seem to be worthwhile.

Direct evidence for the possible overactivity of opioid peptides by their measurement in the biological fluids of schizophrenic patients is limited to the studies of Terenius and colleagues (1976). By means of gel filtration of CSF samples, this group have demonstrated that certain fractions ('fractions 1 and 11') have opiate activity in displacing [³H]-dihydromorphine in a radio-receptor assay. The compounds with opiate activity in fractions 1 and 11 have yet to be identified although it is clear that they are not β-endorphin or met-enkephalin. Gunne *et al.*, (1977) have reported that CSF samples from schizophrenic and manic-depressive patients have elevated levels of fractions 1 and 11. These provocative findings offer support for the endorphin excess theory of schizophrenia. However, it is clear these results need to be replicated by other groups and the chemical identity of the fractions established.

If overstimulation of opiate receptors is involved in the aetiology of schizophrenia, naloxone might be expected to have antipsychotic activity. My colleagues (T. J. Crow and C. D. Frith) and I investigated the effects of 0.4 mg naloxone in a striking case of catatonic schizophrenia at Northwick Park Hospital. The patient was immobile and almost mute with increased muscle tone and catalepsy. These signs were strikingly similar to those produced by β-endorphin in animal studies (see above) and the potency of naloxone in reversing the latter effects bode well for a similar effect in reversing catatonia in this patient. Muscle rigidity and negativism were quantified by means of an EMG recording of the wrist flexors and other aspects of her mental state were rated. Naloxone and saline were administered intravenously on three occasions each and EMG and ratings were made by a 'blind' observer. The results are shown in Figure 3 and it is clear that naloxone had no effect on her rigidity or negativism, nor were other aspects of her mental state affected.

A number of trials of naloxone in schizophrenia have now been carried out (details of which are summarized in Table 4) and these confirm that standard doses of naloxone have no demonstrable antipsychotic effects. These findings seem particularly strong since all the studies were double blind cross-over studies; that is to say, all patients received naloxone and placebo and neither patients nor clinicians knew in advance which was being injected. Furthermore, in two of the studies the diagnosis was confirmed according to Schneiderian first rank symptoms and the Feighner criteria and symptoms were rated on standard psychiatric rating scales (Janowsky *et al.*, 1977; Volvaka *et al.*, 1977). The study by Gunne *et al.*, (1977) is an unsuccessful attempt to replicate their earlier results in an

Table 4 Evidence that low dose naloxone is not antipsychotic

Authors*	Patients (N)	Assessments	Dose
Janowsky et al. (1977)	(8) Schneider positive. Medicated. (6) Hallucinating	BPRS 60 min	1.2 mg
Volavka et al. (1977)	(7) Feighner positive. Frequent hallucinations. Medicated	BPRS 42 h	0.4 mg
Davis et al. (1977)	(14) Criteria? Most unmedicated	Ratings 60 min	0.4 mg (6) 1.2 mg (1) 6–10 mg (3)
Kurland et al. (1977)	(12) Chronic Criteria? Medicated	Ratings	0.4 and 1.2 mg
Gunne et al. (1979) (i)	(10) Criteria?	Self report at 4 h	0.8 mg
Gunne et al. (1979) (ii)	(10) Criteria?	BPRS NOSIE	100 mg naltrexone per day for 2 weeks

*All double blind cross-over studies, comparing single intravenous injections of naloxone with placebo except Gunne et al. (1979) (ii).
BPRS – Brief Psychiatric Rating Scale
NOSIE – Nurses' observational scale for inpatient evaluation

uncontrolled trial in which a beneficial effect of naloxone was claimed (Gunne et al., 1977; see Table 5).

While the doses of naloxone used in these studies are quite sufficient to antagonize the effects of an overdose of morphine, it may be that much larger doses are required to antagonize endogenous opioid peptides because of their greater receptor affinity and local concentration at synapses. In addition there is evidence for multiple receptor actions of opiates and opioid peptides, some of which are resistant to blockade with naloxone (Martin et al., 1976; Lord et al., 1977). The two studies which have so far been carried out with high doses of naloxone do indeed report some limited but encouraging antipsychotic effects (Table 5). Watson et al., (1978) investigated the effects of naloxone 10 mg i.v. in a double

Table 5 Evidence that high dose naloxone may be antipsychotic

Authors*	Patients (N)	Assessments	Dose	Outcome
Gunne et al. (1977)	(10) Criteria? Medicated Frequent hallucinations	clinical	0.8 mg	Hallucinations greatly reduced but non-placebo controlled, 'non-blind' and non-replicated
Watson et al. (1978)	(11) Medicated. Frequent hallucinations	BPRS	10 mg	Decreased hallucinations. No other significant changes.
Emrich et al. (1979) (i)	(20) 1 week drug free, including schizo-affectives and alcoholics	IPMS	4 mg	Hallucination related scores, improved for 2–7 h postdose
Emrich et al. (1979) (ii)	(12) Schizophrenics	IPMS	24.8 mg	Ditto but improvement not greater

* Single intravenous injections of naloxone and placebo, except for Gunne et al. (1977)

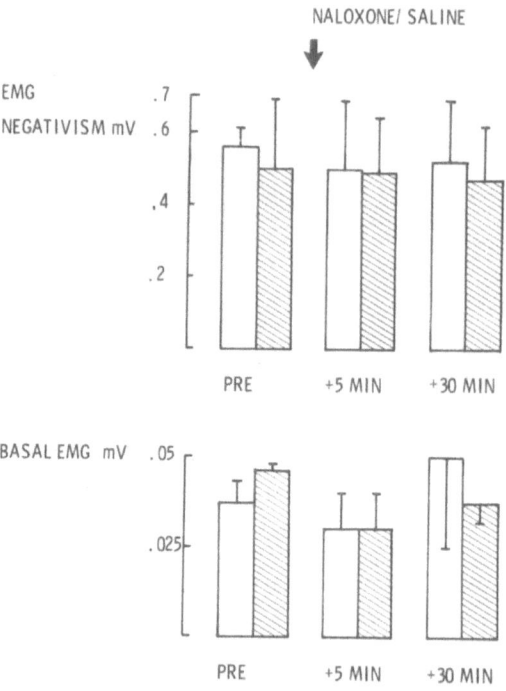

EFFECTS OF NALOXONE ON E. M. G. IN A CASE OF CATATONIA

Figure 3 EMG recorded from forearm flexors with silver-silver chloride electrodes. A Devices high gain amplifier and chart recorder were used for recording. Basal EMG = resting EMG peak to peak amplitude. EMG negativism = peak to peak EMG amplitude during passive extension of the wrist. Open columns = EMG values before and after saline; shaded columns = EMG values before and after naloxone 0.4 mg i.v.

blind, placebo controlled crossover study of eleven Feighner positive schizophrenic subjects selected for their stable, frequent, auditory hallucinations. Ratings of hallucinations were significantly diminished following naloxone injections but not after placebo; however other aspects of their mental state were not significantly altered.

Emrich *et al.* (1977) investigated the effects of 4 mg naloxone in twenty subjects with paranoid psychoses and frequent auditory hallucinations. Ratings of hallucinations and 'key symptoms' on selected subscales of the Inpatient Multidimensional Psychiatric Scale (IMPS) were significantly reduced following naloxone but not placebo in a double blind cross-over design. A curious feature of the results is that significant naloxone effects were not observed until at least two hours following injection, at which time plasma levels of naloxone would have been less than 25% of their peak values. Emrich *et al.* (1979) have repeated this study using a higher dose of naloxone (24.8 mg) in twelve schizophrenic subjects. In contrast to their previous results, the higher dose of naloxone was less effective, key symptom ratings being unaffected and IMPS ratings failing to show improvements until 5 hours after injection. However, the authors point out that the latter results are preliminary and were obtained with a smaller patient group.

CONCLUSION

It seems clear that overstimulation of morphine (μ)-type opiate receptors is not an immediate cause of schizophrenia since these receptors are by definition highly susceptible to naloxone blockade yet standard doses of naloxone are not antipsychotic (Table 4). Nevertheless, the studies reporting a limited antipsychotic effect of high dose naloxone (Table 5) suggest excessive stimulation of non-morphine type opiate receptors by opioid peptides may play an aetiological role in schizophrenia. Thus a major need of further research is to characterize receptors of endogenous opioid peptides and to develop antagonists which can then be tested for antipsychotic activity. On the other hand, the neuroleptic-like properties of opiates and opioid peptides summarized in Table 2 suggest these substances are worthy of well controlled clinical trials in schizophrenia although it is difficult to see how problems of tolerance and withdrawal can be avoided.

Determining the relevance of opioid peptides to schizophrenia will require not only clinical trials but also the direct measurement of these substances in postmortem brains and in the biological fluids of schizophrenic subjects and there can be little doubt that the results of several such studies will be appearing in the next few years.

References

Babbini, M. and Davis, W. M. (1972). Time-dose relationships for locomotor activity effects of morphine after acute or repeated treatment. *Br. J. Pharmacol.*, **46**, 213

Bloom, F., Battenberg, E., Rossier, J., Ling, N. and Guillemin, R. (1978). Neurons containing Beta Endorphin in rat brain exist separately from those containing Enkephalin: immunocytochemical studies. *Ann. NY Acad. Sci. USA*, **75**, 1591

Bradbury, A. F., Smyth, D. G. and Snell, C. R. (1975). Biosynthesis of Beta-MSH and ACTH. In *Chemistry: Structure and Biology*, pp. 609–615. (Ann. Arbor: Sci. Inc.)

Bradbury, A. F., Smyth, D. G., Snell, C. R., Birdsall, N. J. H. and Hulme, E. C. (1976). C fragment of lipotropin has a high affinity for opiate receptors. *Nature (London)*, **260**, 793

Bradbury, A. F., Smyth, D. G., Snell, C. R., Deakin, J. F. W. and Wendlandt, S. (1977). Comparison of the analgesic properties of lipotropin C-fragment and stabilized enkephalins in the rat. *Biochem. Biophys. Res. Commun.*, **74**, 748

Connell, P. H. (1958). *Amphetamine Psychosis*. (London: Oxford University Press)

Creese, I., Burt, D. R. and Snyder, S. H. (1976). Dopamine receptor binding predicts clinical and pharmacological potencies of antischizophrenic drugs. *Science*, **192**, 481

Crow, T. J., Deakin, J. F. W., Johnstone, E. C. and Longden, A. (1976). Dopamine and schizophrenia. *Lancet*, **2**, 563

Davis, G. C., Bunney, W. E. Deraites, E. G., Kleinman, J. E. and Wyatt, R. J. (1977). Intravenous naloxone administration in schizophrenia and affective illness. *Science*, **197**, 74

De Wied, D., Kovacs, G. L., Bohus, B., Van Ree, J. M. and Greven, H. M. (1978). Neuroleptic activity of the neuropeptide BLPH 62–77. *Eur. J. Pharmacol.*, **49**, 527

Elde, R., Hökfelt, T., Johansson, O. and Terenius, L. (1976). Immunohistochemical studies using antibodies to leucine-enkephalin. Initial observations on the nervous system of the rat. *Neuroscience*, **1**, 349

Emrich, H. M., Cording, C., Pirée, S., Möller, H-J., von Zerssen, C. and Herz, A. (1977). Actions of naloxone in different types of psychoses. In Usdin, E., Bunney, W. W. and Kline, N. S. (eds.) *Endorphins and Mental Health Research*, pp 452–460. (London: Macmillan)

Emrich, H. M., Cording, C., Kolling, A., von Zerssen, D. and Herz, A. (1979). Induction of an antipsychotic action of the opiate antagonist naloxone. *Pharmakopsychiatrie*, **10**, 265

Enna, S. J., Bennet, J. P., Burt, D. R., Creese, I. and Snyder, S. H. (1976). Stereospecificity of interaction of neuroleptic drugs with neurotransmitters and correlation with clinical potency. *Nature (London)*, **263**, 338

Feldberg, W. and Smyth, D. G. (1976). The C-fragment of lipotropin – a potent analgesic. *J. Physiol.*, **260**, 30

Fukui, K., and Takagi, H. (1972). Effect of morphine on the cerebral contents of metabolites of dopamine and normal and tolerant mice: its possible relation to analgesic action. *Br. J. Pharmacol.*, **44**, 45

Geisow, M. J., Deakin, J. F. W., Dostrovsky, J. O. and Smyth, D. G. (1977). Analgesic activity of lipotropin C fragment depends on carboxyl terminal tetrapeptide. *Nature*, **269**, 167

Gunne, L. M., Lindstrom, L. and Terenius, L. (1977) Naloxone-induced reversal of schizophrenic hallucinations. *J. Neural Transmission*, **40**, 13

Gunne, L. M., Lindstrom, L. and Widerlov, E. (1979) Possible role of endorphins in schizophrenia and other psychiatric disorders. In Usdin, E., Bunney, W. W. and Kline, N. S. (eds.) *Endorphins and Mental Health Research*, pp. 547–560. (London: Macmillan)

Halliwell, J. V. and Kumar, R. (1977). Influence of morphine dependence and withdrawal on circling behaviour in rats with unilateral nigral lesions. *Br. J. Psychol.*, **59**, 454

Hambrook, J. M., Morgan, B. A., Rance, M. T. and Smith, C. F. C. (1976). Mode of deactivation of the enkephalins by rat and human plasma and rat brain homogenates. *Nature (London)*, **262**, 782

Hughes, J. (1975). Isolation of an endogenous compound from the brain with pharmacological properties similar to morphine. *Brain Res.*, **88**, 295

Hughes, J., Smith, T. W., Kosterlitz, H. W., Fothergill, L. A., Morgan, B. A. and Morris, H. R. (1975). Isolation of two related pentapeptides from brain with potent opiate agonist activity. *Nature (London)*, **258**, 577

Jaffe, J. H. and Martin, W. R. (1975). Narcotic analgesics and antagonists. In Goodman, L. S. and Gilman, A. (eds.) *The Pharmacological Basis of Therapeutics*, Chapter 15. (New York: Macmillan)

Jaquet, Y. F. and Marks, N. (1976). Endorphins: profound behavioural effects in rats suggest new aetiological factors in mental illness. *Science*, **194**, 630

Janowsky, D. S., Segal, D. S., Bloom, F., Abrams, A. and Guilleman, R. (1977). Lack of effect of naloxone in chronic schizophrenia. *Am. J. Psychiatry*, **134**, 926

Jasinski, D. R., Martin, W. R. and Haertzen, C. A. (1967). The human pharmacology and abuse potential of N-allyl noroxymorphone (naloxone). *J. Pharmacol. Exp. Ther.*, **157**, 420

Jorgensen, A., Fog, R. and Veilis, B. (1979). Synthetic enkephalin analogues in treatment of schizophrenia. *Lancet*, **1**, 935

Kline, N. S., Li, C. H., Lehman, H. E., Lajtha, A., Laski, E. and Cooper, T. (1977). Beta-endorphin induced changes in schizophrenic and depressed patients. *Arch. Gen. Psychiatry*, **34**, 1111

Kurland, A. A., McCabe, O., Hanlon, T. E. and Sullivan, D. (1977). The treatment of perceptual disturbances in schizophrenia with naloxone hydrochloride. *Am. J. Psychiatry*, **134**, 1408

Kushinsky, K. (1976). Actions of narcotics on brain dopamine metabolism and their relevance for psychomotor effects. *Arzneim. Forsch.*, **26**, 563

Lord, J. A. M., Waterfield, A. A., Hughes, J. and Kosterlitz, H. W. (1977). Endogenous opioid peptides: multiple agonists and receptors. *Nature (London)*, **267**, 495

Martin, W. R., Eades, C. G., Thompson, J. A., Huppler, R. E. and Gilbert, P. E. (1976). The effects of morphine and nalorphine-like drugs in the non-dependent and morphine dependent chronic spinal dog. *J. Pharmacol. Exp. Ther.*, **197**, 517

Minneman, K. P. and Iversen, L. L. (1977). Morphine selectively blocks dopamine stimulated cyclic AMP formations in rat neostriatal slices. *Br. J. Pharmacol.*, **59**, 480

Owen, F., Cross, A. J., Crow, T. J., Longden, A., Poulter, M. and Riley, G. J. (1978). Increased dopamine receptor sensitivity in schizophrenia. *Lancet*, **2**, 223

Pert, A., De Wald, A., Liao, H. and Sivit, C. (1979). Effects of opiates and opioid peptides on motor behaviours: sites and mechanisms of action. In Usdin, E., Bunney, W. W., and Kline, N. S. (eds.) *Endorphins in Mental Health Research*, pp. 45–61. (London: Macmillan)

Pollard, H., Llorens-Cortes, C. and Schwartz, J. C. (1977). Enkephalin receptors on dopaminergic neurones in rat striatum. *Nature (London)*, **268**, 745

Rivier, C., Vale, W., Ling, W., Brown, M. and Guillemin, R. (1977). Stimulation *in vivo* of the secretions of prolactin and growth hormone by Beta-endorphin. *Endocrinology*, **100**, 238

Schwartz, A. S. and Marchok, P. L. (1974). Repression of morphine-seeking behaviour by dopamine inhibition. *Nature (London)*, **248**, 257

Segal, D. S., Browne, R. G., Bloom, F., Ling, N. and Guillemin, R. (1977). Beta-endorphin: endogenous opiate or neuroleptic? *Science*, **198**, 411

Smith, G. M. and Beecher, H. K. (1961). Subjective of heroin and morphine in normal subjects. *J. Pharmacol. Exp. Ther.*, **136**, 47

Terenius, L., Lindstrom, L. and Widerlov, E. (1976). Increased levels of endorphins in chronic psychosis. *Neurosci. Lett.*, **3**, 157

Van Ree, J. M., Verhoeven, W., Van Praag, H. M. and De Weid, D. (1978a). Antipsychotic action of (DES-TYR^f) γ-endorphin (BLPH 62–77). In Van Ree, J. M., and Terenius, L. (eds.) *Characteristics and Functions of Opioids*, pp. 181–184. (Amsterdam: Elsevier/North-Holland Biomedical Press)

Van Ree, J. M., Witter, A. and Leysen, J. E. (1978b). Interaction of des-tyrosine-beta-endorphin (DTBetaE, BLPH 62–77) with neuroleptic binding sites in various areas of rat brain. *Eur. J. Pharmacol.*, **52**, 411

Volvaka, J., Mallya, A., Baig, S. and Perez-Cruet, J. (1977). Naloxone in chronic schizophrenia. *Science*, **196**, 1227

Watson, S. J., Berger, P. A., Akil, H., Mills, M. J. and Barchas, J. D. (1978). Effects of naloxone in schizophrenia: reduction in hallucinations in a subpopulation of subjects. *Science*, **201**, 73

4

The possible actions of peptides with opioid activity derived from pepsin hydrolysates of wheat gluten and of other constituents of gluten in the function of the central nervous system

W. A. KLEE and C. ZIOUDROU

Over the last few years evidence has accumulated to suggest that about a dozen or more peptides may be involved as transmitters or synaptic modulators in the CNS (Prange *et al.*, 1978). Neurotransmitting substances are characterized by (a) their distribution in the different regions of the CNS and the enzymes required for their biosynthesis and catabolism; (b) their binding to the specific receptors on the target cells; and (c) the biochemical and behavioural effects of drugs that inhibit the binding to the specific receptors or the enzymes, involved in the expression of the physiological effect.

The regulatory peptides of the hypothalamus, thyrotropin releasing factor (TRH), luteinizing hormone releasing factor (LHRH), growth hormone releasing factor (somatostatin) and other peptides synthesized in the hypothalamus and other regions of the CNS such as angiotensin II, the antidiuretic hormone (ADH), substance P, and neurotensin, in addition to their hormonal roles, may function as neurotransmitters (Vale *et*

53

al., 1977; Walker, 1978). Some peptides with activity in the CNS are responsible for promoting sleep; they were isolated from the CSF of sleep deprived animals (Monnier and Schoenenberger, 1974). Other peptides active in the CNS are responsible for the acquisition and preservation of learning and other behaviours (Ungar, 1975). De Wied (1977) has demonstrated that ACTH, vasopressin and related peptides influence behaviour by direct action on the brain.

The number of examples of neuropeptides is increasing exponentially but their physiological roles are only beginning to be understood. Many neuropeptides are found in tissues other than brain. For instance, substance P is not only found in the CNS but it has also been shown to be localized in the enterochromaffin cells of the gastrointestinal tract. Somatostatin, first isolated from the hypothalamus, has been detected by radio-immunoassay in the stomach and pancreas, and has been shown to inhibit the release of glucagon and insulin as well as of growth hormone. On the other hand, gastrin which was believed to exist only in the G cells of the stomach has been found, by radio-immunoassay, in extracts of human and animal brains. Similarly the intestinal peptides, the vasoactive intestinal peptide and cholecystokinin, are found in parts of the brain as well (Pearse, 1977). Recently, the neuropeptide enkephalin has also been found in the intestine (Polak *et al.*, 1977) and insulin was detected in rat brain in high amounts (Havrankova *et al.*, 1978). Many, if not most, peptides are found both in the brain and in the periphery. Another source of biologically active peptides could derive from ingestion of food proteins.

The present report describes the isolation, from pepsin hydrolysates of wheat gluten and α-casein, of peptides with opioid activity, the exorphins, as well as the characterization of an ingredient present in wheat gluten, the nucleoside adenosine which counteracts the effects of the exorphins.

OPIOID PEPTIDES AND THEIR BIOLOGICAL ROLES

In 1964, Li isolated from the pituitary gland the polypeptide β-lipotropin, the major function of which seemed to be the mobilization of fat *in vivo*. In 1973 Pert and Snyder, Simon *et al.*, and Terenius demonstrated stereospecific binding of morphine and its derivatives and their antagonists to homogenates of animal and human brain. Because it was thought unlikely that the human brain contained stereospecific receptor sites designed to interact with opium alkaloids, scientists hypothesized that most receptors for pain relieving drugs would be receptors for endogenous compounds. The search for endogenous opiates led to the discovery of the opioid peptides, the enkephalins, by Hughes *et al.*, (1975) and the pituitary endorphins by Goldstein (1976). Recently evidence continues to mount that endorphins in the pituitary gland are derived from a larger peptidic precursor of molecular weight 31 000 by the pathway: 31 K precursor→ β-lipotropin→ β-endorphin→ γ-endorphin→ α-endorphin (Roberts and Herbert, 1977). Met-enkephalin may be derived from the degradation of the endorphins or other precursors by the action of brain peptidase whereas the origin of the leu-enkephalin remains still unknown. The enkephalins, endorphins and β-lipotropin are extremely potent in their morphine-like actions; in addition they evoke potent and divergent behavioural responses (Snyder, 1978). Exogenously administered endorphins and enkephalins in animals and humans produce analgesia, euphoria, catatonia, hypermotility and other opiate actions which are reversed by the opiate antagonist, naloxone. The putative neurotransmitting actions of the opioid peptides are covered in Volume 18 of the Advances in Biochemical Pharmacology (Costa and Trabucchi (eds.), 1978).

In hybrid cells derived from fusion of mouse neuroblastoma and rat glial cell lines (NG-108-15) (Klee and Nirenberg, 1974), binding of morphine results in a rapid inhibition of basal and PGE_1- or adenosine-stimulated adenylate cyclase and a decrease in cAMP. Continuous exposure to morphine causes an increase in adenylate cyclase activity restoring cAMP levels to normal. This process renders cells tolerant to morphine and dependent upon the opiate (Sharma et al., 1975). Withdrawal of morphine or addition of the specific antagonist naloxone raises cAMP to normal levels. The enkephalins and many analogues of enkephalins resistant to hydrolysis mimic these effects (Lampert et al., 1976). One of the characteristic effects of the opiates in human is the production of a state of indifference and emotional detachment. This could possibly be explained by suppression of endogenously synthesized endorphins due to the administration of exogenous opiates. The removal of the exogenous stimulus can expose the individual to an acute abstinence syndrome and one can hypothesize that opiate withdrawal symptoms in man may be related to an endorphin deficiency.

Considerable interest is expressed recently in the possibility that endorphins may well be related to the symptomatology of psychotic patients (Lindstrom et al., 1978; Verebey et al., 1978). Bloom et al. (1976) have shown that intracisternal injection of β-endorphin in rats elicits a profound catatonic state and the same effect was produced by injection of β-endorphin in the periaqueductal grey in rats (Jacquet and Marks, 1976). Elevated levels of endorphins have been detected with rats under stressful (Mata et al., 1977) or painful (Madden et al., 1977) conditions. Endorphin effects are not easily shown in man (Grevert and Goldstein, 1977, 1978). A number of trials of the opiate antagonist naloxone, in the treatment of schizophrenic patients have been unsuccessful or ambiguous

(Herz *et al.*, 1978) following the early report of success by Gunne *et al.*, (1977). There is thus little evidence that an excess of endorphins may be a causative factor in most schizophrenias. On the other hand, there is a preliminary, and as yet unconfirmed, report which indicates that some schizophrenic patients may be helped by renal dialysis and that the dialysates of these patients contain a peptide related to β-endorphin (Palmour *et al.*, 1977). This work needs to be confirmed with a larger number of patients and the incorporation of suitable controls, particularly since a negative report has already appeared (Kroll *et al.*, 1978). The alternative hypothesis, that too little endorphin may cause schizophrenia, has recently been tested in a preliminary, non-blind study of six schizophrenic patients (Kline *et al.*, 1977). Four of the six responded to intravenous administration of β-endorphin with significantly improved symptoms. This work, too, needs replication in a larger study under double-blind conditions. From the existing data to date it is logical to assume that alternations in the homeostatic regulation of the endogenous opioid peptides could have a profound significance in mental illness.

It has long been recognized that the exact composition and structure of a biologically active peptide is not absolutely essential for its activity (Woolley and Merrifield, 1963). Replacement of one amino acid by another may result in an increase, decrease or no change in the activity of the peptide. Occasionally, a synthetically prepared peptide analogue such as the D-ala^2-met-enkephalin is more active *in vivo* than its naturally occuring peptide (Pert *et al.*, 1976). Many recent reports continue to show a great deal of compositional and conformational mobility for enkephalins. Beddell *et al.* (1977) studied a series of enkephalin analogues using the mouse vas deferens bioassay and binding to receptors of brain homogenates and constructed a map for the allowable structural alterations for opiate activity and degree of potency. Klee *et al.* (1978) studied the potencies of a series of enkephalin analogues using their inhibitory action on the adenylate cyclase of the NG 108-15 hybrid cells. These two studies and many others conclude that D-amino acids can replace glycine in position 2 and methionine in position 5 with little or no change in potency. The analogues with D-amino acids resist hydrolysis by various proteinases and are suitable for studies of the physiological actions of enkephalins. Because of the extraordinary potency of the enkephalin analogues a peptide with 100- or 1000-fold decrease in potency could still be a highly active substance. For example the concentration of met-enkephalin for half-maximal inhibition of adenylate cyclase of the NG 108-15 hybrid cells is of the order of 10^{-8} mol/l whereas a concentration of 10^{-6} mol/l of the N-terminal arginine-met-enkephalin is needed to produce the same effect (Klee *et al.*, 1978).

CAN EXOGENOUS BIOLOGICALLY ACTIVE PEPTIDES REACH THE BRAIN?

The biological activity of peptide analogues *in vivo* reflect many properties including transport, degradation rates, receptor binding affinity and efficacy. If enkephalin or endorphin analogues administered exogenously are to reach the brain they should (a) survive hydrolysis by the peptidases of the gastro-intestinal tract and lysosomal enzymes and (b) cross the blood-brain barrier.

Despite the classical hypothesis that proteins are converted to free amino acids before absorption from the gastro-intestinal tract, work in several laboratories has provided strong evidence that protein absorption involves mucosal uptake of intact peptides followed by hydrolysis in the absorptive cell (Matthews and Path, 1977). It has also been demonstrated that amino acids can be absorbed more rapidly from peptides than in the free form (Crampton *et al.*, 1971). The percentage absorption of individual amino acids in a mixture of a total hydrolysate of a protein was reduced when the enzymatic hydrolysate of the protein was used (Nixon and Mawer, 1970a,b). Furthermore, it has been documented that peptides compete for uptake with one another (Addison *et al.*, 1974; Adibi and Soleimanpour, 1974).

Dietary alteration (protein deprivation) in rats (Lis *et al.*, 1972) reduces the intestinal absorption of free amino acids of a mixture simulating casein but had no effect on the absorption of oligopeptides of a tryptic hydrolysate of casein. Studies of the absorption of amino acids and peptides by the intestine of individuals with hereditary intestinal defects, like cystinuria, Hartnup disease (Milne and Asatoor, 1975) and coeliac sprue (Adibi *et al.*, 1974; Silk *et al.*, 1974) showed that the carrier-mediated intestinal absorption of peptides was unaltered, whereas the absorption of free amino acids was severely impaired. The intestinal absorption of peptides also depends on their size, lipophilicity and their resistance to hydrolysis. Hydrophobic peptides are likely to be absorbed by diffusion through membrane lipids.

Although the bulk of dietary protein normally reaches the portal blood in the form of amino acids, peptides also are absorbed into the bloodstream without prior degradation. Peptides which are resistant to degradation by pancreatic and intestinal enzymes such as gly-gly, proline containing peptides, β-alanylhistidine (carnosine) and those containing D-amino acids are efficiently absorbed into the bloodstream from the intestinal lumen (Matthews and Path, 1977). Thus, peptide hydrolysis by intestinal enzymes is not a necessary part of the mechanism of peptide uptake. Biologically active peptides, particularly those which are relatively resistant to proteolysis are also absorbed from the gastro-intestinal tract. Evidence for the absorption of orally presented proteins or large fragments of such proteins exists for insulin (Danforth and Moore, 1959), botulinus toxin (Heckly *et al.*, 1960) and a number of other proteins (Warshaw *et al.*, 1974; Hemmings *et al.*, 1977). In neonatal animals, large amounts of proteins, particularly immunoglobulins, are absorbed from the intestine without prior degradation (Hemmings *et al.*, 1977). This massive protein uptake apparently ceases within a few weeks of birth, but it is interesting to wonder what the consequences might be if this uptake mechanism were only partially shut down. Large molecular breakdown products of ferritin-labelled IgG and α-gliadin have been demonstrated to cross the gut wall and the cell membranes of other body tissues, (Hemmings and Williams, 1978).

Essential nutrients cross the blood–brain barrier through specific carrier-mediated transport (Rapaport, 1976). A variety of substances diffuse into the brain at rates that are a function of their lipophilicity and size. Biologically important peptides have been shown to cross the blood–brain barrier (Greenberg *et al.*, 1976; Hemmings, 1978). Hemmings (1978) provided direct evidence that after feeding a number of different ^{131}I-labelled proteins to rats, labelled peptides, as well as products with very high molecular weights, are found in the brain and other parts of the body. Much of this incorporated radioactivity was recognized by antibodies directed against the ingested proteins and they must therefore have been reasonably intact. Interestingly, the proteins tested by Hemmings included α-gliadin which has been implicated in the aetiology of coeliac disease and perhaps of schizophrenia. Recently it has been shown that gluten given orally to rats potentiates the behavioural stereotypy of amphetamine (Taylor, 1978). These findings were confirmed by Williams *et al.* (1979) who also showed that oral administration of IgG had a lesser effect than wheat gluten on the behaviour of rats treated with amphetamine.

Biologically active peptides administered extracerebrally may affect brain functions. Intravenously injected $ACTH_{4-10}$ in man influences attention and memory (Miller *et al.*, 1974) and L-prolyl- L-leucyl-glycine amide potentiates the effect of levodopa in man after i.v. injection (Barbeau, 1975). Current experiments with D-ala^2-endorphin showed that the opioid peptides pass readily the blood–brain barrier (Rapaport *et al.* in preparation), although Cornford *et al.* (1978), have recently reported that only a small amount of met-enkephalin reaches the brain from the carotid blood. A number of synthetic enkephalin or endorphin analogues that resist proteolysis have been shown to produce analgesia after i.v. injection (Bajusz *et al.*, 1977; Tseng *et al.*, 1976; Yamashiro *et al.*, 1977) or by oral administration (Roemer *et al.*, 1977).

WHEAT GLUTEN AND SCHIZOPHRENIA

The primary environmental cause of coeliac disease or gluten entero-pathy is attributed to a number of cereal grain proteins, particularly in wheat gluten or its major constituents, the gliadins (Hekkens and Pena, 1974). The major symptoms of coeliac disease are massive diarrhoea associated with characteristic intestinal lesions. Patients with the disease may also present psychotic symptoms (Pauley, 1959; von Käser, 1961). The similarities between the behavioural anomalies of coeliac patients and those of schizophrenics led Dohan (1966a) to examine the role of cereal proteins and especially wheat gluten in the pathology of schizophrenia. Dohan's findings can be summarized as follows:

(1) The psychotic effects of gluten were confirmed in controlled trials with schizophrenics of a cereal grain-free and milk-free diet with and without added gluten (Dohan and Grasberger, 1973). These findings were also confirmed on a double-blind basis by Singh and Kay (1976), who showed that schizophrenic patients deteriorated when wheat gluten was substituted for soy flour in their diets.
(2) Hospital admissions of schizophrenics and the length of stay in the hospital are highly correlated with cereal grain consumption (Dohan, 1966b).
(3) Intracerebral injection of some gluten peptide fractions (derived from pepsin-pancreatic hydrolysis) in rats produce stereotyped movements, catalepsy, prolonged chewing in air, and seizures (Dohan et al., 1978).
(4) Coeliac disease occurs in schizophrenics and vice versa far more often than might be expected on the basis of chance (Graff and Handford, 1961; Dohan, 1976). Also intestinal lesions similar to those seen in untreated coeliac disease have sometimes been found in schizophrenics on autopsy, although these were not found in more recent post-mortem examinations of neuroleptic-treated schizophrenics (Dohan, 1969, 1976). A recent report shows that 54% of a group of mental patients have antibodies to cereal proteins compared with 19% of control group (Mascord et al., 1978).

These observations led Dohan to conclude that schizophrenia and gluten enteropathy share one or more common genes and that the differences in the two diseases are determined by the dissimilar components of the genotypes.

OPIOID PEPTIDES FROM FOOD PROTEINS

The behavioural effects of endogenous peptides and gluten peptides produced by the gastro-intestinal peptidases and the reports relating gluten and possibly casein consumption with mental illness stimulated us to examine the biological activities of peptides derived from wheat gluten and α-casein by the action of the stomach peptidase, pepsin.

Wheat gluten and α-casein were subjected to pepsin hydrolysis at pH 2 and 37 °C, conditions which resemble those in the stomach. These digests and some peptides purified from them were shown to have morphine-like activity in several biochemical and biological assays. The assays used routinely were (a) the inhibition of adenylate cyclase of neuroblastoma × glioma hybrid cells (Sharma *et al.*, 1975); (b) the inhibition of contractions of the mouse vas deferens (Henderson *et al.*, 1972); and (c) the binding to rat brain membrane opiate receptors by measuring the competition with [³H]dihydromorphine (Klee and Streaty, 1974). The opioid activity generated as a function of time when wheat gluten and α-casein were treated with pepsin are shown in Figures 1 and 2 (Zioudrou

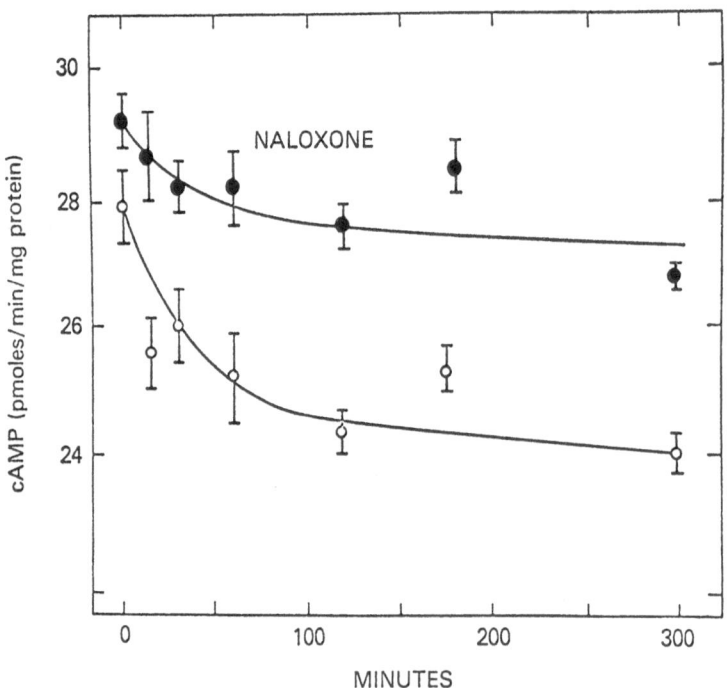

Figure 1 Exorphin activity in a pepsin digest of gluten as a function of time of treatment with pepsin. Activity was determined as the effect of the gluten digest upon the adenylate cyclase activity of homogenates of neuroblastoma × glioma hybrid NG-108-15 cells assayed in the presence (filled circles) or in the absence (open circles) of 0.1 mol/l naloxone

and Klee, 1978). It should be noticed that the activities of both hydrolysates are reversed by the opiate antagonist (−)-naloxone. The purification of fractions with opiate activity was achieved by several
chromatographic methods and the opioid activity was followed by the
inhibition of adenylate cyclase (Zioudrou *et al.*, 1979). The opioid activity
of highly purified materials was lost after treatment with pronase. Other
proteinases such as subtilisin, thermolysin and chymotrypsin are less
effective and the opioid activity is practically not affected by the action of
trypsin. We named these peptides 'exorphins', because of their exogenous origin and their opioid activities. Casein exorphin was totally inactivated by pronase whereas gluten exorphin was inactivated 70%. The
potency of the exorphins is shown in Figure 3. Small amounts of exorphin
inhibit adenylate cyclase to the same extent as do saturating amounts of
morphine.

The exorphins also inhibit the contractions of electrically stimulated

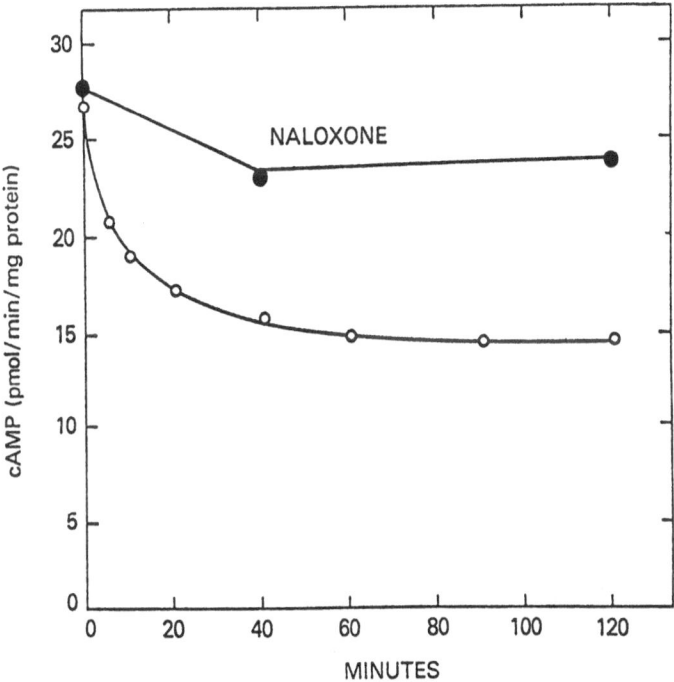

Figure 2   Exorphin activity in a pepsin digest of α-casein as a function of time of treatment
with pepsin. Activity was determined as the effect of the α-casein digest upon the adenylate
cyclase activity of homogenates of neuroblastoma × glioma hybrid cells NG-108-15, assayed
in the presence (filled circles) or in the absence (open circles) of 0.1 mol/l naloxone

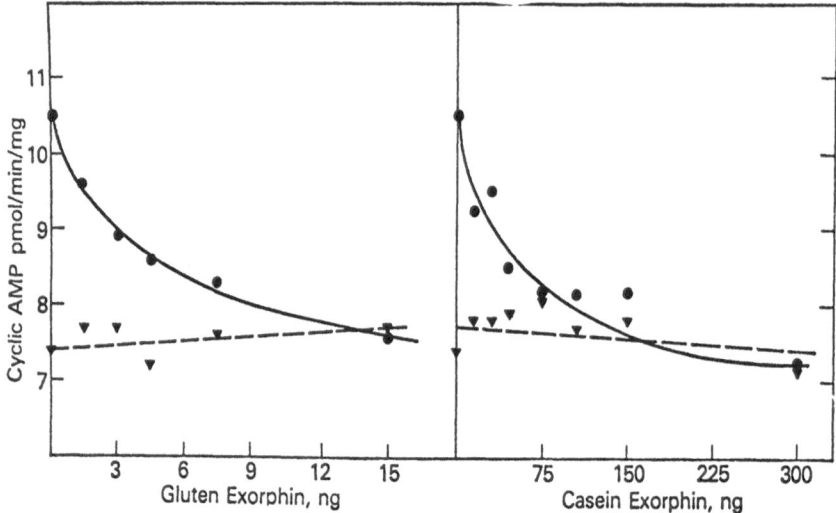

Figure 3   Effect of varying concentrations of exorphins on the activity of NG-108-15 adenylate cyclase at the concentrations indicated in the absence (filled circles) and in the presence (triangles) of 2×10^{-5} mol/l morphine

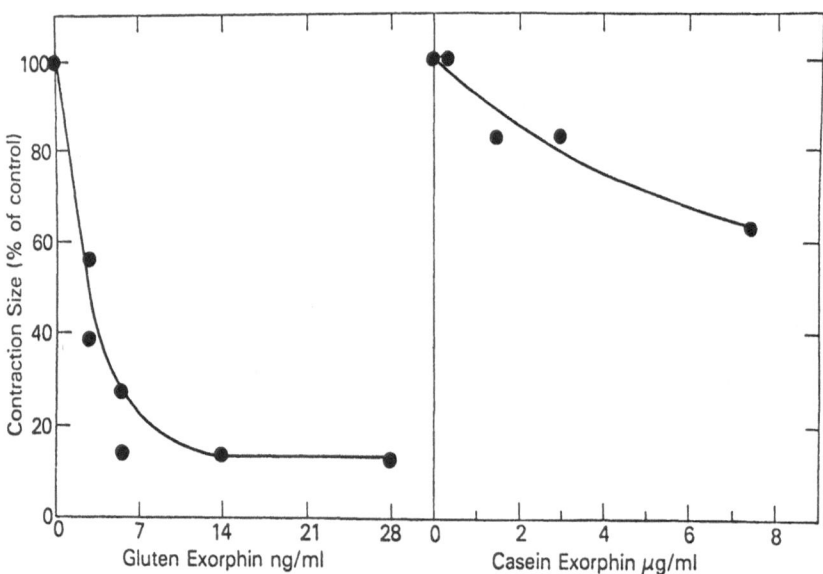

Figure 4   Effect of varying concentrations of exorphins on the contraction size of the mouse vas deferens

mouse vas deferens in a concentration dependent way and the inhibition is reversed by (−)-naloxone. These effects are shown in Figure 4. In both assays, the inhibition of adenyl cyclase and the vas deferens, gluten exorphin is much more potent than casein exorphin. However the potency of casein exorphin is only 1/4000 that of gluten exorphin in the mouse vas deferens assay whereas it is 1/10 that of gluten exorphin in the adenylate cyclase assay.

The binding of the exorphins to the specific opiate receptors to rat brain membrane homogenates, is shown in Figure 5 by the displacement of [³H]dihydromorphine. The results with [³H]D-ala-met-enkephalin are similar.

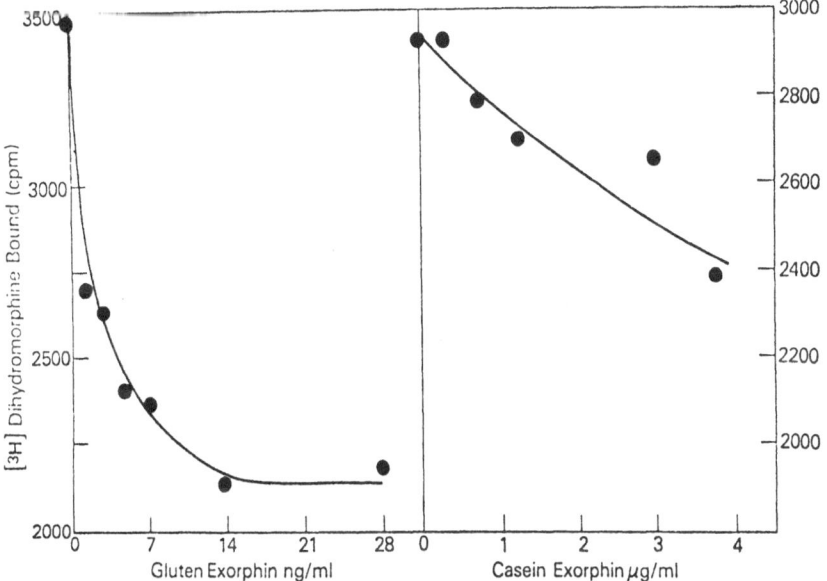

Figure 5 Displacement of [³H]dihydromorphine from rat brain opiate receptors by varying concentrations of exorphins

A comparison of the potency of the exorphins with met-enkephalin and morphine in the three opiate assays is presented in Table 1. The potency of gluten exorphin in each of the assays is comparable to that of met-enkephalin. Casein exorphin, on the other hand, is much less potent in all assay systems used, and the relative opioid potencies of gluten and casein exorphins vary with the assay. Thus, gluten exorphin is least active in the adenylate cyclase assay where casein exorphin is most active. The results in Table 1 are expressed in nanograms per ml required for half-maximal effects. Preliminary calculations of the molecular weights of the exorphins based on amino acid analysis data, show that the molar concentrations of gluten exorphin for half-maximal effects on the adenylate cyclase and vas deferens assays as well as the binding to brain opiate receptors range between 10^{-9} to 10^{-8} mol/l and are almost identical to those for met-enkaphalin. In fact gluten exorphin is one hundred times more potent than morphine in inhibiting adenylate cyclase and the electrically stimulated vas deferens. The molar concentration of casein exorphin needed to produce half maximal effects ranges between 10^{-7} and 10^{-6} mol/l. Casein exorphin seems to be equipotent with morphine in the adenyl cyclase and vas deferens assays. The amino acid sequence, the synthesis of the exorphins and the study of their conformation may explain the potency differences. Work is in progress for the determination of the chemical composition of the exorphins and their synthesis.

Table 1 Concentrations of exorphins (nanograms/ml) for half-maximal inhibitions in several opiate assays

	Brain receptor binding	Adenylate cyclase	Vas deferens
Gluten exorphin	2	30	2
Casein exorphin	3500	320	8000
Met-enkephalin	20	7	7*
Morphine sulphate	1	570	190*

* Calculated from the data of Lord et al. (1976)

The opioid peptides isolated from wheat gluten and α-casein were resistant to the intestinal proteinases trypsin and chymotrypsin. In addition their high binding affinity (KD approximately 10^{-9} and 10^{-6} mol/l) for gluten and casein exorphins respectively) for the specific opiate receptor of rat brain homogenates which are rich in aminopeptidases, suggests that the exorphins may also be resistant to exopeptidases. The exorphins behave as small hydrophobic peptides as they have been characterized by several chromatographic systems. Thus, the exorphins may be expected to survive extensive degradation in the intestine, and to some extent, be absorbed without prior degradation, from the gastro-intestinal tract into the bloodstream, and subsequently, they could reach the brain in functionally significant amounts where they could be expected to exhibit central effects.

A CONSTITUENT OF WHEAT GLUTEN THAT OPPOSES THE INHIBITORY ACTIVITIES OF THE EXORPHINS

Pepsin hydrolysates of wheat gluten are extremely complex mixtures and along with the peptides with opioid activity they also contain a material which stimulates both the adenylate cyclase of the NG-108-15 cells and the electrically induced contractions of the mouse vas deferens. A partially purified stimulatory fraction (by column chromatography on DE-52-cellulose and Biogel P-6) stimulates the contractions of the mouse vas deferens by 150% and the effect was not reversed by naloxone. The same material stimulates the adenylate cyclase of the NG-108-15 cell in a bell-shaped concentration-dependent curve, i.e. low concentrations were stimulatory and high concentrations inhibited strongly the production of cAMP. Neither stimulation or inhibition were affected by naloxone (Zioudrou and Klee, 1979).

The stimulatory actions of gluten were not affected by proteolytic enzymes such as pronase, trypsin, chymotrypsin or subtilisin. However, the activity was destroyed by periodate oxidation. The existence of the stimulatory material could also be detected in the zero time samples of pepsin digests of gluten and in neutralized extracts of gluten with 0.1 N acetic acid or 0.1 N hydrochloric acid. Purification of these extracts was achieved by gel filtration on Sephadex G-25 and finally the stimulatory material was monitored on a Waters high pressure liquid chromatographer using a Bondapak C-18 column and an ammonium acetate (10 mmol/l, pH 7.5)–methanol (0–70%) gradient.

The structure of this material was determined by mass spectrometry and ultra violet spectra. Both analyses revealed that the compound is the nucleoside adenosine and both spectra were identical with those of authentic adenosine.

The stimulatory action of authentic adenosine and adenosine isolated from gluten on the adenylate cyclase of NG-108-15 cells is shown in Figure 6. The stimulation is not affected by naloxone and shows a bell-shape concentration dependence. Adenosine does not bind to opiate receptors but is antagonized by methylxanthines such as theophylline. The effect of theophylline is shown in Figure 7. Theophylline inhibits the stimulation of adenylate cyclase by adenosine only at the side of low concentrations and has practically no effect in the presence of high concentrations of adenosine.

It has also been shown that liver adenylate cyclase is stimulated by gluten-adenosine and the activity is abolished by the action of adenosine deaminase and inhibited by theophylline. In addition the stimulatory action of liver adenylate cyclase was shown to be strongly GTP dependent. Gluten-adenosine also inhibits the isoproterenol-stimulated adenylate cyclase of fat cell (Zioudrou, Londos and Klee, in preparation). Some

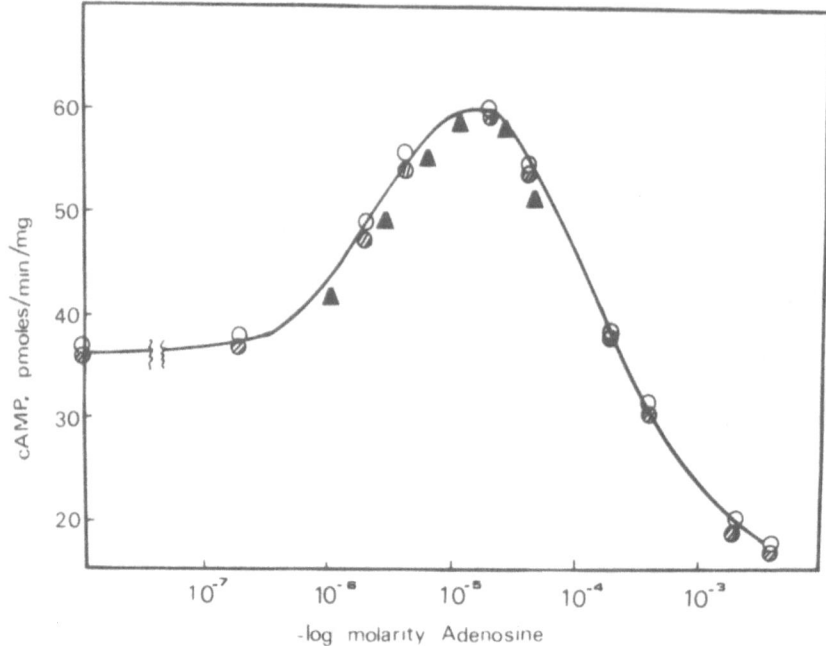

Figure 6 Effect of varying concentrations of adenosine on the activity of NG-108-15 adenylate cyclase, authentic adenosine (open circles), authentic adenosine in the presence of 0.1mmol/l naloxone (striped circles) and adenosine isolated from wheat gluten (triangles)

of these effects are shown in Table 2. An estimate of the amount of adenosine present in 0.1 N acetic acid extracts of gluten (gluten used in these

Table 2 Effects of adenosine deaminase (ADA) and GTP on the stimulation of adenylate cyclase of rat liver plasma membranes by adenosine*

Additions	Adenylate cyclase activity (cAMP, pmoles/min mg protein)			
	Control	ADA†	−GTP	+GTP‡
None	58.6	60.0	29.8	50.6
Adenosine (gluten)¶	106.0	58.9	30.1	88.6
Adenosine (authentic)¶	96.0	60.2	–	–

* Adenylate cyclase activity was assayed as described by Salomon et al. (1974)
† Adenosine deaminase, 2 units per ml
‡ GTP 10^{-5} mol/l
¶ Concentrations of adenosine 5×10^{-7} mol/l

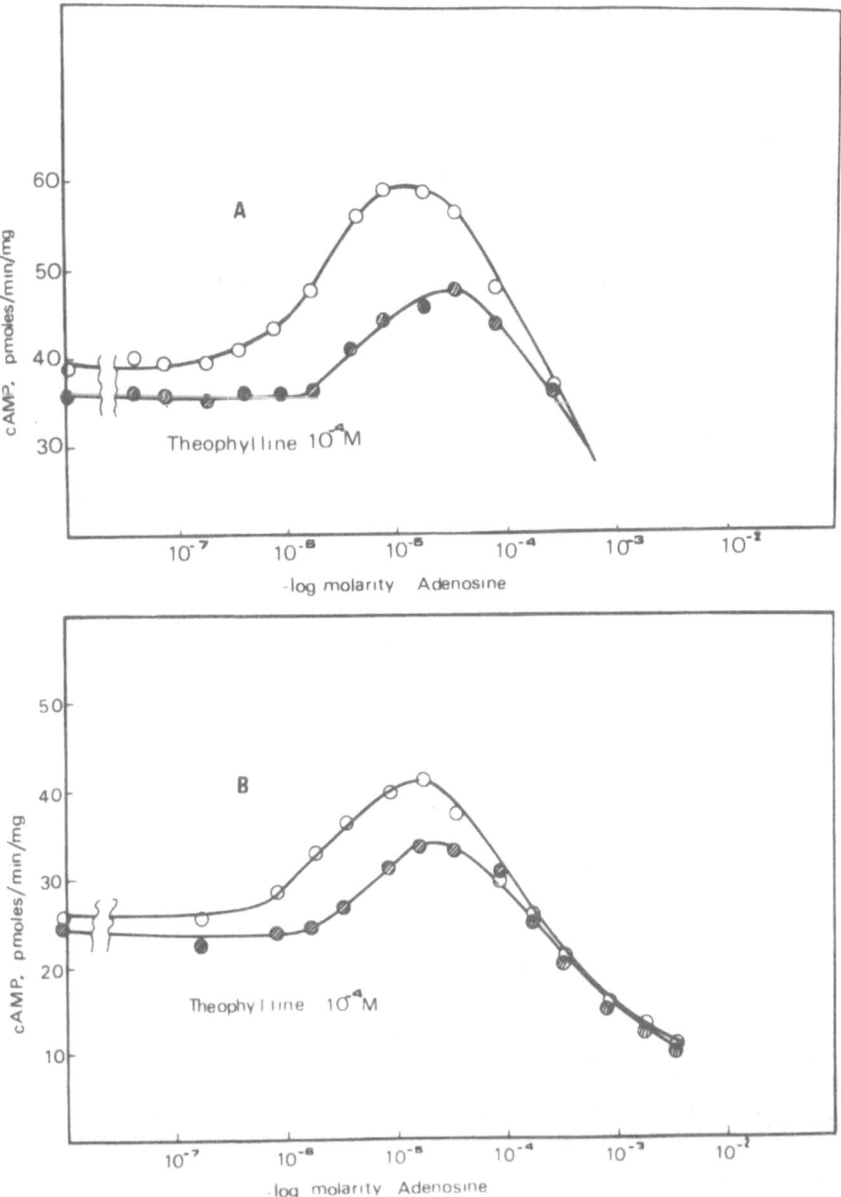

Figure 7 Effect of varying concentrations of adenosine in absence (open circles) and presence (striped circles) of 10^{-4} mol/l theophylline: (A) adenosine isolated from wheat gluten; (B) authentic adenosine

experiments was purchased from ICN) gave approximately 50 mg per kilogram of gluten. Adenosine was identified in onion extracts and was the factor which inhibited platelets aggregation (Weisenberger *et al.*, 1972).

During the course of this work we tested pepsin hydrolysates of a number of other proteins using the effect of the hydrolysates on the NG-108-15 adenylate cyclase activity (Zioudrou *et al.*, 1979). The hydrolysates of grain protein zein and hordein showed stimulation mixed with naloxone-reversible inhibition, whereas avenin and secalin showed only stimulation.

SOME BIOLOGICAL EFFECTS OF ADENOSINE

Adenosine and some of its derivatives are toxic to mammalian and bacterial cells. The major biological properties of adenosine are coronary vasodilatation, inhibition of platelet aggregation, inhibition of the immune response, delayed neurotransmission and inhibition or stimulation of hormone secretion (Fox and Kelley, 1978). The vasomotor and other autonomic actions of adenosine as well as the release of adenosine from tissues in response to various stimuli led Burnstock (1975) to propose the existence of purinergic nerves which use adenosine and some of its derivatives as neurotransmitters. The effects of adenosine on the intracellular production of cAMP of different tissues are attributed to the interaction of adenosine with a specific receptor on the external cell surface (Burnstock, 1977). For example, adenosine stimulates the adenylate cyclase in liver cells (Londos and Wolff, 1977, and references cited therein), in cerebral cortex slices (Sattin and Rall, 1970; Huang and Daly, 1974; Phillis and Kostopoulos, 1975), in C-1300 murine neuroblastoma cells (Green and Stanberry, 1977), and inhibits the adenylate cyclase in fat cells (Fain *et al.*, 1972; Londos *et al.*, 1978).

The major roots of adenosine metabolism in mammalian cells are its conversion to inosine by the action of adenosine deaminase or its phosphorylation to AMP by the action of ATP:adenosine 5'-phosphotransferase. For normal cell function in man a normal level of both enzymes is required, which compete for the same substrate. Deficiency of adenosine deaminase resulting in increased levels of adenosine, is associated with increased intracellular concentration of adenine nucleotides. Adenosine deaminase acts at concentrations of substrate above 3 μ mol/l whereas at low concentrations adenosine is converted to its nucleotides (Fox and Kelley, 1978). Immunodeficiency diseases (van der Weyden and Kelley, 1977) and cardiovascular effects (Stein, 1975) have been shown to be associated with loss of or reduced activity of adenosine deaminase and accumulation of adenosine. Adenosine and ATP have depressive activities in the peripheral nervous system such as relaxation of smooth muscle, slowing of the heart and potent depressive action on neurons of the cerebral cortex (Ribeiro, 1978). Compounds which inhibit adenosine deaminase or adenosine uptake potentiate the effects by adenosine. Theophilline and caffeine antagonize the effects (Burnstock, 1975). Adenosine, cAMP or adenine have been shown to antagonize the analgesic action of morphine (Gourley and Beckner, 1973).

There are some interesting observations which relate adenosine or adenosine nucleotides to mental illness. Abdulla and Hamadah (1975) reported a strong stimulation of PGE_1 synthesis in platelets of normal individuals in response to ADP but not in the platelets of 20 diagnosed schizophrenics. Recently Horrobin (1977) has suggested that mental disorders may be due to prostaglandin deficiency. High levels of adenosine and ATP were determined in the whole blood of diagnosed schizophrenics, psychotic and neurotic patients and very high erythrocyte adenosine concentrations were measured in a few young schizophrenics (Hansen, 1972).

Adenosine has been shown to inhibit transmethylation reactions stimulated by a brain enzyme. It was proposed that adenosine acts by inhibiting the hydrolysis of S-adenosylhomocysteine by S-adenosylhomocysteinase (Deguchi and Barchas, 1971). A recent report shows that adenosine forms a tight complex (K_D 5 × 10^{-8} mol/l) with S-adenosylhomocysteinase from yellow lupin seed (Yakubowski and Guronowski, in press).

POSSIBLE BIOLOGICAL SIGNIFICANCE OF EXORPHINS AND ADENOSINE

In the present report we described the isolation and partial purification of peptides with opioid activity, the exorphins, derived from wheat gluten and α-casein. Also we showed that the material in wheat gluten which antagonizes the opiate actions of the exorphins by stimulating the adenylate cyclase of the NG-108-15 hybrid cells and the contractions of the mouse vas deferens is the nucleotide, adenosine. The pepsin hydrolysates of wheat gluten (which are a partially digested gluten) show mixed opiate agonist–antagonist activities and it is known that the opiates with mixed activities such as nalorphine and cyclazocine, often produce profound dysphoria and psychotic symptoms (Martin, 1967; Jaffé and Martin, 1975). Thus, if the cause of schizophrenia is due to a deficiency of endorphins (Jacquet and Marks, 1976) a functional deficiency could be produced by high levels of adenosine, which antagonizes the effects of the opioid peptides. On the other hand, from Figures 6 and 7, it can be seen that high concentrations of adenosine reduce strongly the production of cAMP and therefore could possibly act in a synergistic way with opioid peptides, inhibiting the action of adenylate cyclase. In the presence of high concentrations of adenosine, theophylline is without effect. Similar biphasic effects of adenosine concentration on the activity of adenylate cyclase have been demonstrated in liver plasma membranes and most other cell systems. In addition agents that stimulate adenylate cyclase in the intestinal mucosa are known to cause diarrhoea and this symptom of gluten-sensitive enteropathy may possibly be related to the effects of adenosine present in wheat gluten.

Wheat gluten products do not produce psychotic symptoms when ingested by normal individuals. Presumably genetic factors determine whether or not gluten will exert toxic or psychotic symptoms. Research today has revealed that schizophrenia is not a single disease due to a single biochemical disorder, but probably it is the result of many unknown biochemical aberrations that predispose to inheritance of the disease. Some of the biochemical factors which could contribute to the exacerbation of psychotic symptoms by ingestion of gluten and possibly other proteins are the following: (1) deficiencies in intestinal proteinases so that larger than normal amounts of toxic peptides are present (Cornell and Townley, 1973) or abnormal secretion of gastrointestinal peptides (Besterman et al., 1978; Konturcks et al., 1978); (2) defects in the intestinal mucosa which allow abnormally large amounts of peptides to be absorbed into the bloodstream (Walker and Isselbacher, 1974); (3) deficiencies in peptidase activity in lysosomes in the liver or in the capillary walls of the lungs which lead to a decreased rate of peptide loss from the bloodstream; (4) increased permeability at the blood–brain barrier; (5) deficiencies in peptidase activities in the target organs, the brain for example, so that peptides have a longer lifetime of action at their receptor sites; (6) increased sensitivity of the receptors to the action of the peptides; (7) deficiency of adenosine deaminase or adenosine kinase resulting in high levels of adenosine in the circulation or intracellularly. These considerations revolve around the tacit assumption that peptides, to affect behaviour, must necessarily act in the central nervous system. Although this assumption is correct in many cases, it is not difficult to imagine mechanisms whereby primary effects on peripheral organs, the endocrine system for example, may liberate substances which, in turn, enter the brain and modify behaviour. Alternatively, chemosensory neurons may transmit information about peptides directly from the periphery to the central nervous system by a feedback signal similar to information that the brain receives from the ACTH-stimulated glucocorticoids when ACTH is released by the pituitary.

Thus, peptides derived from food proteins need not necessarily ever leave the gastrointestinal tract in order to influence behaviour. Much work remains to be done in order to establish the role of either the endorphins or the exorphins or the adenosine present in gluten in a disease as complex and elusive as schizophrenia. Evidence is being accumulated that genetic factors are importantly involved in coeliac disease and schizophrenia (Kessler, 1976; Pena *et al.*, 1978). However, the importance of environmental influences and in particular of nutrition merit further examination.

The effects of the exorphins have not yet been studied *in vivo*; however the present report provides a plausible mechanism in support of Dohan's hypothesis of common features in the aetiology of coeliac disease and schizophrenia.

References

Abdulla, Y. H. and Hamadah, K. (1975). Effect of ADP on PGE formation in blood platelets from patients with depression, mania and schizophrenia. *Br. J. Psychiatry*, **127**, 591

Addison, J. M., Matthews, D. M. and Burston, D. (1974). Competition between carnosine and other peptides for transport by hamster jejunum *in vitro*. *Clin. Sci. Mol. Med.*, **46**, 707

Adibi, S. A., Fogel, M. R. and Agranal, R. M. (1974). Comparison of free amino acid and dipeptide absorption in the jejunum of sprue patients. *Gastroenterology*, **67**, 586

Adibi, S. A. and Soleimanpour, M. R. (1974). Functional characterization of dipeptide transport system in human jejunum. *J. Clin. Invest.*, **53**, 1368

Bajusz, S., Rónai A. Z., Székely, J. I., Graf, L., Dunai-Kovács, Z., and Berzétei, I. (1977). A superactive antinociceptive pentapeptide (D-Met^2, Pro^5)-enkephalinamide. *FEBS Lett.*, **76**, 91

Barbeau, A. (1975). Potentiation of levodopa effect by intravenous L-prolyl-L-leucyl-glycine amide in man. *Lancet*, **2**, 683

Beddell, C. R., Clark, R. B., Hardy, G. W., Lowe, L. A., Ubatuba, F. B., Vane, J. R., Wilkinson, S., Chang, K. J., Guatrecasas, P. and Miller, R. J. (1977). Structural requirements for opioid activity of analogues of the enkephalin. *Proc. R. Soc. (London)*, **198B**, 249

Besterman, H. S., Sarson, D. L., Johnston, D. I., Stewart, J. S., Guerin, S., Bloom, S. R., Blackburn, A. M., Patel, H. R., Modigliani, R. and Mallinson, C. N. (1978). Gut hormone profile in coeliac disease. *Lancet*, **1**, 785

Bloom, F., Segal, N., Ling, H. and Guillemin, R. (1976). Endorphins: Profound behavioral effects in rats suggest new etiological factors in mental illness. *Science*, **194**, 630

Burnstock, G. (1975). Purinergic transmission. In Iversen, L. L., Iversen, S. D. and Snyder, S. H. (eds.) *Handbook of Psychopharmacology*. Vol. 5, pp. 131–194. (New York: Plenum Press)

Burnstock, G. (1977). The purinergic nerve hypothesis. In *Purine and Pyrimidine Metabolism*. Ciba Foundation Symposium, 48, pp. 295–314. (Amsterdam: Elsevier-North Holland)

Cornell, H. J. and Townley, R. R. W. (1973). Investigation of possible intestinal peptidase deficiency in coeliac disease. *Clin. Chim. Acta*, **43**, 113

Cornford, E. M., Braun, L. D., Crane, P. D. and Oldendorf, W. H. (1978). Blood-brain barrier restriction of peptides and the low uptake of enkephalin. *Endocrinology*, **103**, 1297

Costa, E., and Trabucchi, M. (eds.) (1978). *The Endorphins*, Vol. 18, *Advances in Biochemical Psychopharmacology*. (New York: Raven Press)

Crampton, R. F., Gangolli, S. D., Simson, P. and Matthews, D. M. (1971). Rates of absorption by rat intestine of pancreatic hydrolysates of proteins and their corresponding amino acid mixtures. *Clin. Sci. Mol. Med.*, **41**, 409

Danforth, E., Jr. and Moore, R. O. (1959). Intestinal absorption of insulin in the rat. *Endocrinology*, **65**, 118

Deguchi, T. and Barchas, J. (1971). Inhibition of transmethylation of Biogenic Amines by S-adenosylhomocysteine. *J. Biol. Chem.*, **246**, 3175

De Wied, D. (1977). Peptides and behaviour. *Life Sci.*, **20**, 195

Dohan, F. C. (1966a). Cereals and schizophrenia data and hypothesis. *Acta Psychiatr. Scand.*, **42**, 125

Dohan, F. C. (1966b). Wheat 'consumption' and hospital admissions for schizophrenia during World War II. *Am. J. Clin. Nutr.*, **18**, 7

Dohan, F. C. (1969). Schizophrenia: Possible relationship to cereal grains and coeliac disease. In Sankar, S. (ed.) *Schizophrenia: Current Concepts and Research*, pp. 539–551. (Hicksville: PJD Publications)

Dohan, F. C. (1976). The possible pathogenic effect of cereal grains in schizophrenia, celiac disease as a model. *Acta Neurol. (Napoli)*, **31**, 195

Dohan, F. C., Grasberger, J., Lowell, F., Johnston, H., Jr. and Arbegast, A. (1969). Relapsed schizophrenics: more rapid improvement on a milk and cereal-free diet. *Br. J. Psychiatry*, **115**, 595

Dohan, F. C. and Grasberger, J. C. (1973). Relapsed schizophrenics: earlier discharge from the hospital after cereal-free, milk-free diet. *Am. J. Psychiatry*, **130**, 685

Dohan, F. C., Levitt, D. R. and Kushmir, L. D. (1978). Abnormal behavior after intracerebral injection of polypeptides from wheat gliadin – possible relevance to schizophrenia. *Pavlovian J. Biol. Sci.*, **13**, 73

Fain, Y. N., Pointer, R. H. and Ward, W. F. (1972). Effects of Adenosine nucleotides on Adenylate Cyclase, Phosphodiesterase, cAMP accumulation and lipolysis in fat cells. *J. Biol. Chem.*, **247**, 6866

Fox, I. H. and Kelley, W. N. (1978). The role of adenosine and 2'-deoxy-adenosine in mammalian cells. *Annu. Rev. Biochem.*, **47**, 655

Goldstein, A. (1976). Opioid peptides (endorphins) in pituitary and brain. *Science*, **193**, 1081

Gourley, D. R. H. and Beckner, S. K. (1973). Antagonism of morphine analgesia by adenine, adenosine and adenine nucleotides. *Proc. Soc. Exp. Biol. Med.*, **144**, 774

Graff, H. and Handford, A. (1961). Celiac syndrome history of five schizophrenics. *Psychiatr. Q.*, **35**, 306

Green, D. R. and Stanberry, L. R. (1977). Elevation of cAMP in C-1300 murine neuroblastoma by adenosine and related compounds and the antagonism of this response by methylxanthines. *Biochem. Pharmacol.*, **26**, 37

Greenberg, R., Whalley, C. E., Jourdikian, F., Mendelson, I. S., Walter, R., Nikolics, K., Coy, D. H., Schally, A. V. and Kastin, A. J. (1976). Peptides readily penetrate the blood-brain barrier: uptake of peptides by synaptosomes in passive. *Pharmacol. Biochem. Behav. (Suppl.)* **5**, 151

Grevert, P. and Goldstein, A. (1977). Effects of naloxone on experimental induced ischemic pain and on mood in human subjects. *Proc. Natl. Acad. Sci. USA*, **74**, 1291

Grevert, P. and Goldstein, A. (1978). Endorphins: naloxone fails to alter experimental pain or mood in humans. *Science*, **199**, 1093

Gunne, L. M., Lindstrom, L. and Terenius, L. (1977). Naloxone-induced reversal of schizophrenic hallucinations. *J. Neural Transmission*, **40**, 13

Hansen, O. (1972). Blood nucleoside and nucleotide studies in Mental Disease. *Br. J. Psychiatry*, **121**, 341

Havrankova, J., Schmechel, D., Roth, J. and Brownstein, M. (1978). Identification of insulin in rat brain. *Proc. Natl. Acad. Sci. USA*, **75**, 5737

Heckly, R. J., Hildebrand, G., Jr., and Lamanna, C. (1960). On the size of the toxic particle passing the intestinal barrier in botulism. *J. Exp. Med.*, **111**, 745

Hekkens, W. Th. J. M. and Pena, A. S. (1974). *Coeliac Disease*. (Leiden: M. Stenfert and B. V. Kroese)

Hemmings, C., Hemmings, W. A., Patey, A. L. and Wood, C. (1977). The ingestion of dietary proteins as large molecular mass degradation products in adult rats. *Proc. R. Soc.*

(London), **198B**, 439

Hemmings, W. A. and Williams, E. W. (1978). Transport of large breakdown products of dietary protein through the gut wall. *Gut*, **19**, 715

Hemmings, W. A. (1978). The entry into the brain of large molecules derived from dietary protein. *Proc. R. Soc. (London)*, **200B**, 175

Henderson, G., Hughes, J. and Kosterlitz, H. W. (1972). A new example of a morphine-sensitive neuro-effector junction: Adrenergic transmission in the mouse vas deferens. *Br. J. Pharmacol.*, **46**, 764

Herz, A., Bläsig, J., Emrich, H. M., Cording, C., Pirée, S., Kolling, A. and Zerssen, D. V. (1978). Is there some indication from behavioral effects of endorphins for their involvement in psychiatric disorders? *Adv. Biochem. Psychopharmacol.*, **18**, 333

Horrobin, D. F. (1977). Schizophrenia as a prostaglandin deficiency disease. *Lancet*, **1**, 936

Huang, M. and Daly, J. W. (1974). Adenosine-elicited accumulation of cAMP in brain slices: Potentiation by agents which inhibit uptake of adenosine. *Life Sci.*, **14**, 489

Hughes, J., Smith, W. T., Kosterlitz, H. W., Fothergill, L. A., Morgan, B. A. and Morris, H. R. (1975). Identification of two related pentapeptides from brain with potent opiate agonist activity. *Nature*, **258**, 320

Jacquet, Y. and Marks, N. (1976). The C-fragment of β-lipotropin. An endogenous neuroleptic or antipsychotogen? *Science*, **194**, 632

Jaffé, J. H., and Martin, W. R. (1975). Narcotic analgesics and antagonists. In Goodman, L. S. and Gilman, A. (eds.) *The Pharmacological Basis of Therapeutics*, Fifth Edition, pp. 245–283. (New York: MacMillan Publishing Co)

von Käser, H. (1961). Diagnose und Klinik der coeliake, *Ann. Paediatr.*, **197**, 320

Kessler, S. (1976). Progress and regress in the research on the genetics of schizophrenia. *Schizophrenia Bull.*, **2**, 434

Klee, W. A. and Nirenberg, M. (1974). A neuroblastoma × glioma hybrid cell line with morphine receptors. *Proc. Natl. Acad. Sci. USA*, **71**, 3474

Klee, W. A. and Streaty, R. A. (1974). Narcotic sites in morphine dependent rats. *Nature*, **248**, 61

Klee, W. A., Zioudrou, C. and Streaty, R. A. (1978). Exorphins: peptides with opioid activity isolated from wheat gluten and their possible role in the etiology of schizophrenia. In Usdin, E., Bunney, W. E. and Kline, N. S. (eds.) *Endorphins in Mental Health Research*, pp. 209–218. (New York: MacMillan)

Kline, N. S., Li, C. H., Lehmann, H. E., Lajtha, A., Laski, E. and Cooper, T. (1977). β-Endorphin-induced changes in schizophrenic and depressed patients. *Arch. Gen. Psychiatry*, **34**, 1111

Konturcks, S. J., Tasler, J., Cieszkowski, M., Jaworek, J., Coy, D. H. and Schally, A. V. (1978). Inhibition of pancreatic secretion by enkephalin and morphine in dogs. *Gastroenterology*, **74**, 851

Kroll, P., Port, F. K. and Silk, K. R. (1978): Hemodialysis and schizophrenia. A negative report. *J. Nerv. Ment. Dis.*, **166**, 291

Lampert, A., Nirenberg, M. and Klee, W. A. (1976). Tolerance and dependence evoked by an endogenous opiate peptide. *Proc. Natl. Acad. Sci. USA*, **73**, 3165

Li, C. H. (1964). Lipotropin: a new active peptide from human pituitary gland. *Nature*, **201**, 924

Lindstrom, L. H., Widerlow, E., Gunne, L. M., Wahlstrom, A. and Terenius, L. (1978). Endorphins in human cerebrospinal fluid: Clinical correlations to some psychotic states. *Acta Psychiatr. Scand.*, **57**, 133

Lis, M. T., Matthews, D. M. and Crampton, R. F. (1972). Effects of dietary restriction and protein deprivation on intestinal absorption of protein digestion products in the rat. *Br. J. Nutr.*, **28**, 443

Londos, C. and Wolff, J. (1977). Two distinct adenosine-sensitive sites of adenylate cyclase *Proc. Natl. Acad. Sci. USA*, **74**, 5482

Londos, C., Cooper, D. M. F., Schlegel, W. and Rodbell, M. (1978). Adenosine analogs inhibit adipocyte adenylate cyclase by a GTP-dependent process: Basis for action on adenosine and methylxanthines on cAMP production and lipolysis. *Proc. Natl. Acad. Sci. USA*, **75**, 5362

Lord, J. A. H., Waterfield, A. A., Hughes, J. and Kosterlitz, H. W. (1976). Multiple opiate receptors. In Kosterlitz, H. W. (ed.) *Opiates and Endogenous Opioid Peptides*, pp. 275–280. (Amsterdam: Elsevier–North Holland)

Madden, J., Akil, H., Patrick, R. L. and Barchas, J. D. (1977). Stress-induced parallel changes in central opioid levels and pain responsiveness in rat. *Nature*, **265**, 359

Martin, W. R. (1967). Opioid antagonists. *Pharmacol. Rev.*, **19**, 463

Mascord, I., Freed, D. and Durrant, B. (1978). Antibodies to foodstuffs in schizophrenia. *Br. Med. J.*, **1**, 1351

Mata, M. M., Gainer, H. and Klee, W. A. (1977). Effect of dehydration on the endogenous opiate content of the rat neurointermediate lobe. *Life Sci.*, **21**, 1159

Matthews, D. and Path, F. R. C. (1977). Memorial lecture: Protein absorption – then and now. *Gastroenterology*, **73**, 1267

Miller, L. H., Kastin, A. J., Sandman, C. A., Fink, M. K. and van Veen, W. J. (1974). Polypeptide influence on attention, memory and anxiety in man. *Pharmacol. Biochem. Behav.*, **2**, 663

Milne, M. D. and Asatoor, A. M. (1975). Peptide absorption in disorders of amino acid transport. In Matthews, D. M. and Payne, J. W. (eds.) *Peptide Transport in Protein Nutrition*, pp. 167–182. (Amsterdam: Elsevier–North Holland)

Monnier, M. and Schoenenberger, G. A. (1974). Neurohormonal coding of sleep and physiological sleep factor delta. In Myers, R. D. and Drucker-Collin, R. P. (eds.) *Neurohormonal Coding of Brain Function*, pp. 207–232. (New York: Plenum Press)

Nixon, S. E. and Mawer, G. E. (1970a). The digestion and absorption of protein in man. *Br. J. Nutr.*, **24**, 227

Nixon, S. E. and Mawer, G. E. (1970b). The digestion and absorption of protein in man. The form in which digested protein is absorbed. *Br. J. Nutr.*, **24**, 241

Palmour, R. M., Ervin, F. R., Wagenmaker, H. and Cade, R. (1977). Characterization of a peptide derived from serum of psychiatric patients. *Soc. Neurosci. Abstr.*, **3**, 320

Paulley, J. W. (1959). Emotion and personality in the etiology of steatorrhea. *Am. J. Digest. Dis.*, **4**, 352

Pearse, A. G. E. (1977). Diffuse neuroendocrine system: Peptides common to brain and intestine and their relationship to the APUD concept. In Hughes, J. (ed.) *Centrally Acting Peptides*, pp. 49–57. (Baltimore: University Park Pres)

Pena, A. S., Mann, D. L., Hague, N. E., Heck, J. A., van Leeuwen, A., van Rood, J. J. and Strober, W. (1978). Genetic basis of gluten-sensitive enteropathy. *Gastroenterology*, **75**, 230

Pert, C. B., Pert, A. and Chang, J. R. (1976). D-Ala²-met-enkephalinamide: a potent long lasting synthetic analgesic. *Science*, **194**, 330

Pert, C. B. and Snyder, S. H. (1973). Opiate receptor: Demonstration in nervous tissue. *Science*, **179**, 1011

Phillis, J. W. and Kostopoulos, G. K. (1975). Adenosine as a putative transmitter in the cerebral cortex. Studies with potentiators and antagonists. *Life Sci.*, **17**, 1085

Prange, A. J. Jr., Nemeroff, C. B., Lipton, M. S., Breese, G. R. and Wilson, I. C. (1978). Peptides in the central nervous system. In Iversen, L. L. Iversen, S. D., and Snyder, S. H. (eds.) *Handbook of Psychopharmacology*, Vol. 13 pp. 1–107 (New York: Plenum Press)

Polak, J. M., Sullivan, S. N., Bloom, R. S., Facer, P. and Pearse, A. G. E. (1977). Enkephalin like immunoreactivity in the human gastrointestinal tract. *Lancet*, **1**, 972

Rapaport, S. M. (1976). *Blood–Brain Barrier in Physiology and Medicine*, pp. 177–206. (New York: Raven Press)

Ribeiro, J. A. (1978). ATP: Related nucleotides and adenosine on neurotransmission. *Life Sci.*, **22**, 1373

Roberts, J. L. and Herbert, E. (1977). Characterization of a common precursor to corticotropin and β-lipotropin. *Proc. Natl. Acad. Sci. USA*, **74**, 5300

Roemer, D., Buescher, H. H., Hill, R. C.,, Pless, J., Bauer, W., Cardinaux, F., Closse, A., Hauser, D. and Huguenin, R. (1977). A synthetic enkephalin analogue with prolonged parenteral and oral analgesic activity. *Nature (London) 268*, 547

Salomon, Y., Londos, C. and Rodbell, M. (1974). A highly sensitive adenylate cyclase assay method. *Anal. Biochem.*, **58**, 541

Sattin, A. and Rall, T. W. (1970): The effect of adenosine and adenosine nucleotides on the cAMP content of Guinea Pig cerebral cortex slices. *Mol. Pharmacol.*, **6**, 13

Sharma, S. K., Nirenberg, M. and Klee, W. A. (1975). Morphine receptors as regulators of adenylate cyclase activity. *Proc. Natl. Acad. Sci. USA*, **72**, 590

Singh, M. M., and Kay, S. R. (1976). Wheat gluten as a pathogenic factor in schizophrenia, *Science*, **191**, 401

Silk, D. B. A. Kumar, P. J., Perrett, D., Clark, M. L. and Dawson, A. M. (1974). Amino acid and peptide absorption in patients with coeliac disease and dermatitis herpetiformis. *Gut*, **15**, 1

Simon, E. J., Hiller, J. M. and Edelman, I. (1973). Stereospecific binding of the potent narcotic analgesic ^{3}H-etorphine to rat brain homogenate. *Proc. Natl. Acad. Sci. USA*, **70**, 1947

Snyder, S. H. (1978). The opiate receptor and morphine-like peptides in the Brain. *Am. J. Psychiatry*, **135**, 645

Stein, H. H., Somani, P. and Prasad, N. (1975). Cardiovascular effect of nucleoside analogs. *Ann. N. Y. Acad. Sci.*, **255**, 380

Taylor, M. (1978). A preliminary investigation on dietary constituents and amphetamine induced abnormal behavior. In Hemmings, G. and Hemmings, W. A. (eds.) *The Biological Basis of Schizophrenia.* (Lancaster: MTP Press)

Terenius, L. (1973). Stereospecific interaction between narcotic analgesics and a synaptic membrane fraction of rat cerebral cortex. *Acta Pharmacol. Toxicol.*, **32**, 317

Tseng, L. F., Loh, H. H. and Li, C. H. (1976). β-Endorphin as a potent analgesic by intravenous injection. *Nature (London)*, **263**, 239

Ungar, G. (1975). Peptides and behavior. *Int. Rev. Neurobiol.*, **17**, 37

Vale, W., Rivier, C. and Brown, M. (1977). Regulatory peptides of the Hypothalamus. *Annu. Rev. Physiol.*, **39**, 473

Verebey, K., Volavka, J. and Clouet, D. (1978). Endorphins in psychiatry. *Arch. Gen. Psychiat.*, **35**, 877

Walker, W. A. and Isselbacher, K. J. (1974). Uptake and transport of macromolecules by the intestine. Possible role in clinical disorders. *Gastroenterology*, **67**, 531

Walker, R. J. (1978). Polypeptides as central transmitters. *Gen. Pharmacol.*, **9**, 129

Warshaw, A. L., Walker, W. A. and Isselbacher, K. J. (1974). Protein uptake by the intestine: evidence for absorption of intact macromolecules. *Gastroenterology*, **66**, 987

Weisenberger, H., Grube, H., Koenig, E. and Pelzer, H. (1972). Isolation and identification of the platelet aggregation inhibitor present in the onion *Allium Cepa*. *F.E.B.S. Lett.*, **26**, 105

van der Weyden, M. B. and Kelley, W. N. (1977). Adenosine deaminase deficiency and severe combined immunodeficiency disease. *Life Sci.*, **20**, 1645

Williams, E. W., Laidlaw, H. and Lowe, C. F. (1979). Behaviour elicited by low doses of d-amphetamine after oral administration of proteins to adult rats. *IRCS Med. Sci.* **7**, 241

Woolley, D. W. and Merrifield, R. B. (1963). Anomalies of the structural specificity of peptides. *Ann. N. Y. Acad. Sci.*, **104**, 161

Yamashiro, D., Tseng, L. F. and Li, C. H. (1977). (D-Thr^2, Thz^3)- and (D-Met^2, Thz^5)- enkephalinamides: Potent analgesic by intravenous injection. *Biochem. Biophys. Res. Commun.*, **78**, 1124

Zioudrou, C. and Klee, W. A. (1978). Exorphins-peptides with opioid activity derived from α-casein and wheat gluten. In van Ree, J. M. and Terenius, L. (eds.) *Characteristics and Function of Opioids*, pp. 243–244. (Amsterdam: Elsevier–North Holland)

Zioudrou, C. and Klee, W. A. (1979). Possible roles of peptides derived from food proteins in brain function. In Wurtman, R. J. and Wurtman, J. J. (eds.) *Nutrition and the Brain*, Vol. 4, pp. 125–158. (New York: Raven Press)

Zioudrou, C., Streaty, R. A. and Klee, W. A. (1979). Opioid peptides derived from food proteins: the exorphins. *J. Biol. Chem.*, **254**, 2446

5
Preliminary studies of the identification of brain peptides in relation to the genesis and expression of schizophrenia

H. R. MORRIS, A. DELL and A. T. ETIENNE

Shortly after the structure elucidation of enkephalin in 1975, which led to the synthesis and subsequent physiological testing of opioid peptides, H. R. Morris, J. Edwardson and T. Crow began work on testing a new hypothesis of whether 'incorrect' levels of brain peptides were responsible for the genesis or expression of schizophrenia. This work involves characterizing peptides from very complex biological sources and quantifying them. Ideally one would require a chemical characterization of all known (and even unknown) brain peptides and a quantitative estimate for each of them in one and the same experiment. The magnitude of this problem or indeed only part of it – characterization – is appreciated only when we reflect that the structure elucidation of thyrotropin releasing hormone (TRH) took two research teams ten years, and hundreds of thousands of animal hypothalami were used (Burgus *et al.*, 1970: Nair *et al.*, 1970).

The development of modern analytical techniques such as mass spectrometry has revolutionized this structural work and for the structure elucidation of enkephalin only 100 pig brains were used to isolate sufficient material for study (approximately 50 μg) (Hughes *et al.*, 1975a). Clearly the job of defining unknown structures is more difficult than the task of screening known structures, and a true structural characterization of a peptide still requires similar amounts of material at the 1979 level of technology. At this stage the problem of quantitation cannot even be addressed in chemical terms. In medical studies we cannot normally pool brains etc. and therefore the amount of peptide available is even less than that obtained from animal preparations. We can thus appreciate the magnitude of the problem before us – how to get a chemically accurate analysis (identification and quantitation) from just one patient, either as cerebrospinal fluid (CSF) and post-mortem brain or (perhaps less relevantly in the case of neuropeptides) blood and urine. Because of the restricted volume/weight) of fluid/tissue obtainable from each patient, peptide levels will be very low and chemical identification seemingly impossible.

However, are we not forgetting radio-immunoassay(RIA)? Is this not a sensitive and specific method for the analysis of known brain peptides? Certainly no-one will deny the sensitivity of the method which is accurate in the picogram range, but the basic reason for our own development work, presented below, was a belief, based only on intuition in 1975, that the specificity of some radio-immunoassays would be found to be lacking. If this is true – and we now have evidence to corroborate our intuition – then the physiological conclusions based upon RIA of crude biological extracts are without meaning. This lack of specificity may be cross-reactivity with other known peptides (a common phenomenon e.g. in the opioid area) which can be corrected for, or more disturbingly, with unknown substances.

Our objective has been to develop a reliable method for chemical characterization and quantitation. This involves the use of a high resolution purification step to give a partial chemical characterization coupled with RIA which provides high sensitivity quantitation. A particular advantage of the method lies in the ability to assay over ten component peptides from a single sample (e.g. of CSF).

Table 1 Protocol for high pressure liquid chromatography

(I) Columns	(1) μ Bondapak C_{18}; 0.39 × 30 cm
	(2) μ Bondapak C_{18}; 0.78 × 30 cm
(II) Eluents	(A) 5% acetic acid
	(B) propan-1-ol
(III) Conditions	Column 1: 20 min linear gradient from 90:10 (v/v) to 60:40 (v/v) A:B at 1 ml/min
	Column 2: 30 min concave gradient from 90:10 (v/v) to 60:40 (v/v) A:B at 1 ml/min

METHODS AND DISCUSSION

Micro ion-exchange

A long established method for peptide purification is ion-exchange chromatography. This was developed for the separation of peptides at > 10 nanomol/l level for sequencing studies. For our neuropeptide work it was therefore necessary to ascertain the applicability of the method at the sub-nanomolar level. We have examined several ion-exchange procedures for brain peptide separation using micro columns and special 6μ spherical resins giving high resolution separations on very small quantities of material (Morris *et al.*, 1978). Our early attempts concentrated on (i) developing a volatile buffer system, since salts (and especially salt gradients) are not compatible with bioassay or RIA techniques and (ii) the examination of fluorometric detection of the eluted peptides. Using pyridine/acetic acid gradients good separation of a number of neuropeptides was obtained (for example, see Figure 1) and the resolution of the peaks at the sub-nanomolar level was preserved even after the necessary mixing with the fluorescamine reagent which was used to generate the fluorescent derivative. This has proved to be a good method for peptide separation but has two disadvantages: (a) removal of all traces of pyridine prior to assay and (b) the length and complexity of the run requiring constant skilled operator attention. For these reasons we have developed a complementary high pressure liquid chromatography (HPLC) procedure.

High pressure liquid chromatography (HPLC)

In the original enkephalin work (Hughes *et al.*, 1975b), a HPLC system was used for purification, but did not (as the structural work revealed) separate the two enkephalins. In contrast our new procedure, summarized in Table 1, gives an excellent separation of these two peptides and indeed of all the known opioid peptides (see Figure 2). The method is rapid and gives good separation of most of the known neuropeptides. Figure 3 shows the chromatography of a mixture of 17 important neuropeptides, the majority of which are well resolved. The few which co-chromatograph are either those which could be readily separated using the ion-exchange procedure described above or where cross-reactivity in RIA is not a problem.

Excellent reproducibility of this system is found even when very crude brain extracts are loaded onto the column and CSF can be directly injected without any prepurification. Many of the HPLC procedures for peptide separation reported in the literature have stated that yields off the

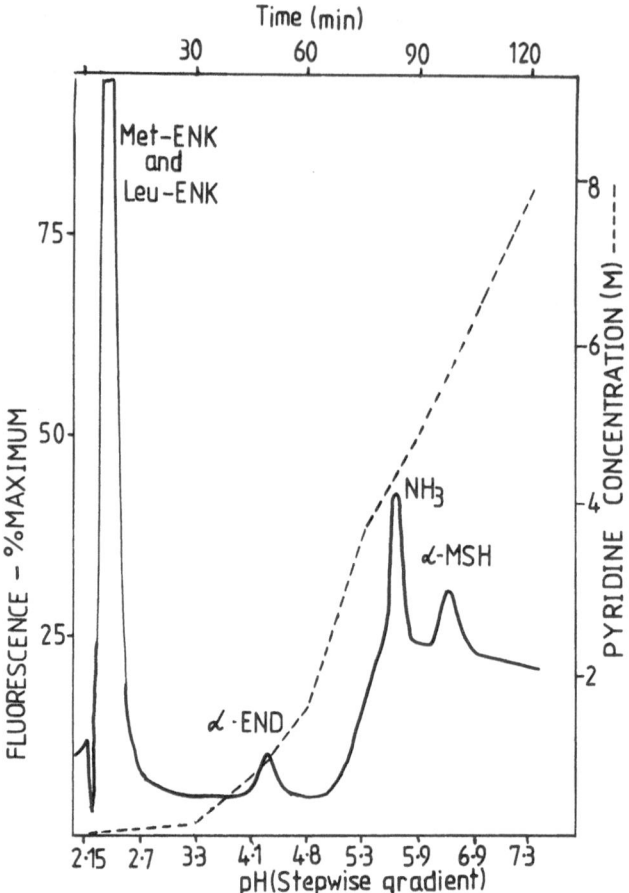

Figure 1 Ion-exchange chromatography of met-enkephalin (2.8 nmol), leu-enkephalin (3.0 nmol), α-endorphin (2.7 nmol) and α-melanocyte stimulating hormone (2.5 nmol) using sulphonated polystyrene beads. Operating conditions were: resin bed, 0.4 × 6.0 cm; column temperature, 60 °C; flow rate, 0.38 ml/min. The eluate was stream-split and 20% was reacted with fluorescamine; the resulting fluorophor was detected at $\lambda_{excitation}$ = 365 nm and $\lambda_{emission}$ = 450 nm

column have been poor when reverse phase chromatography is used; e.g. Gentleman *et al.* (1978) were unable to recover opioid activity after injection of < 10 nmol of β-endorphin. In contrast 85–90% recoveries of β-endorphin are obtained from our system at the sub-nanomolar level and even at the 2–4 picomolar level, yields of 85% of radioactive vasoactive intestinal polypeptide (VIP) were preserved.

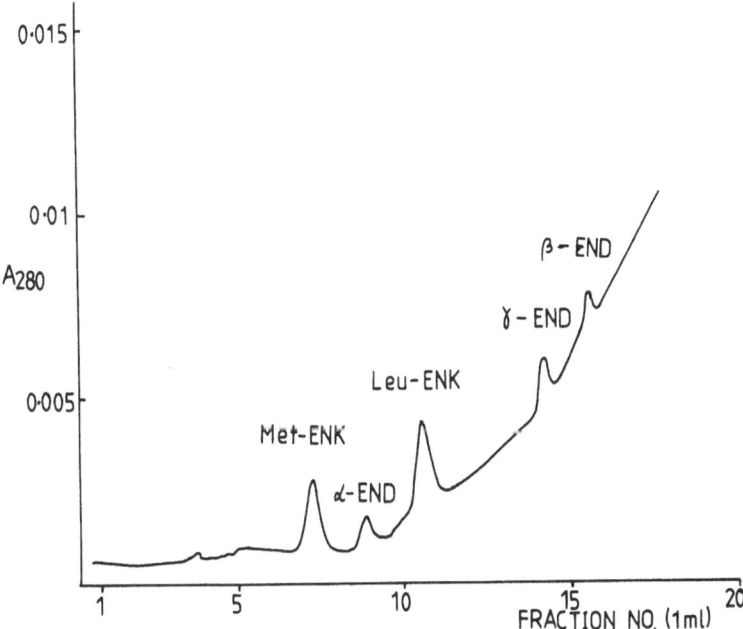

Figure 2 Resolution of a mixture of met-enkephalin, leu-enkephalin, α-endorphin, γ-endorphin and β-endorphin on Column 1 (see Table 1). The rising baseline is due to a buffer viscosity effect with increasing propan-1-ol and does not interfere with the analysis. The vertical axis gives u.v. absorbance at 280 nm

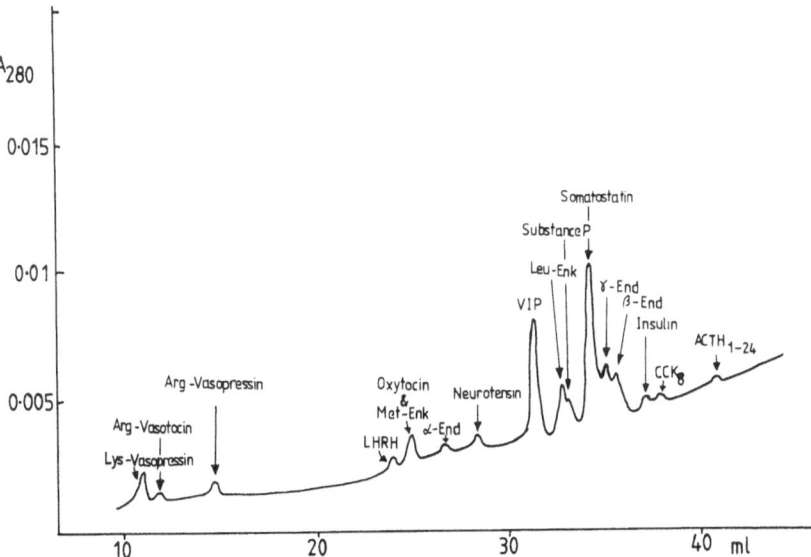

Figure 3 Resolution of a complex mixture of neuropeptides on Column 2 (see Table 1). The vertical axis gives u.v. absorbance at 280 nm

Table 2 Opioid activity in met-enkephalin equivalents (pmol/ml) of lumbar CSF*

Patient	Control	0.5 h	6 h
KP	3.6	13.2	2.1
VH	3.8	5.8	2.8
FA	1.7	90.0	3.3
RW	28.0	108.0	15.0

* Data from four patients who were given electrical stimulation for the treatment of pain. The control value is the pre-stimulation level, and post-stimulation CSF was taken after 0.5 h and 6 h. Opiate activity was determined using the mouse vas deferens.

An example of the use of this HPLC system in work on neurological disorders involves patients suffering from chronic pain. This is collaborative work which we are carrying out with Dr J. Miles (Liverpool) and Dr J. Hughes (London). Here we can demonstrate the point made earlier about the specificity of the method, i.e. its partial chemical characterization. Table 2 shows pre- and post-electrical stimulation values for the total opioid bioactivity of CSF from a number of patients. Although the increase in opioid activity on stimulation is clearly apparent from the data, we have no information on the chemical nature of the opioid peptides present in the CSF. Using the HPLC system, coupled with bioassay,

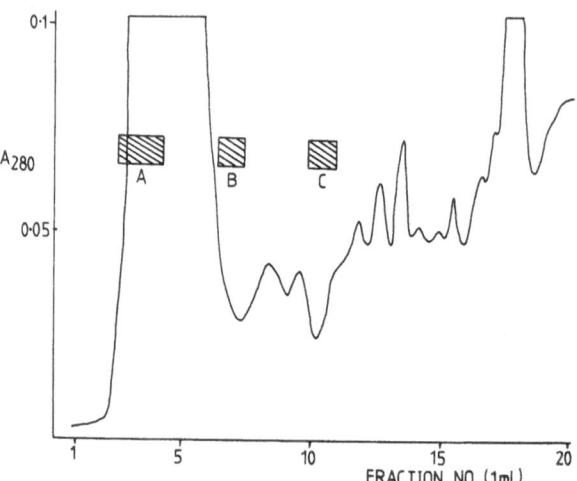

Figure 4 U.v. absorbance profile at 280 nm (vertical axis) and opioid activity (hatched areas) of post-stimulation CSF after chromatography on Column 1. B and C correspond to the elution positions of met- and leu-enkephalins respectively

we are able to answer the question as to which endorphins are present in the post-stimulation sample or whether new opioid peptides are giving the bioactivity. A typical result for one CSF sample is shown in Figure 4. Three regions of opioid activity are present – two correspond to the enkephalin elution positions but the third elutes earlier than any of the known opiates.

We are currently studying schizophrenic and control CSF provided by Dr T. Crow and Dr J. Edwardson and are now at a stage where from a single CSF run we can screen a number of peptides by RIA. This work is now in progress and some preliminary results on VIP are presented in Table 3. As yet too few patients have been screened for any conclusions to be drawn from the data but it is interesting to note that the level of VIP in the schizophrenic CSF is consistently higher than in the controls. The VIP studies have corroborated the suspicion mentioned above with regard to the specificity of a purely RIA approach to neuropeptide quantitation. In addition to obtaining activity at the true VIP elution position we have found VIP-like immunoreactivity at other elution positions after chromatography of the CSF samples. Hence quantitation of VIP by RIA of neat CSF would have given incorrect results.

Table 3 Levels of vasoactive intestinal polypeptide (VIP) in schizophrenic (S) and control (C) CSF*

CSF type	VIP in CSF (pg/ml)
S	98
S	165
S	42
S	173
S	98
C	29
C	60
C	0

* Data determined by radio-immunoassay of fractions corresponding to the VIP elution position; high pressure liquid chromatography was performed on Column 1 (see Table 1)

CONCLUSION

We have developed high resolution purification procedures which, when coupled with radio-immunoassay quantitation, have allowed us to take the first steps towards a proper chemical characterization of neuropeptides. The methods are being used to screen for a number of neuropeptides in CSF and post-mortem brain to ascertain whether they are involved in the expression of schizophrenia.

Acknowledgements

The authors wish to thank The Wellcome Trust for financial support and R. Albuquerque for VIP radio-immunoassays.

References

Burgus, R., Dunn, T. F., Desiderio, D., Ward, D. N., Vale, W. and Guillemin, R. (1970). Characterisation of bovine hypothalamic hypophysiotropic TSH-releasing factor. *Nature*, **226**, 321

Gentleman, S., Lowney, L. I., Cox, B. M. and Goldstein, A. (1978). Rapid purification of β-endorphin by high performance liquid chromatography. *J. Chromatogr.*, **153**, 274

Hughes, J., Smith, T. W., Kosterlitz, H. W., Fothergill, L. A., Morgan, B. A. and Morris, H. R. (1975a). Identification of two related pentapeptides from the brain with potent opiate agonist activity. *Nature*, **258**, 577

Hughes, J., Smith, T., Morgan, B. A. and Fothergill, L. A. (1975b). Purification and properties of enkephalin – the possible endogenous ligand for the morphine receptor. *Life Sci.*, **16**, 1753

Morris, H. R., Etienne, A. T. and Dell, A. (1978). Brain peptides: high pressure column/ fluorescence screening procedure. In Simpkins, M. A. (ed.) *Sixth International Symposium on Medicinal Chemistry*, p. 31. (Brighton: University of Sussex)

Nair, R. M. G., Barrett, J. F., Bowers, C. Y. and Schally, A. V. (1970). Structure of porcine thyrotropin releasing hormone. *Biochemistry*, **9**, 1103

6

The role of the dopamine system in schizophrenia

C. W. ABELL

This chapter describes certain steps in the synthesis and degradation of dopamine and how alterations in them may lead to changes in neurotransmission and behaviour. The ideas discussed here reflect the collective efforts of many of my colleagues at The University of Texas Medical Branch at Galveston, who have contributed significantly to an integrated programme of biochemical, pharmacological, psychiatric, and behavioural studies of schizophrenic patients, paralleled by correlative studies in animal models. My discussion will include well established principles in the process of neurotransmission, and some innovative hypotheses which are currently being tested.

The primary elements of the dopamine neurosystem as it is understood at the present time are shown in Figure 1 (for review see Molinoff and Axelrod, 1971). Dopamine is synthesized from phenylalanine and tyrosine in a series of steps requiring several enzymes, including the aromatic amino acid hydroxylases, dihydropteridine reductase, and dihydroxyphenylalanine decarboxylase. The rate limiting step in the synthetic pathway is the hydroxylation of tyrosine, which requires tyrosine hydroxylase, dihydropteridine reductase, reduced pteridine cofactor, and oxygen. Once dopamine has been synthesized, it can be stored or sent along three or four alternative paths: it can cross the synapse to transmit its message to the postsynaptic membrane; it can be degraded intraneuronally by monoamine oxidase (MAO) or extraneuronally by catechol-O-methyl transferase; it can be converted into the neurotransmitter norepinephrine in a reaction catalyzed by dopamine-β-hydroxylase; and, as shown recently in Parkinsonian patients treated with L-dopa (Coscia *et al.*, 1977) or in phenylketonurics (Lasala and Coscia, 1979), it

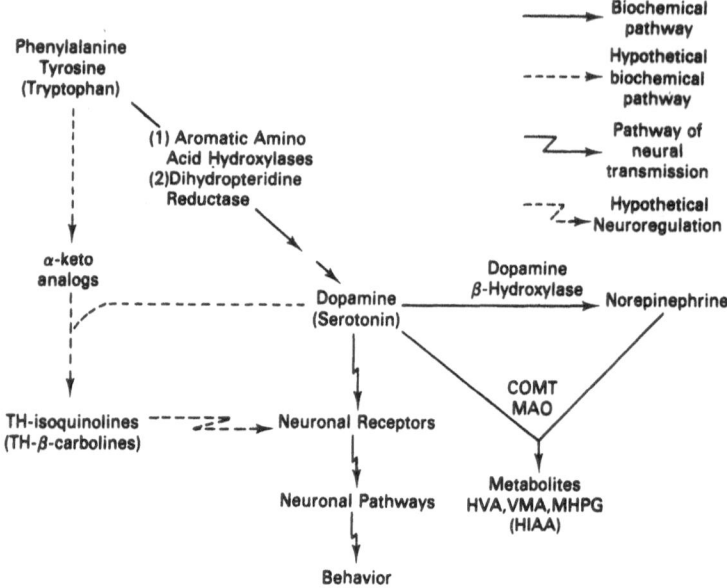

Figure 1   Synopsis of dopamine system

can condense with α-keto analogues derived from transamination of the aromatic amino acids to form tetrahydroisoquinolines. Derivatives in this class of compounds have been implicated as possible false neuroregulators of dopaminergic transmission (Cohen, 1976).

Previous studies by several groups of investigators have shown that the concentration of neurotransmitters in the brain (see Wurtman and Fernstrom, 1976, for review) may be altered by manipulating the plasma levels of amino acids from which they are derived by either oral loading or dietary restriction. When dietary restriction is applied, however, a period of 6–8 weeks is needed to achieve a reduction of plasma levels of that amino acid to 70–80% of the control. An alternative method of reducing phenylalanine is to inject phenylalanine ammonia-lyase (PAL), an enzyme that catalyzes the rapid deamination of phenylalanine and tyrosine to cinnamic acid and coumaric acid, respectively (Fritz et al., 1976). When PAL is injected intraperitoneally into a mammal, it is transported into the circulation and reaches a maximum level within 4–8 hours, decreasing subsequently with a biological half-life of approximately 21 hours (Shen et al., 1977).

As the enzyme reaches the plasma, phenylalanine and tyrosine are rapidly converted to their deaminated products. Consequently, the circulating activity of PAL corresponds inversely to the concentration of phenylalanine and tyrosine in the plasma. When PAL is injected repeatedly (once every 2 days for 5 days), the half-life of the enzyme decreases from approximately 21 hours to less than 2 hours (Shen *et al.*, 1977). This change in rate of clearance is caused by the appearance of antibodies that effectively remove PAL from the host. In recent studies, we found that the host can be immunosuppressed indefinitely when cyclophosphamide is given at the same time or within a 24 hour interval of PAL, making it possible to manipulate plasma levels of phenylalanine and tyrosine at different periods of time during the entire life span of the host (Shen *et al.*, 1979).

Previous studies employed a single administration of PAL to examine the effects of decreasing phenylalanine and tyrosine levels on behaviour in trained monkeys (Barratt *et al.*, 1976). Three types of tests were performed: sleep pattern measurements, a simple behavioural task, and a multi-chained complex behavioural task. PAL had a marked effect on the sleep–wakefulness patterns of squirrel monkeys, causing an increase in the awake stage, decreases in stages 2–4 of slow wave sleep, and a pronounced decrease in rapid eye movement (REM) sleep. Within 72 hours after PAL administration, however, the stages of the sleep–wakefulness pattern approached normal patterns. PAL had no statistically significant effect on the performance of a simple operant task, but markedly affected the ability of the squirrel monkey to perform proficiently a complex operant task. Within 2 hours after the administration of PAL, there was a pronounced decrease in the number of correct trials that were performed, with a related increase in the length of the session needed to achieve these correct trials.

Analyses of the common amino acids in the brains of rats, performed 4 hours after PAL treatment to approximate the time of the observed behavioural disruption of squirrel monkeys on the complex operant task, revealed significant decreases in tyrosine and phenylalanine and an increase in tryptophan (Abell *et al.*, 1978). Analysis of the three biogenic amines, dopamine, norepinephrine, and serotonin in the brain of these animals after PAL injection showed that serotonin increased approximately 3-fold (with a subsequent decrease to normal values within 24 hours), while dopamine and norepinephrine remained unchanged within 4 hours but were reduced to approximately 18% and 50%, respectively, of the levels in controls within 8 hours and remained low for at least 24 hours. The 3-fold increase in serotonin levels within 4 hours after PAL injection suggests that it may have been derived from increased biosynthesis as well as from increased transport of tryptophan into brain cells. Collectively, these studies strongly support the concept that nutrition contributes significantly to the determination of behaviour.

The rate limiting steps for neurotransmitter synthesis and degradation are ultimately determined by enzymes in interrelated biochemical pathways in neuronal systems. If psychiatric disorders such as schizophrenia have a multi-factorial genetic basis, as several geneticists have proposed (see Gottesman and Shields for review, 1976), then more than one primary biochemical defect might contribute to the complex behavioural and physiological symptomatology of this disease. I propose here to focus on two hypotheses of dopamine malfunction which in combination could explain the major evidence for a disorder in the dopamine system in schizophrenic patients. The first hypothesis proposes a defect at the dopaminergic synapse, which has been implicated by previous studies showing that neuroleptic drugs block dopamine receptors. The theory is consistent with the existence of hypothetical lesions either in presynaptic neurons or at postsynaptic receptor sites (see Crow, 1979, for review). Precise localization of the defect has proved difficult, however, and the dopamine hyperactivity hypothesis itself has been criticized because CSF studies of homovanillic acid have shown no increase in dopamine turnover in schizophrenics. Furthermore, prolactin secretion, which presumably is inversely proportional to dopamine levels, is the same in unmedicated acute and chronic schizophrenic patients as in control subjects. Recent studies, however, have found elevated dopamine levels in the nucleus accumbens in 50 patients who died with a hospital diagnosis of schizophrenia (Bird et al., 1979).

One possible explanation of dopamine hyperactivity which has persisted in the literature is that monoamine oxidase (MAO) is low or defective in schizophrenics (see Wyatt et al., 1979, for review). MAO presumably controls dopamine levels in the presynaptic neurons. The molecular structure of the enzyme, however, and the mechanisms by which it inactivates neurotransmitters are not yet fully understood (see Achee et al., 1977, for review). The activity of this enzyme has been measured many times in platelets from schizophrenics, and the majority of studies (19 out of 26), agree that activity levels are low in this patient group, although several studies have failed to confirm these results. A wide variety of factors contribute to this confusion. MAO preparations from separate tissues within the same species have different affinitives for various substrates, and also exhibit different sensitivities to certain drugs (Johnston, 1968). These differences for the most part have been explained by the observation that MAO exists in two different forms, A and B. MAO A preferentially deaminates serotonin and norepinephrine, and is selectively inhibited by clorgyline. MAO B, however, preferentially deaminates phenylethylamine and benzylamine and is inhibited by deprenyl. Other amines, such as dopamine, tyramine, and tryptamine serve as substrates for either MAO A or MAO B.

The activities of these two enzymes vary independently among different tissues and also among different cell types within a tissue. The molecular weight of MAO varies considerably in range, and multiple bands have been resolved by electrophoresis. Furthermore, to add to the confusion, the kinetic properties of the enzyme change during purification, rendering molecular weight determinations difficult to interpret (Achee et al., 1977). Studies by Dennick and Mayer (977) and Russell et al. (1979), however, found that human liver MAO could be purified to a single band on polyacrylamide gels, and antisera prepared against this preparation cross-reacted with MAO from liver, brain cortex, platelets, and placenta. These results were interpreted to imply that the apparently functionally different MAO activities found in different tissues are immunologically related and may be identical.

Several different possibilities can be offered to explain the basic differences between MAO A and MAO B. These apparently different activities may arise from complexing of different lipid components to the protein in the mitochondrial membrane. Since the substrates studied differ in hydrophobicity, the amount and type of lipid attached to MAO could influence its activity. Another possibility is that the difference in MAO activities are a result of post-transcriptional modification of the enzyme. This notion is supported by studies suggesting that MAO A may be a precursor form of MAO B (Suzuki and Yagi, 1977). Still another possibility is that these enzyme activities represent two different enzymes coded by different structural genes. This hypothesis can be examined by studying the primary structure of MAO A and MAO B by direct methods or indirectly by immunological techniques.

In sum, it has been difficult to obtain consistent results on MAO activities in comparative studies between normal subjects and patients with schizophrenia. Psychiatrists generally attribute these inconsistencies to problems in selecting diagnostically homogeneous subject groups, and in controlling for the effects of chronic illness and long-term neuroleptic therapy. Undoubtedly, the problems associated with assay reproducibility for a membrane bound enzyme have also contributed to the different patterns that have emerged from the extensive studies performed in different laboratories.

Our approach to reduce one of these problems is to measure the amount of MAO protein rather than its activity in platelets, using monospecific and monoclonal antibodies. We have purified MAO approximately 40-fold from human blood platelets obtained from outdated platelet rich plasma (Landowski et al., 1979). MAO was solubilized from the membrane with 1.5% Triton X-100 and purified by chromatography sequentially on DEAE, cellulose, Sepharose, and DEAE-cellulose columns. The purification achieved was about 40-fold with an overall yield of about 10%. Purified MAO gave a single band of activity (stained with benzylamine or tyramine and tetrazolium) and protein (stained with Coomassie blue) on standard polyacrylamide gels. One major band and two minor bands of protein were resolved by SDS-polyacrylamide gel electrophoresis. The properties of platelet homogenates of MAO, Triton

X-100 solublized enzyme, and purified MAO were compared using benzylamine, tyramine, phenylethylamine, and tryptamine. The results demonstrated that the kinetic properties of MAO B in platelet homogenates remained virtually the same throughout the purification procedure. Furthermore, studies with the inhibitors deprenyl (selective for MAO B) and clorgyline (selective for MAO A) supported the contention that the B form of MAO had been purified.

Antibodies to purified MAO have been raised in rabbits using standard procedures for immunization (Fritz *et al.*, unpublished). Based on the methodology established by Laurell (1966), we have developed a quantitative electroimmunoassay to determine the amount of MAO protein in platelets, an approach which promises to reduce much of the variability which has confused earlier activity measurements. Using this method, we hope to resolve the issue of whether MAO protein is, in fact, reduced in platelets from patients with schizophrenia and to examine further the primary structure of MAO protein to probe for possible altered sequences in this enzyme. By simultaneously measuring the levels of the MAO substrates, dopamine and norepinephrine, and their metabolites, in fluid specimens from schizophrenic subjects and controls, it should be possible to examine the whole biochemical system of dopamine and norepinephrine metabolism as a unit to clarify the functional relationship between its component parts.

If schizophrenia has a multifactorial genetic basis, then a defect in MAO alone would not explain the basis of this disease. A second contributing factor could be a defect in one of the enzymes involved in the rate limiting step for dopamine synthesis, the hydroxylation of tyrosine to DOPA, which would result in a loss of physiological control of this neurotransmitter. At first glance, the hydroxylation hypothesis appears to be diametrically opposed to the hypothesis of dopamine hyperactivity because a defect in hydroxylation should result in decreased levels of dopamine. Since dopamine synthesis is controlled by feedback inhibition by dopamine at the tyrosine hydroxylation step, however, the effect of a partial blockage at this point is difficult to predict. It is likely that a defect in one of the components required for hydroxylation of tyrosine to DOPA causes a loss in regulation of the rate of dopamine synthesis, resulting in the formation of dopamine at irregular intervals, independent of physiological control. The possibility of a hydroxylation deficiency in schizophrenics has not been systematically studied, but some evidence gives preliminary support to this hypothesis.

Phenylalanine load studies were performed in control subjects and schizophrenic patients in collaboration with Potkin and Wyatt, St. Elizabeth's Hospital, Washington, D.C. Plasma levels of phenylalanine and tyrosine were determined by the enzymatic method of Shen and Abell (1977). These preliminary studies show that some but not all schizophrenics metabolize oral loads of phenylalanine to tyrosine at lower rates than normal controls. In contrast, no difference in the rate of metabolism of phenylalanine to tyrosine in patients with affective disorders was found (Targum *et al.*, 1979). Studies have also revealed increased levels of phenylethylamine in some schizophrenics (Fischer *et al.*, 1972), suggesting but not proving that in these patients phenylalanine or tyrosine may be metabolized less rapidly through the dominant metabolic pathways.

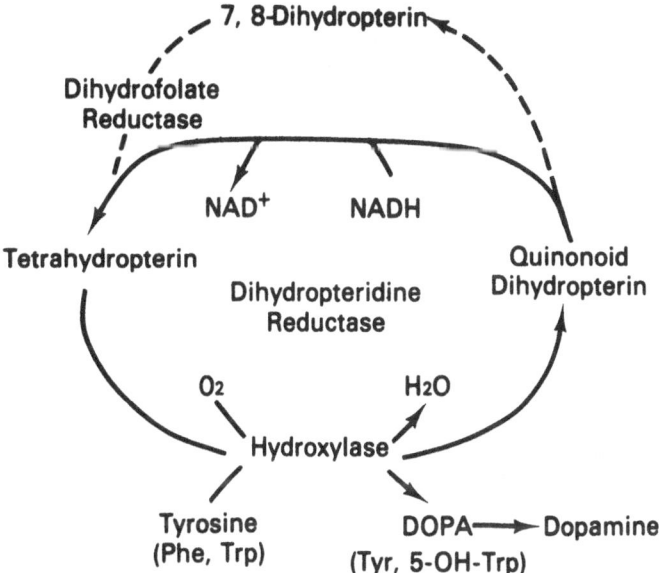

Figure 2 Pterin cycle

The hydroxylation of aromatic amino acids requires at least four essential components: the enzymes, hydroxylase and reductase, and the cofactors, tetrahydrobiopterin and reduced pyridine nucleotide (see Kaufman, 1976, for review). A defect in either of the two enzymes or the two systems that generate the reduced cofactors will alter the hydroxylation reaction. A possible candidate for the defect in schizophrenia is dihydropteridine reductase. This enzyme is responsible for regenerating the tetrahydro form of biopterin, the required cofactor for the hydroxylation of the three aromatic amino acids, phenylalanine, tyrosine, and tryptophan (see Figure 2). During the hydroxylation reaction, quinonoid dihydrobiopterin, an unstable form of biopterin, is produced. If this compound is not rapidly reduced to tetrahydrobiopterin by dihydropteridine reductase, it rearranges by tautomerization to a more stable isomer, 7, 8-dihydrobiopterin. This derivative, however, is converted to tetrahydropterin by dihydrofolate reductase. The ratio between dopamine and tetrahydrobiopterin is critical because dopamine inhibits its own synthesis by competing with endogenous tetrahydrobiopterin for the cofactor binding site on tyrosine hydroxylase.

A second reason for a special interest in dihydropteridine reductase is the fact that it has been shown to be essential for neurological function *in vivo*. A variant form of phenylketonuria was discovered that is deficient in dihydropteridine reductase rather than phenylalanine hydroxylase (Koslow and Butler, 1977). This patient was diagnosed early in life as a classical phenylketonuric and was placed on a low phenylalanine diet. Despite good control of serum phenylalanine levels, this individual experienced seizures and retardation. Dihydropteridine reductase activity was found to be less than 1% of that usually found in liver, and little or no detectable tetrahydrobiopterin could be demonstrated in the liver of this patient. Dihydropteridine reductase is detectable in normal human fibroblasts at a level of 20–30% of the activity in liver, but fibroblasts isolated from the patient's skin had no detectable reductase activity (Kaufman, 1977). Furthermore, the synthesis of certain neurotransmitters was found to be defective in the patient; lower than normal levels of homovanillic acid and 5-hydroxy-indoleacetic acid were found in CSF, suggesting a decreased turnover of dopamine and serotonin.

As a corollary to a defect in dihydropteridine reductase, one would expect to find the presence of tetrahydroisoquinolines in patients. Compounds of this class can be formed by the spontaneous condensation of aldehydes or keto-containing compounds with dopamine or other biogenic amines. Circumstances favouring the formation of these compounds would be present if a defect in hydroxylation occurs. The search for such substances in psychiatric or neurological disorders is not new; several of these derivatives have been found in alcoholics and presumably contribute to their clinical symptomatology (Cohen, 1976). The possibility that α-keto analogues of the aromatic amino acids, which increase to significant levels in patients with hyperhyenylalaninaemia and tyrosinaemia, condense with dopamine, however, has not previously been investigated in schizophrenics. Two of these derivatives, 3'-O-methyl-norlaudanosolinecarboxylic acid (MNLCA) and 3',4'-deoxy-norlaudanosolinecarboxylic acid (DNLCA) have recently been found at 2- to 3-fold elevated levels in Parkinsonian patients treated with L-dopa (Coscia *et al.*, 1977) and in phenylketonurics (Lasala and Cosicia, 1979).

Tetrahydroisoquinolines are generally thought to be psychoactive or to act as false neuroregulators by competing with dopamine for receptors on neurons. In theory, defects in both tyrosine hydroxylation and the degradation of dopamine by MAO would produce concentrations of α-keto analogues and dopamine which would favour the formation of tetrahydroisoquinolines. A relatively high concentration of these potential false neuroregulators and a low concentration of dopamine available for physiologically controlled neurotransmission could produce many of the complex symptoms that have been observed in patients with schizophrenia.

In conclusion, I have proposed a two-defect hypothesis of schizophrenia which argues that the rate limiting step for dopamine synthesis and the catabolic step for its degradation may be genetically altered in schizophrenic patients. Evidence for the first defect has yet to be obtained; decreases in MAO have been observed, but the significance of this finding remains to be determined. Comprehensive clinical and biochemical studies are in progress which should result in adoption or rejection of this hypothesis.

Acknowledgements

This work was supported by the Multidisciplinary Research Program on Schizophrenia. I express my sincere appreciation to Dr Constance Denney for her critical evaluation of this manuscript.

References

Abell, C. W., Fritz, R. R., Poffenbarger, P. L., Adams, P. M. and Barratt, E. S. (1978). A novel nutritional approach to probe the molecular basis of behavior. In *Birth Defects: Original Artic. Ser.* Volume XIV Number 5 pp. 323–332 (Alan R. Liss New York)

Achee, F. M., Gabay, S. and Tipton, K. F. (1977). Some aspects of monoamine oxidase activity in brain. *Prog. Neurobiol.*, **8**, 325

Barratt, E. S., Adams, P. M., Poffenbarger, P. L., Fritz, R. R. and Abell, C. W. (1976). Effects of rapid depletion of phenylalanine and tyrosine on sleep and behavior. *Pharmacol. Biochem. Behav.*, **5**, 47

Bird, E. D., Spokes, E. G. and Iversen, L. L. (1979). Brain norepinephrine and dopamine in schizophrenia. *Science*, **204**, 93

Cohen, G. (1976). Alkaloid products in the metabolism of alcohol and biogenic amines. *Biochem. Pharmacol.*, **25**, 1123

Coscia, C. J., Burke, W., Jamroz, G., Lasala, J. M., McFarlane, J., Mitchell, J., O'Toole, M. M. and Wilson, M. L. (1977). Occurrence of a new class of tetrahydroisoquinolin alkaloids in L-dopa-treated parkinsonian patients. *Nature* (London) **269**, 617

Crow, T. J. (1979). What is wrong with dopaminergic transmission in schizophrenia. *Trends in Neuroscience*, **2**, 52

Dennick, R. G. and Mayer, R. J. (1977). Purification and immunochemical characterization of monoamine oxidase from rat and human liver. *Biochem. J.*, **161**, 167

Fischer, E., Spatz, H. and Reggiani, H. (1972). Phenylethylamine content of human urine and rat brain, its alterations in pathological conditions and after drug administration. *Experientia*, **28**, 307

Fritz, R. R., Hodgins, D. S. and Abell, C. W. (1976). Phenylalanine ammonia-lyase induction and purification from yeast and clearance in mammals. *J. Biol. Chem.*, **251**, 4646

Fritz, R. R., Landowski, J. and Abell, C. W. (1980). Quantitative electroimmuno assay of monoamine oxidase. (In preparation)

Gottesman, I. I. and Shields, J. (1976). A Critical Review of Recent Adoption, Twin, and Family Studies of Schizophrenia: Behavioral Genetics Perspectives. *Schizophr. Bull.*, **2**, 360

Johnston, J. P. (1968). Some observations upon a new inhibitor of MAO in brain tissue. *Biochem. Pharmacol.*, **17**, 1285

Kaufman, S. (1976). The phenylalanine hydroxylating system in phenylketonuria and its variants. *Biochem. Med.*, **15**, 42

Koslow, S. H. and Butler, I. J. (1977). Biogenic amine synthesis defect in dihydropteridine reductase deficiency. *Science*, **198**, 522

Landowski, J., Fritz, R. R. and Abell, C. W. (1979). Purification and characterization of human platelet monoamine oxidase. *Fed. Proc.*, **38**, 514

Lasala, J. M. and Coscia, C. J. (1979). Accumulation of a tetrahydroisoquinoline in phenylketonuria. *Science*, **203**, 283

Laurell, C.-B. (1966). Quantitative estimation of proteins by electrophoresis in agarose gel containing antibodies. *Anal. Biochem.*, **15**, 45

Molinoff, P. B. and Axelrod, J. (1971). Biochemistry of Catecholamines. *Annu. Rev. Biochem.*, **40**, 465

Russell, S. M., Davey, J. and Mayer, R. J. (1979). Immunochemical characterization of monoamine oxidase from human liver, placenta, platelets and brain cortex. *Biochem. J.*, **181**, 15

Shen, R.-S., Fritz, R. R. and Abell, C. W. (1977). Clearance of phenylalanine ammonia-lyase from normal and tumor-bearing mice. *Cancer Res.*, **37**, 1051

Shen, R.-S. and Abell, C. W. (1977). Phenylketonuria: A new method for the simultaneous determination of plasma phenylalanine and tyrosine. *Science*, **197**, 665

Shen, R.-S., Fritz, R. R. and Abell, C. W. (1979). Biochemical properties and immunogenicity of phenylalanine ammonia-lyase: effects on tumor-bearing mice. *Cancer Treatment Reports*, **63**, 1063

Suzuki, O. and Yogi, K. (1977). Multiple forms of monoamine oxidase in the human cerebral cortices at different ages. In A. Vernadakis and G. Filogamo (eds.). *Maturation of Neurotransmission*, p. 100. (Basel: S. Karger)

Targum, S. D., Gershon, E. S., Shen, R.-S. and Abell, C. W. (1979). Screening for PKU heterozygosity in bipolar affectively ill patients. *Biol. Psychiatry* (In press)

Wurtman, R. J. and Fernstrom, J. D. (1976). Commentary: Control of brain neurotransmitter synthesis by precursor availability and nutritional state. *Biochem. Pharmacol.*, **25**, 1691

Section 2:
IMMUNOLOGY

7
The relevance of immuno-pathology to research into schizophrenia

A. M. DENMAN

INTRODUCTION

Immune responses have been implicated in a variety of chronic inflammatory and degenerative disorders (Holborow and Reeves, 1977). These undoubtedly contribute to tissue damage and indeed may be the major factors which initiate and perpetuate many inflammatory diseases. Nevertheless, whilst the immunological investigation of many chronic diseases of unknown aetiology has helped elucidate the mechanisms leading to tissue damage, this approach has been less successful in pinpointing the initiating causes. The inflammatory events in many allergic disorders are rather non-specific and do not help to distinguish between, for example, the immunopathological consequences of persistent virus infections on the one hand and hypersensitivity to environmental allergens on the other (Denman, 1977). Thus, in considering the relevance of immunology to seeking the cause of schizophrenia it is unlikely that this discipline will prove decisive in terms of the techniques that are available now. However, there are three ways in which immunology may help us to understand the pathogenesis of schizophrenia by providing additional means of testing hypotheses proposed on other grounds.

Firstly, immunological techniques can help to diagnose hypersensitivity reactions to allergens implicated by clinical and other evidence.

Secondly, if an infective agent such as a persistent viral infection should prove to be the cause of schizophrenia, immune processes may be

97

involved in the persistence of such infection. Defects in the host response may allow agents to penetrate the central nervous system which are normally eliminated at other sites or alternatively could permit normally transient infections to persist indefinitely in the central nervous system. In addition the immune response against infected cells bearing virus-coded antigens on the surface could provoke an inflammatory reaction which is primarily allergic in nature.

Thirdly we should consider the possibility that schizophrenia is a form of auto-immune disease and that a primary abnormality in the immune system could lead to an immune response against brain antigens analogous to that which leads to the destruction of acetylcholine receptors in myaesthenia gravis. Of course these possibilities are not mutually exclusive and it is always possible that allergic reactions initiated by an external allergen could be potentiated by an auto-immune response.

POSSIBLE ALLERGIC CAUSES OF PSYCHIATRIC DISORDERS

There has been much speculation that food allergy can induce protean diseases with ill-defined physical and mental symptoms (Mackarness, 1976). It is essential to test the possibility that psychiatric disturbances in individual patients can be attributed to food allergy in an objective, controlled manner. This can be achieved by challenging patients with a random sequence of suspected allergens and placebos in double-blind fashion and assessing their clinical state and their immune reactions after each challenge.

The most important method of assessing the response is to document the clinical features provoked by the suspected allergen. However laboratory methods are helpful in verifying clinical impressions and include tests for detecting complement activation, rises in specific IgE, and circulating immune complexes (Platts-Mills and Denman, 1976).

The suggestion that unsuspected allergy can provoke mental symptoms has provoked several scientific and popular publications few of which contain scientifically verified evidence to support such assertions. Credence can only be given to those reports in which double-blind provocation studies have been assessed by objective clinical and laboratory measurements. However in some patients bizarre symptoms can be caused by dietary allergens. For example we recently studied a fourteen year old schoolgirl with a history of milk sensitivity in childhood producing gastro-intestinal symptoms. Initially she kept to a milk-free diet and on this regime her symptoms settled, she gained weight and height normally, and her intellectual development was also normal. However this diet later lapsed and she began to develop mental disturbance principally in the form of irrational bouts of crying and hysteria, and episodes when

Table 1 Controlled provocation tests in the diagnosis of food allergy

Phase[1]	Challenge[2]	Disodium cromoglycate[3]	Symptoms[4]	IgE (iu/ml)[5]	Complement activation[6]
1	–	–	nil	350	–
2	milk	–	+++	750	+
3	milk	+	+	480	–
4	placebo	–	nil	350	–
5	placebo	–	nil	90	–
6	–	–	nil	100	–

Data from 14 year old girl with milk hypersensitivity

[1] Each phase lasted 14 days
[2] Double-blind challenge, 30 ml by mouth
[3] 600 mg disodium cromoglycate (Intal) given immediately after challenge
[4] Summary of double-blind assessments by physician and psychiatrist
[5] Normal laboratory range: 0–200 iu/ml
[6] Determined by two-dimensional immunoelectropheresis

she would withdraw from her family and seek the privacy of her own room. There were also episodes in which she would hear voices and develop similar illusions. She also developed weakness and nausea. In association with our Psychiatric Department (Dr T. J. Crow), our Dietetics Department (Miss Pam Brereton), and the Department of Clinical Immunology (Dr Gerald Loewi) the patient was put on a diet excluding not only milk and dairy products but also other foods which would be likely to contain milk proteins. At regular two weekly intervals she was challenged with milk or placebo and during one period of exposure to milk she also received disodium cromoglycate (Intal, Fisons Pharmaceuticals Limited) as a drug for specifically blocking immediate hypersensitivity reactions. During the course of each challenge she was assessed by standard clinical and psychiatric methods and also by laboratory tests for detecting immediate hypersensitivity reactions (Table 1). Only milk precipitated the physical and psychological abnormalities and this reaction was blocked by oral disodium cromoglycate. Moreover laboratory tests indicated that exposure to milk precipitated complement activation and a rise in serum IgE.

IMMUNOPATHOLOGICAL REACTIONS AND PERSISTENT VIRUS INFECTIONS

It is now well recognized that persistent viral infections account for degenerative disorders of the central nervous system in both experimental animals and man (Weiner et al., 1973). Recent evidence suggests that such an agent may cause schizophrenia (see Chapter 2). These observations focus attention on the ways in which immunopathological processes provided by persistent virus infections may induce tissue damage. The extent to which the immune response accounts for tissue damage in viral infections of the central nervous system varies with different viruses. In some infections such damage can be attributed exclusively to the cytopathic effect of the virus. In contrast other viruses are not themselves cytopathic but the host response to virus-infected cells is entirely responsible for the resulting tissue damage.

This distinction is well illustrated by comparing the effects of immunosuppressive agents on different virus infections (Hirsch and Murphy, 1968). Antilymphocyte serum for example is only effective in preventing tissue damage when the pathological effects result entirely from the immune and inflammatory responses to the infected cells. Another good example is the natural history of lymphocytic choriomeningitis virus infections (Oldstone and Dixon, 1969). This virus is not cytopathic and it is the immune and inflammatory response against persistently infected cells which produces tissue damage. Intracerebral inoculation provokes an intense encephalitis which is commonly fatal, but can be prevented by a variety of immunosuppressive manoeuvres. These reactions are initiated by the proliferation of specifically sensitized T lymphocytes which react with virus altered antigens on the surface of the infected cell (Doherty et al., 1976). Following the generation of a specific antibody response, antibody and complement also damage the membranes of the infected cells. The reaction between surface antigens and antibody or cytotoxic T lymphocytes initiates a series of non-specific inflammatory events involving mononuclear cell populations, complement, and cells of the granulocyte series.

In contrast there are experimental models of virus infection of the central nervous system, in which infecting viruses either provoke no immune response or at best a feeble, ineffective response. It is the failure of the immune system to eliminate these agents which leads to the perpetuation of the infection. Nevertheless this continued, abortive response contributes to the chronic inflammatory reaction within the central nervous system. A consideration of the many ways in which the immune response normally operates both to limit the extent of viral infection and often to achieve its eventual elimination, also indicates the variety of defects which could interrupt this process. In particular there are several ways in which lymphocytes contribute to host defence in virus infections (Table 2). Firstly, specifically sensitized T lymphocytes eliminate infected cells which display viral antigens and there is considerable evidence both in animal experiments and also in man that the cytotoxic T lymphocytes recognize histocompatibility antigens or other 'self' antigens in association with viral antigens (Doherty et al, 1976). Secondly, other lymphocyte populations which are not specifically sensitized to antigens of the invading virus are cytotoxic for infected cells which have become sensitized by specific antibodies. Thirdly, lymphocytes and cells of the monocyte–macrophage series produce interferon which limits the spread of virus to susceptible cells. It is also likely that products of monocytes and lymphocytes other than interferon have antiviral activity. Fourthly lymphocytes with 'helper' function are also needed to initiate antibody responses against a variety of viruses.

There are, in general terms, two kinds of abnormality which might increase the virulence of neurotropic viruses in susceptible human hosts. On the one hand disease could be provoked by exaggerated cell-mediated responses to virus infected cells, and such hypersensitivity is clearly relevant to acute demyelinating conditions and encephalitis following exanthematous virus infections. It is unlikely however that such mechanisms would operate in persistent virus infection. Although there is little information on this in man, in experimental animal models genetically controlled susceptibility to acute encephalitis induced by agents

Table 2   Contribution of lymphocytes to host defence against virus infections

Function	Population
(1) Eliminating virus-infected cells	(a) Specific T lymphocytes (b)* 'Natural killer' (NK) cells (c)* 'Killer' (K) cells
(2) Protecting susceptible cells	(a) Interferon (b) Other mediators
(3) Synthesizing anti-viral antibody	(a) 'Helper' T lymphocytes (b) Antibody-producing B lymphocytes

* Non-specific mechanisms – see Holborow and Reeves (1977) for further details

such as lymphocytic choriomeningitis virus appears to operate only in the short term. Alternatively, various forms of immunodeficiency may lead to persistent virus infection. These may antedate the infection or be induced by the virus itself. Such defects characteristically give rise to chronic immune complex disease.

There are two principal factors which determine the severity of the immunopathological sequelae. Firstly there are genetic factors which determine the extent to which the virus will replicate in various cells and tissues and secondly the character of the immune response. The available evidence suggests that damage to the central nervous system resulting from persistent virus infection is most likely to result from defects in the host response which result in failure to eliminate the infecting organism.

There are many strategies for viral persistence which enable the virus to evade elimination by the immune and inflammatory response of the host. One experimental model which illustrates these features is visna virus which causes a demyelinating disorder in Icelandic sheep (Figure 1). During the acute infection, virus can readily be recovered both from peripheral organs and also from the central nervous system (Petursson *et al.*, 1976). As the disease progresses it becomes increasingly difficult to isolate virus from the central nervous system or from other sites. In the early stages of infection there is a brisk immune response against the invading organism. Neutralising antibody in high titre can be detected in the blood and cerebrospinal fluid. As the disease progresses this titre falls, a decline which has been variously attributed to the central de-

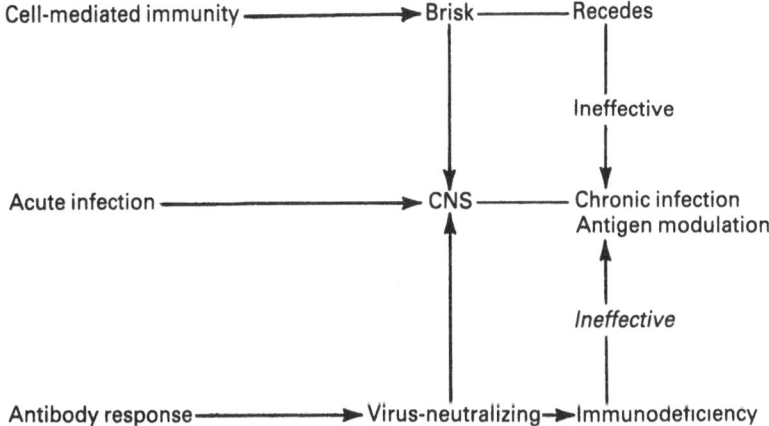

Figure 1   Visna virus persistence in infected sheep

pletion of specifically reactive B lymphocytes or to antigenic variations of
the virus which render the antibody increasingly ineffective. When infection is first established, specific cell-mediated immune reactions against
visna-infected cells can readily be demonstrated, and viral antigens
induce specific lymphocyte transformation *in vitro*. These reactions also
recede as the infection progresses. Visna is also insensitive to interferon
so that the combined failure of lymphocytes to protect host cells at risk
from infection and to react specifically with virus infected cells contributes to viral persistence. Thus this animal model of a persistent viral
infection in the central nervous system illustrates how the nature and distribution of the infecting agent and the progressive suppression of the
host immune response lead to the perpetuation of a chronic, demyelinating disease.

There is no example of a persistent viral infection in man which has
yet been proven to cause schizophrenia or related disorders. Nonetheless
the principle is well established that a loss of intellectual ability occurs in
virus infections of the kuru or Creuzfeldt–Jacob varieties which fail to
induce any obvious immune response (Manuelidis *et al.*, 1978). This is an
obvious example of virus which may persist largely because of its failure
to provoke any kind of immune response.

Intellectual deterioration is also part of the clinical picture of subacute
sclerosing panencephalitis, a disease caused by measles virus infection.
Despite much investigation there is no clear evidence that immune
responses in general or to measles virus in particular are depressed in this
disorder. High titre antibody to measles virus can be detected in the
blood and cerebrospinal fluid and specific cell-mediated immune
responses against measles virus can also be detected. This is therefore an

example of virus infection which persists despite an ostensibly normal immune response and clearly other factors must determine the occasional ability of measles virus to persist in the central nervous system of susceptible individuals.

The possibility that Epstein–Barr (EB) virus infections may be implicated in the aetiology of schizophrenia has been stimulated by clinical observations that depressive illnesses of unusual severity may follow isolated examples of infectious mononucleosis (Liberman, personal communication). Lethargy and depression are common symptoms of infectious mononucleosis and may persist for up to a year. Moreover EB virus infection may have an unusually severe course in susceptible individuals (Figure 2). In the majority of individuals this virus is acquired either as a silent infection or as the benign, self-limited lymphoproliferative disorder, infectious mononucleosis. Various forms of host defence control the proliferation of the specifically infected B lymphocytes of which T lymphocyte responses are probably the most important.

The characteristic atypical mononuclear cells in the blood of patients with infectious mononucleosis are cytotoxic T lymphocytes able to eliminate B lymphocytes infected by EB virus. Interferon and other mediators produced by T lymphocytes are also highly efficient in protecting suscep-

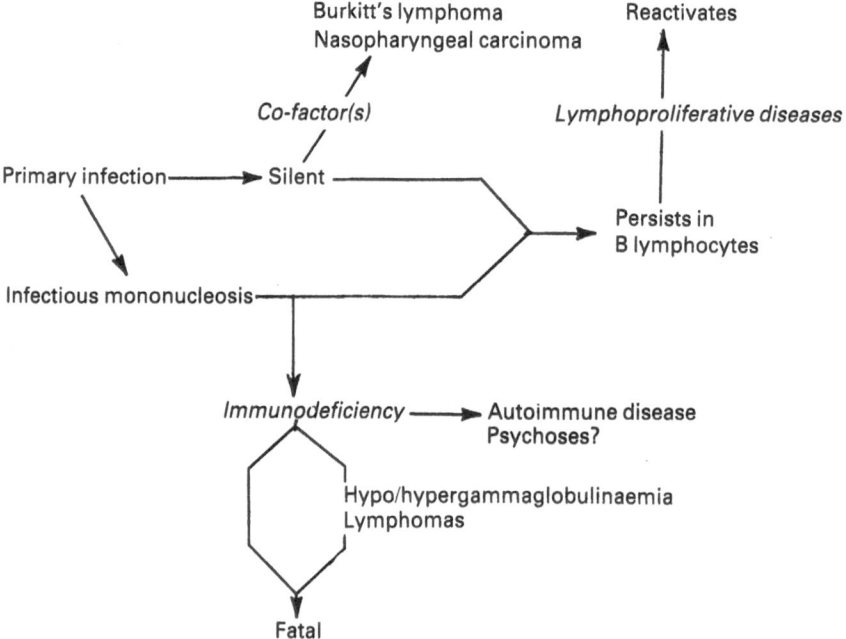

Figure 2   Natural history of Epstein-Barr (EB) virus infections

tible mononuclear cells from virus transformation (Rickinson *et al.*, 1977). However, despite the ability of normal individuals to control the proliferation of EB virus infected cells whether in asymptomatic infection or in infectious mononucleosis, EB virus persists throughout life in a small percentage of B lymphocytes and can become reactivated in subsequent lymphoproliferative disorders.

In susceptible individuals EB virus has an unusually severe clinical course during the primary infection and indeed the infection may terminate in fatal dysproteinaemias such as hypergammaglobulinaemia or hypogammaglobulinaemia (Purtilo *et al.*, 1978). Specific immune defects have been described which predispose towards an unusually severe course. For example a deficiency in the production of interferon by T lymphocytes in patients with primary EB virus infections may lead to a progressive lymphoproliferative disorder (Virelizier *et al.*, 1978). Similarly a patient lacking cytotoxic T lymphocytes for EB virus infected cells developed severe autoimmune disease with Coombs-positive haemolytic anaemia requiring steroid treatment (Smith and Denman, 1978). In other patients the lymphoproliferative process may be extremely intense or even fatal despite the lack of any obvious failure to produce cytotoxic T lymphocytes in the blood and lymphoid tissues (Britten *et al.*, 1978; Crawford *et al.*, 1979).

Thus EB virus infections illustrate how variations in host resistance determine the clinical outcome. In addition to the realization that this virus may cause severe depression of long duration, organic involvement of the central nervous system in infectious mononucleosis is well recognized (Carter and Penman, 1969).

AUTOIMMUNE DISEASE AND DEGENERATIVE CHANGES OF THE CENTRAL NERVOUS SYSTEM

It is now well accepted that primary autoimmune diseases account for many forms of acute and chronic human disease. The best documented instances of autoimmune reactions leading to disease are those directed against circulating cells in the blood such as platelets, red cells, and white cells.

Autoimmune phenomena accompany a variety of chronic inflammatory disorders, but in most instances it is less certain that these autoantibodies are directly responsible for the clinical disorder. However in one disorder of the nervous system, myaesthenia gravis, there is good evidence that autoimmune reactions may be of primary pathogenic importance since autoantibodies against acetylcholine receptors are readily detected and it is the cumulative depletion of these receptors which produces the clinical features (Mittag *et al.*, 1976).

It is possible therefore that autoimmunity could produce psychoses such as schizophrenia. Such abnormalities undoubtedly arise in patients with undisputed autoimmune diseases and one clear example is systemic lupus erythematosus. In this disease there is autoantibody production against a variety of tissues. Psychiatric disturbances in the form of disorientation, hallucinations, paranoia, and other symptoms resembling schizophrenia occur and indeed may be the presenting clinical feature (Sergent *et al.*, 1975). There is controversy concerning the pathogenesis of these features and it is sometimes difficult to distinguish psychiatric features which are part of the disease from those induced by steroid therapy or by intercurrent infections. However two lines of evidence indicate that the pathogenesis of the neuropsychiatric features of systemic lupus erythematosus is similar to that operating in other tissues: firstly, there is complement activation in the cerebrospinal fluid (Hadler *et al.*, 1973); secondly, autoantibodies which cross react with brain antigen are particularly prominent in patients with neurological involvement.

The nature of the primary abnormality in autoimmune systemic lupus erythematosus is still unknown. It is now well recognized that in man as in other species autoreactive B lymphocytes normally exist with specificity for self-antigens (Bankhurst and Williams, 1975). These lymphocytes could proliferate as a primary uncontrolled process which escapes the normal regulatory mechanisms of the immune system and could result from an acquired or congenital defect in the regulatory population. On this basis systemic lupus erythematosus is attributed to the uncontrolled proliferation of a variety of B lymphocytes with specificity for a wide spectrum of self-antigens including those of the central nervous system.

Alternatively autoimmune disease has been attributed to changes in the antigens normally borne on the surface of different host cells. This is thought to be either a primary somatic mutation leading to the expression of abnormal antigens or the expression of antigens which are normally repressed. Alteration of membrane antigens by persistent virus infection could achieve the same effect. These altered antigens induce the proliferation of B lymphocytes with specific receptors. The recognition that T lymphocytes are heterogeneous populations with both helper and suppressor function has introduced an experimental basis for such speculations. T lymphocytes are required for the induction of an antibody response against a variety of exogenous antigens. These sensitized T lymphocytes give a signal to reactive B lymphocytes whose proliferation leads to the synthesis and release of specific antibody. T lymphocytes recognize altered self-antigens and thereby initiate a response by populations of potentially autoreactive B lymphocytes. This process is usually limited by regulatory T lymphocyte populations. However these control mechanisms could be by-passed by the response to self-antigens seen in combination with viral or other antigens ('associative recognition'). Auto-reactive B lymphocytes can readily be detected in patients with systemic lupus erythematosus and there have also been claims that defects of regulatory T lymphocyte populations can also be detected (Sagawa and Abdou, 1978).

Characterizing the defect in systemic lupus erythematosus, an extreme example of autoimmunity, should help us to understand the nature of other degenerative inflammatory disorders associated with autoimmunity. There is one disease producing transient abnormality of the central nervous system which is initiated by bacterial infection, namely chorea in association with rheumatic fever following streptococcal infections. Involvement of the central nervous system is attributed to cross-reaction between streptococcal antigens and antigens in the basal ganglia of the cerebral hemispheres leading to the proliferation of autoreactive B lymphocytes with specificity for brain antigens. Such observations stimulate speculation that similar factors might result in persistent degenerative changes in the brain after a variety of infections.

Behçet's syndrome is another inflammatory disorder characterized by vasculitis, the formation of autoantibodies and, frequently, involvement of the central nervous system (O'Duffy and Goldstein, 1976). Families have been described in which several members have suffered severe psychoses as well as the commoner features of the syndrome (Goolamali *et al.*, 1976). As with all chronic inflammatory disorders involving peristent vasculitis, there has been considerable speculation about the role of the autoimmune phenomena reported in this disorder (Lehner, 1979) but it is not clear whether these are of primary importance or are secondary to vascular damage. Recent studies of viral replication in the blood lymphocytes of patients with this disease have suggested that these cells may be persistently infected with defective virus particles (Denman *et al.*, 1979).

CONCLUSIONS

There is no firm evidence that immunological factors are involved in the pathogenesis of schizophrenia. Nevertheless immunological techniques can be used to support and amplify data from other sources that a particular aetiological factor may cause schizophrenia. In particular, should schizophrenia prove to be a disorder caused by persistent infection by a virus or other microbe commonly encountered in normal individuals, it will be vital to characterize the nature of the host defect in susceptible individuals. This is not merely of theoretical interest but could point the way to specific manoeuvres which might reverse the defect in host responses.

Acknowledgement

The author wishes to thank Fisons Pharmaceuticals Ltd., for generously providing Intal samples.

References

Bankhurst, A. D. and Williams, Jr., R. C. (1975). Identification of DNA-binding lymphocytes in patients with systemic lupus erythematosus. *J. Clin. Invest.*, **56**, 1378

Britten, S., Andersson-Anvret, M., Gergely, P., Henle, W., Jondal, M., Klein, G., Sandstedt, B. and Svedmyr, E. (1978). Epstein–Barr virus immunity and tissue distribution in a fatal case of infectious mononucleosis. *N. Engl. J. Med.*, **298**, 89

Carter, R. L. and Penman, H. G. (eds.) (1969). *Infectious Mononucleosis*. (Oxford: Blackwell, Scientific Publications

Crawford, D. H., Epstein, M. A., Achong, B. G., Finerty, S., Newman, J., Liversedge, S., Tedder, R. S. and Stewart, J. W. (1979). Virological and immunological studies on a fatal case of infectious mononucleosis. *J. Infect.*, **1**, 37

Denman, A. M. (1977). Viruses, poisons and arthritis. *Rheumatism and Rehabilitation*, **16**, 205

Denman, A. M., Fialkow, P. J., Pelton, B. K., Salo, A. C. and Appleford, D. J. (1979). Attempts to establish a viral aetiology for Behcet's syndrome. In Lehner, T. and Barnes, C. G. (eds.) *Behcet's Syndrome*, p. 91. (London: Academic Press).

Doherty, P. C., Götze, D., Trinchieri, G. and Zinkernagel, R. M. (1976). Models for recognition of virally modified cells by immune thymus-derived lymphocytes. *Immunogenetics*, **3**, 517

Goolamali, S. K., Comaish, J. S., Hassanyeh, F. and Stephens, A. (1976). Familial Behçet's syndrome. *Br. J. Dermatol.*, **95**, 637

Hadler, N. M., Gerwin, R. D. Frank, M. M., Whitaker, J. N., Baker, M. and Decker, J. L. (1973). The fourth component of complement in the cerebrospinal fluid of systemic lupus erythematosus. *Arthritis Rheum*, **16**, 507

Hirsch, M. S. and Murphy, F. A. (1968). Effects of anti-lymphoid sera on viral infections. *Lancet*, **2**, 37

Holborow, E. J. and Reeves, W. G. (1977). *Immunology in Medicine*. (London: Academic Press)

Lehner, T. (1979). Immunological aspects of Behçet's Disease. In Dilşen, N. and Koniçe, M. (eds.) *Behçet's Disease*, p. 203. Excerpta Medica, International Congress Series, No. 467

Mackarness, R. (1976). *Not all in the mind*. (London: Pan Books)

Manuelidis, E. E., Gorgacz, E. J. and Manuelidis, L. (1978). Viraemia in experimental Creutzfeld–Jakob disease. *Science*, **200**, 1069

Mittag, T., Kornfeld, P., Tormay, A. and Woo, C. (1976). Detection of anti-acetylcholine receptor factors in serum and thymus from patients with myasthenia gravis. *N. Engl. J. Med.*, **294**, 691

O'Duffy, J. D. and Goldstein, N. P. (1976) Neurologic involvement in seven patients with Behçet's disease. *Am. J. Med.*, **61**, 170

Oldstone, M. B. A. and Dixon, F. J. (1969). Pathogenesis of chronic disease associated with persistent lymphocytic choriomeningitis viral infection. *J. Exp. Med.*, **129**, 483

Petursson, G., Nathanson, N., Georgsson, G., Panitch, H. and Palsson, P. A. (1976). Pathogenesis of Visna. I. Sequential virologic, serologic and pathologic studies. *Lab. Invest.*, **35**, 402

Platts-Mills, T. A. E. and Denman, A. M. (1976). Hypersensitivity to food and immune reactions. *J. Hum. Nutr.*, **30**, 141

Purtilo, D. T., Hutt, L., Bhawan, J., Yang, J. P. S., Cassel, C., Allegra, S. and

Rosen, F. S. (1978). Immunodeficiency to the Epstein–Barr virus in the X-linked recessive lymphoproliferative syndrome. *Clin. Immunol. Immunopathol.*, **9**, 147

Rickinson, A. B., Crawford, D. and Epstein, M. A. (1977). Inhibition of the *in vitro* outgrowth of Epstein-Barr virus transformed lymphocytes by thymus-dependent lymphocytes from infectious mononucleosis patients. *Clin. Exp. Immunol.*, **28**, 72

Sagawa, A. and Abdou, A. I. (1978). Suppressor-cell dysfunction in systemic lupus erythematosus. *J. Clin. Invest.*, **62**, 789

Sergent, J. S., Lockshin, M. D., Klempner, M. S. and Lipsky, B. A. (1975). Central nervous system disease in systemic lupus erythematosus. *Am. J. Med.*, **58**, 644

Smith, H. and Denman, A. M. (1978). A new manifestation of infection with Epstein-Barr virus. *Br. Med. J.*, **2**, 248

Virelizier, J. L., Lenoir, G. and Griscelli, C. (1978). Persistent Epstein–Barr virus infection in a child with hypergammaglobulinaemia and immunoblastic proliferation associated with a selective defect in immune interferon secretion. *Lancet*, **2**, 231

Weiner, L. P., Johnson, R. T. and Herndon, R. M. (1973). Viral infections and demyelinating diseases. *N. Engl. J. Med.*, **24**, 1103

8
Some connections between immunoglobulins and schizophrenia

E. PULKKINEN

IMMUNOGLOBULINS, PSYCHOPATHOLOGY AND PROGNOSIS

In the literature, very early reports on the deviations of serum proteins in schizophrenics can be found; for reviews see Fessel (1962) and Solomon and Moos (1964). However, there is very little information so far about how the observed changes are connected with schizophrenic disease, although different opinions have been presented.

Heath and Krupp (1967) suggested that the autoimmunological character of schizophrenia was indicated by findings that a protein fraction, 'taraxein', isolated from the serum of schizophrenics, runs contrary to IgG auto-antibody brain tissue. In the later studies, these observations, however, have been difficult to verify. The possibility of an immunological process has also been reported by Bock et al. (1971), who thought that the IgM and β_{1a}/β_{1c}-globulin concentrations, which were lower in schizophrenic patients than in normal controls, indicated a complement-fixating antigen–antibody reaction. On the other hand, according to these authors, the significant changes in protein verified at acute phase (increase in orosomucoid and haptoglobin, and decrease in α_2HS glycoprotein, β-lipoprotein and transferrin) in schizophrenic and borderline psychotic patients indicated unspecific reflection of stress. Several other workers have also reported on the effects of mental stress. Among these are Solomon et al. (1974), who consider stress to be a possible cause of

111

dys- and hypofunction of the immunological system.

Although deviations in serum immunoglobulins have been found in other psychiatric patients as well as in schizophrenics (Solomon *et al.* (1969)), it appears that the immunology of schizophrenia also has specific characteristics. Strahilevitz and Davis (1970) found that IgA was significantly higher in schizophrenic patients than in normal persons and controls with other psychiatric disorders. Solomon *et al.* (1966) found that in chronic schizophrenics the severity of psychotic symptoms had a negative correlation to the total gammaglobulin concentration and a positive correlation to the 19-S macroglobulin concentration. On the other hand, Solomon *et al.* (1969) were unable to find in schizophrenic patients any significant correlations of immunoglobulins (IgA, IgG and IgM) and severity of symptoms or the classifications process–reactive, paranoid–non-paranoid. Amkraut *et al.* (1973) have published their findings on the connection between the prognosis of recovery and immunoglobulins in a study in which IgA, IgG and IgM concentrations were determined in 80 schizophrenics and 315 controls. Patients with IgA and IgG values below average were more likely to recover during treatment than those with both globulin values above average.

Since a more detailed analysis of psychopathology and prognosis may produce more information concerning the immunology of schizophrenia, the IgA, IgG and IgM determinations have been included as a part of a larger study, which will enable the investigation of the correlations of immunoglobulins to those variables that depict psychopathology, prognosis and background.

The present study attempts to find an answer to the following questions: To what extent do the IgA, IgG and IgM concentrations at the inception of treatment correlate with (1) psychopathology, (2) prognostic background variables, and (3) prognosis?

Material and methods

The present series consisted of 76 schizophrenic patients admitted to Kellokoski Hospital after 5 September 1972, considered in order of admission. These patients had been under psychiatric care at least once before for schizophrenia or schizophreniform psychosis. The system of 10 malignant schizophrenic symptoms was used for diagnostic purposes (Achté, 1967). The average age of the patients was 34.8 years, both sexes being equally represented.

Determination of immunoglobulins

Serum samples for IgA, IgG and IgM determinations were taken from each patient within 1–3 days of admission. The determination of immunoglobulins was performed using the commercial version (Tri.Partigen®, Behringswerke) of the technique developed by Mancini *et al.* (1965). In this version, H-chain specific antiserum has been added to agar gel and the plate protected with sodium azide against bacterial growth (1 mg sodium azide/ml). The determination was standardized by using three immunoglobulin concentrations. A standard straight line was drawn as a square root function of the diameters of diffusion rings, as a basis for determination; if the concentration of the samples occurred outside the standard straight line, redetermination was performed from diluted serum.

Psychopathology The following scales were used in charting psychopathology: PAAS (Premorbid asocial adjustment scale, Gittelman-Klein and Klein (1969)): Schizoid features of premorbid personality were determined on this scale. The version based on the interview is referred to as P1 and relatives' assessments as P2. WBI (Ward Behavior Inventory; Burdock and Hardesty, 1968); this scale was used to determine the degree of severity of the disease on the basis of a 1 week observation in the ward. Paranoid and withdrawal symptoms were determined in accordance with Venables and O'Connor (1959) on the basis of factors obtained from IMPS and WBRS Scales (Goldberg *et al.* (1963)) from medical records for each admission. In addition, the mean of all admissions with paranoid and withdrawal symptoms was calculated. In order to test the reliability of the method, two persons used the medical records to assess paranoid and withdrawal symptoms in 30 periods in hospital. The degree of reliability arrived at by the assessors was 0.81 for paranoid and 0.86 for withdrawal symptoms.

It was exceedingly difficult to exclude other concurrent disease with absolute certainty as this would have caused the patient undue strain. The anamnesis, laboratory findings and status observations for the patients were, however, studied in order to diagnose other possible diseases. The only clear group to emerge was that of infectious diseases, which was included as a separate variable for control purposes.

Prognostic background variables

The background variables were mainly demographic variables and variables depicting the progress of the disease (86 variables); both of these groups of variables, according to the literature, are related to the prognosis of schizophrenia. Because of the great number of variables in the present study only the main features have been described.

The general background variables/groups of variables were: age; sex; education; socio-economic status; marriage (ever married); and residential environment (rural–urban). Variables depicting the onset of disease were: age at onset of disease; precipitating factor; acuteness of onset of

Table 1 Varimax-rotated factor matrix

Variables	h^2				Factors			
		I	II	III	IV	V	VI	VII
Sex (male)	0.432	0.03	0.21	0.10	-0.03	0.61	-0.00	0.08
Place of birth (rural–urban)	0.319	0.46	0.17	0.02	-0.04	0.02	0.11	-0.27
Education	0.391	0.14	0.00	0.01	-0.09	-0.04	0.60	0.03
Age at onset of disease	0.383	-0.40	-0.01	-0.15	0.08	0.12	-0.33	0.27
Acuteness of onset of disease	0.261	0.09	-0.12	-0.17	0.19	0.02	0.41	-0.03
Duration of disease	0.562	-0.26	-0.68	-0.07	-0.05	0.12	-0.01	-0.13
Number of earlier periods in hospital	0.522	0.06	-0.71	-0.05	0.02	0.06	0.08	0.05
Relatives' willingness to receive patient from hospital	0.498	-0.33	0.04	0.08	-0.06	-0.48	0.38	0.03
Availability of accommodation	0.352	-0.47	0.12	0.16	-0.19	0.06	0.11	-0.19
No. of contacts in open care	0.286	-0.08	-0.34	0.14	-0.00	-0.34	0.06	0.16
No. of neuroleptic units in medication	0.406	0.05	-0.10	0.02	-0.61	0.15	-0.03	0.01
No. of tranquilizer units in medication	0.281	0.14	0.18	0.07	0.12	-0.42	-0.17	0.07
Occurrence of obscure attitudes	0.153	-0.02	-0.07	0.08	0.01	0.37	-0.03	0.12
Occurrence of abnormal speech	0.255	-0.04	-0.33	0.07	-0.19	0.19	0.04	0.25
Suicide attempts	0.200	-0.01	0.01	0.32	0.01	-0.05	0.26	-0.16
Occurrence of neurotic features	0.362	-0.19	-0.11	0.00	0.16	0.06	0.53	0.02
Ward Behavior Inventory (WBI)	0.398	0.29	0.05	-0.01	-0.56	0.03	0.00	-0.03
Interests, ages 14–20, P1	0.259	0.05	0.07	0.27	0.20	-0.14	-0.13	-0.32

Continuation of Table 1

Sociosexual adapatation, P1	0.433	0.05	0.03	0.51	0.07	0.19	-0.34	-0.11
Withdrawal, ages 14–20, P2	0.387	0.03	-0.20	0.49	0.05	-0.24	0.05	0.20
Interests, ages 14–20, P2	0.501	0.26	-0.01	0.61	0.06	0.15	-0.05	0.19
Sociosexual adaptation, P2	0.495	0.00	0.01	0.67	-0.18	0.11	-0.01	0.07
Paranoid symptoms on examination	0.425	0.09	0.03	-0.08	-0.63	-0.07	-0.04	0.10
IgA	0.391	-0.51	-0.05	-0.22	0.21	0.16	0.04	0.08
IgM	0.391	-0.18	0.08	-0.22	0.08	0.02	0.27	-0.47
IgG	0.298	-0.40	0.24	-0.07	0.09	-0.24	0.10	0.03
Participation in physiotherapy	0.460	-0.19	0.23	-0.12	0.37	0.24	0.36	0.18
Occupant density in lodgings (persons/room)	0.277	-0.12	0.24	-0.05	0.22	0.08	0.05	0.38
No. of days on leave	0.435	0.41	0.04	0.11	-0.24	-0.13	0.38	0.21
Interval between relatives' visits	0.467	0.42	-0.34	0.10	-0.11	0.34	-0.18	0.09
Mean score of paranoid symptoms for all periods in hospital	0.465	-0.15	0.13	0.12	0.54	0.05	-0.05	0.34
Mean score of withdrawal symptoms for all periods in hospital	0.413	0.10	0.13	0.03	0.19	-0.01	-0.07	-0.59
Length of stay in hospital	0.584	0.70	-0.19	0.03	-0.21	-0.05	-0.08	0.05
Proportion of periods in hospital in relation to duration of disease	0.268	0.42	0.06	0.07	0.03	0.18	0.16	-0.16
Infectious diseases (present–absent)	0.210	0.08	-0.42	0.06	0.09	-0.12	0.02	0.05
Sums of squares	13.22	2.58	1.94	1.80	2.02	1.61	1.77	1.50

disease; and duration of symptoms before treatment. Variables related to hospital and open care were: treatment motivation on admission; participation in different forms of therapy; the patient's contacts with his relatives during stay in hospital; willingness of relatives to receive the patient from hospital; frequency of open care contacts; occurrence of socially embarrassing behaviour in open care (Wing, 1960); and management of medication in open care.

Variables depicting prognosis

For the purposes of prognosis, follow-up studies were carried out on the present subjects for 6 months from the admission date of the last patient. On the basis of length of time in hospital the subjects were divided into four groups: Group A, 0–30 days; Group B, 31–60 days; Group C, 61–180 days; and Group D, 181 days and over. On the basis of the medical records, the proportion of earlier periods in hospital in relation to the duration of disease was also ascertained. The duration of the disease before the patient was granted a National Invalidity Pension was used as a criterion of the ability to cope socially. Furthermore, at the end of treatment each patient's ability to work was determined on a 1–6 rating scale.

Statistical analysis

The statistical analysis of the present material was performed through factor analysis, using Varimax rotation (Überla, 1968).

Results

Immunoglobulins were found to have significant correlations to the groups of variables presented above. However, due to large numbers of the variables related to psychopathology and background, only the correlations at a statistically significant level for these variables were presented. Correlations below this level were considered in the factorizing (Table 1).

Correlations to psychopathology

Only IgM showed statistically significant correlations to psychopathology. Withdrawal symptoms during the first period of admission and the mean of these symptoms during all periods in hospital had a positive correlation ($p < 0.01$) to IgM concentrations. The correlations of the other variables related to psychopathology remained below this level.

Correlations to prognostic background variables

Only IgA showed a statistically significant correlation to the background variables. The age at the time of investigation had a positive correlation ($p < 0.01$) and place of birth (rural–urban) a negative correlation ($p < 0.01$) to IgA concentration. Because age also had a positive correlation with IgG ($p < 0.05$), another correlation matrix was obtained, in which the age was held constant. A separate note was made when the elimination of the effect of age effected a basic alteration in the results.

Correlations to prognosis

The globulin values were found to be highest in patients who had stayed only a short time in hospital. The globulin concentrations (IgA, $p < 0.01$, IgG, $p < 0.05$; IgM, $p < 0.10$) decreased as the length of period spent in hospital increased. After elimination of the effect of age, the correlation coefficients were at: IgA, $p < 0.05$; IgG, $p < 0.10$; IgM, $p < 0.05$). According to these findings, high immunoglobulin concentrations at the beginning of treatment seem to predict short length of stay in hospital (Table 2).

Table 2 Immunoglobulin concentrations (g/l) grouped in accordance with length of stay in hospital

Group	No. of patients	IgA Mean	s.d.	IgG Mean	s.d.	IgM Mean	s.d.
A	14	3.30	1.43	16.1	2.67	2.28	1.25
B	17	2.73	0.97	14.6	3.42	1.87	0.78
C	26	2.56	0.88	14.6	3.22	1.71	0.70
D	19	2.17	0.83	13.7	3.39	1.72	0.72
Total	76	2.64	1.06	14.6	3.25	1.85	0.86

Normal values: IgA, 0.74–3.06 g/l; IgG, 7.2–15.1 g/l; IgM, 0.23–1.33 g/l

The mean duration of disease prior to the present study was 7.0 years, approximately 1.3 years of which had been spent in hospital. As with the observations presented above, IgG was also found to have a negative correlation ($p < 0.05$) to the proportion of earlier periods in hospital in relation to the duration of the disease. After elimination of the effect of age, $r = -0.22$, which was slightly below the 5% limit, $r \geq \pm 0.23$.

At the time of the study, 30 (39.5%) of the subjects were receiving a National Invalidity Pension. The patients who had been able to manage longest without National Invalidity Pensions were those with the highest IgA concentrations ($p < 0.05$) at the time of the study. After elimination of the effect of age, this connection, however, remained insignificant.

Immunoglobulins showed no significant correlations to ability to work as assessed at the end of treatment.

Factor analysis

Variables correlating with immunoglobulins at the level $r \geq 0.180$ were selected from the correlation matrix for factor analysis, excluding, however, variables depicting the same thing either directly or indirectly. The variables thus selected from the initial 119 for factorization totalled 35.

The principal axis model with 12 factors explained 47.1% of the total variance of the variables. On the basis of eigenvalues a solution with six factors would have been the most reliable, but since IgM had a very prominent loading in the seventh factor, the Varimax solution was worked out with seven factors (Table 1), explaining 37.7% of the total variance.

Since immunoglobulins had more significant loadings (≥ 0.30) only in the first and the seventh factors, only these factors are dealt with in detail.

Factor I This factor may be called the institutionalization factor. The length of period in hospital and the proportion of earlier hospital stays in relation to the duration of the disease change in the same direction, depicting proneness either to become institutionalized or, on the other hand, to avoid becoming institutionalized.

The lowest disposition toward institutionalization appears to occur among patients with the highest IgA and IgG concentrations at the time of examination. Availability of accommodation, having been brought up in the country, late onset of the disease and good relations with relatives have a similar effect.

Factor VII This factor may be called the withdrawal–paranoid factor. The oppositive loadings of withdrawal and paranoid symptoms indicate that a rough classification of patients into 'withdrawal' and 'paranoid' is possible.

The withdrawn patients appear to have had very few interests during their premorbid period (aged 14–20 years), whereas the paranoid patients interests were normal. The withdrawn patients had the highest IgM concentrations and the paranoid patients the lowest, and the increase in occupant density also seems to have had a similar effect as the paranoid symptoms.

Factors II–VI In these factors immunoglobulins did not have any noteworthy loadings.

Factor II may be called the duration of disease factor and factor III the factor representing the degree of schizoidism in premorbid personality. In factor IV some of the variables depicting psychopathology receive considerable loadings. Prognostic background variables are primarily loaded in factors V and VI. The control variable, infectious diseases, was found to have its only considerable loading in factor II. Infectious diseases are likely to increase with the duration of the disease.

Discussion

The rather limited material ($N = 76$) and the fact that the immunoglobulin determination was performed only once, limit interpretation of the present results. Owing to a great number of variables even signicant correlations may occur accidentally. The observation, however, that immunoglobulins had correlations with several parallel variables depicting psychopathology and prognosis, speaks for the significance of the present results. With regard to psychopathology the withdrawn patients showed high IgM concentrations and the paranoid patients low. If this finding is investigated on the basis of the hypothesis that stress may cause dys- or hypofunction of the immunological system (Solomon et al., 1974), then it would have been the paranoid schizophrenics who would have been susceptible to stress, which would consequently be reflected in lower IgM concentrations for these patients. This possibility may be supported by the finding that paranoid schizophrenics are 'hyperscanners' and non-paranoid schizophrenics 'hypo-scanners' of their surroundings, blocking the impulse coming from the surroundings (Silverman, 1964). The autonomic nervous system of paranoid patients has also been found to react more sensitively to stress stimuli than that of the non-paranoid patients (Shean et al. (1974)). On the other hand, the increase in level of arousal found in withdrawn patients (Venables and Wing, 1962) leaves open the question of the extent to which these patients suffer from the effects of external stress, in spite of their withdrawal and the narrowing of their range of attention (Venables, 1966). However, the observation that the adrenal glands of apathic schizophrenics respond weakly to physical stress (Poirier and Richer (1963)) could indicate a lesser susceptibility to stress in withdrawn patients, which would then explain the higher IgM concentrations.

A good prognosis for hospital stay appeared to be connected with higher than average IgA and IgG concentrations at the beginning of treatment (factor I). Age at the onset of the disease, as the only biological variable, could be the connection between immunoglobulin concentrations and prognosis. An early age of onset is known to be a sign of poor prognosis in schizophrenia (Cole et al., 1968), whereas age as such does not explain the present findings for prognosis, which became apparent after elimination of the effect of age.

IMMUNOGLOBULINS, AGE FACTOR AND PROGNOSIS

In an earlier study (Pulkkinen, 1977), high IgA, IgG and IgM concentrations at the beginning of treatment were found to predict a short hospital stay. Primarily, it was also found that the connection between prognosis and immunoglobulins is, in part at least, explained on the basis of age at onset of disease and of age. Since the previous observation period was only six months, the aim of the present study was to establish whether globulin concentrations remain predictive even during a longer period. At the same time, a more detailed investigation of how age and age at onset of disease influence the correlations between immunoglobulins and short-term as well as long-term prognosis, was attempted.

Material and methods

The present material is the same as in the previous study, consisting of schizophrenic patients ($N = 76$) admitted to Kellokoski Hospital after 5 September 1972 and considered in the order of admission. On admission, serum samples for IgA, IgG and IgM determinations were taken from each patient. Two of the initial 76 patients had died by the time of the present study: one from cancer and one had committed suicide. Thus the present series consisted of 74 patients, whose average age was 38.4 years. Both sexes were equally represented. For each patient, a short-term prognosis was determined on the basis of the length of hospital stay following the key admission. Long-term prognosis was established by observing each patient for four years starting from the day of admission, and by adding up the hospital stays during that period. For statistical analysis, the patients were classified on the basis of their cumulative hospital stays in two groups: Group A, under 1 year; Group B, 1–4 years. The average age of Group A was 41.1 years and of Group B, 35.7 years. The difference in the means was not statistically significant ($t = 1.92$). The means and standard deviations of the globulins were calculated by groups and the differences in significance were tested with the t-test.

Results

Immunoglobulins and short term prognosis

Since the short term results were already previously presented, it is in this connection sufficient to state that all globulins had a negative correlation to prognosis; IgA, $p < 0.001$; IgG, $p < 0.05$; and IgM, $p < 0.05$.

Immunoglobulins and long term prognosis

The highest immunoglobulin concentrations seemed to accumulate in Group A and the lowest in Group B (Table 3). The differences in significance between the globulin concentrations tested with the *t*-test were: IgA, $t = 1.84$, $p < 0.10$; IgG, $t = 1.82$, $p < 0.10$; and IgM, $t = 0.58$, $p > 0.10$ ($t = 1.67$, $p < 0.10$, $t = 1.99$, $p < 0.05$).

Table 3 Immunoglobulin concentrations (g/l) by group in accordance with cumulative hospital stays

Group	No. of patients	IgA Mean S.D.	IgG Mean S.D.	IgM Mean S.D.
A (0–1 year)	42	2.86 1.19	15.2 3.45	1.90 0.95
B (1–4 years)	32	2.41 0.81	13.8 2.95	1.78 0.71
Total	74	2.67 1.06	14.6 3.29	1.85 0.85

Normal values: IgA, 0.74–3.06 g/l; IgG, 7.2–15.1 g/l; IgM, 0.23–1.33 g/l

Influence of age, and age at onset

Age and age at onset had a negative correlation to short term ($p < 0.01$; $p < 0.05$) and long term prognosis ($p < 0.05$; $p < 0.01$). Of the immunoglobulins, IgA had a positive correlation to age ($p < 0.01$) and age at onset ($p < 0.05$), and IgG also had a positive correlation ($p < 0.05$) to age.

These two variables were held constant, and partial correlations were calculated in order to eliminate the influence of age and age at onset on the results. The effect of the elimination of these variables is shown in Table 4, with the correlations to short term and long term prognosis.

After the elimination of age and age at onset the correlation of IgA to short term prognosis fell from level $p < 0.001$ to level $p < 0.01$, and that of IgG from level $p < 0.01$ to a non-significant level. For IgM the correlation coefficients increased slightly while, throughout, the statistical significance still remained at level $p < 0.01$ (Table 4).

The elimination of the effect of the two variables related to age resulted in similar changes in the correlation coefficients as described in connection with the short term prognosis. However, none of the correlations reached a statistically significant level (Table 4).

Table 4 Correlations (r) of immunoglobulins and partial correlations (r_1, r_2) after elimination of the effect of age and of age at onset of disease to short-term (a) and long-term (b) prognosis

Variables	r	r_1	r_2
(a)			
IgA	−0.395***	−0.328**	−0.332**
IgG	−0.234*	−0.173	−0.191
IgM	−0.241*	−0.257*	−0.270*
(b)			
IgA	−0.211	−0.144	−0.160
IgG	−0.210	−0.160	−0.220
IgM	−0.068	−0.074	−0.113

r_1 – age eliminated; r_2 – age and age at onset of disease, both eliminated; $p < 0.20$, $r \geqslant 0.150$; $p < 0.10$, $r \geqslant 0.192$; *$p < 0.05$, $r \geqslant 0.228$; **$p < 0.01$, $r \geqslant 0.295$; ***$p < 0.001$, $r \geqslant 0.371$, $n = 74$

Discussion

The present results indicate that high IgA and IgG concentrations at the beginning of treatment predict short hospital stays in long term prognosis, thus supporting the previous report with regard to the prognostic significance of the globulins. The observations did, however, not reach a statistically significant level. This in part may be due to the relatively limited material ($n = 74$) and additionally to the fact that a long term prognosis may be influenced by a large variety of factors which did not emerge clearly enough in the short term prognosis made on the basis of the hospital stay following the key admission. An early age at onset predicted poor prognosis. However, on the basis of the elimination of age and age at onset of disease it was found that these two biological variables only in part explained the connection between prognosis and immunoglobulins, indicating the complex character of this connection.

These and other unclarified questions require further investigation. However, the present results already indicate that the psychopathology and progress of schizophrenia are reflected in serum immunoglobulin concentrations, though they leave open the question of the extent to which the changes verified are specific for schizophrenia.

Acknowledgements

I am grateful for the support given by the Foundation for Psychiatric Research in Finland, to the laboratory staff of the Kellokoski Hospital as well as to the Laboratory of Oy Medix Ab for their kind assistance. My special thanks are due to Docent Elosuo and Professor Rimòn for their comments on my manuscript. I am indebted to Jorma Torppa, for carrying out the statistical analysis. In addition, I am grateful for the help provided by my wife.

References

Achté, K. A. (1967). On prognosis and rehabilitation in schizophrenic and paranoid psychoses. *Acta Psychiatr. Scand.*, **196**, (Suppl.), 26

Amkraut, A., Solomon, G. F., Allansmith, M., McCellan, B. and Rappaport, B. (1973). Immunoglobulins and improvement in acute schizophrenic reactions. *Arch. Gen. Psychiatry*, **28**, 673

Bock, E., Weeke, B. and Rafaelsen, O. J. (1971). Serum proteins in acutely psychotic patients. *J. Psychiat. Res.*, **9**, 1

Burdock, E. I. and Hardesty, A. S. (1968). *Ward Behavior Inventory: Manual.* (New York: Springer)

Cole, J. O., Deykin, E., Klerman, G. L., Boothe, H., Goldberg, S. G. and Scholer, N. (1968). Short-term improvement in schizophrenia: The contribution of background factors. *Am. J. Psychiatry*, **124**, 900

Fessel, W. J. (1962). Blood proteins in functional psychoses. *Arch. Gen. Psychiatry*, **6**, 132

Gittelman-Klein, R. and Klein, D. F. (1969). Premorbid asocial adjustment and prognosis in schizophrenia. *J. Psychiatr. Res.*, **7**, 35

Goldberg, S. C., Cole, J. O. and Clyde, D. J. (1963). Factor analyses of ratings of schizophrenic behavior. *Psychopharmacol. Serv. Cent. Bull.*, **2**, 23

Heath, R. G. and Krupp, I. M. (1967). Schizophrenia as an immunologic disorder. *Arch. Gen. Psychiatry*, **16**, 24

Mancini, G., Carbonara, A. O. and Heremans, J. F. (1965). Immunochemical quantitation of antigens by single radial immunodiffusion. *Immunochemistry*, **2**, 235

Poirier, J. L. and Richer, C. L. (1963). Adrenocortical and autonomic reactivity in schizophrenia. *Arch. Gen. Psychiatry*, **8**, 605

Pulkkinen, E. (1977). Immunoglobulins, psychopathology and prognosis in schizophrenia. *Acta Psychiatr. Scand.*, **56**, 173

Shean, G., Faia, C. and Schmaltz, E. (1974). Cognitive appraisal of stress and schizophrenic subtype. *J. Abnorm. Psychol.*, **83**, 523

Silverman, J. (1964). The scanning control mechanism and cognitive filtering in paranoid and non-paranoid schizophrenia. *J. Consult. Psychol.*, **28**, 385

Solomon, G. F., Allansmith, M., McCellan, B. and Amkraut. A. (1969). Immunoglobulins in psychiatric patients. *Arch. Gen. Psychiatry*, **20**, 272

Solomon, G. F., Amkraut, A. and Kasper, P. (1974). Immunity, emotions and stress with special reference to the mechanism of stress effects on the immune system. A lecture at the Psychiatric Department of the Helsinki University, June 26, 1973. *Psychiatrica Fennica*, 289

Solomon, G. F. and Moos, R. H. (1964). Emotions, immunity and disease: A speculative theoretical integration. *Arch. Gen. Psychiatry*, **11**, 657

Solomon, G. F., Moos, R. H., Fessel, W. J. and Morgan, E. E. (1966). Globulins and behavior in schizophrenia. *Int. J. Neuropsychiatry*, **2**, 20

Strahilevitz, M. and Davis, S. D. (1970). Increased IgA in schizophrenic patients. *Lancet*, **2**, 370

Überla, K. (1968). *Faktoranalyse.* (Berlin: Springer)

Venables, P. H. (1966). Psychophysiological aspects of schizophrenia. *Br. J. Med. Psychol.*, **39**, 289

Venables, P. H. and O'Connor, N. (1959). A short scale for rating paranoid schizophrenia. *J. Ment. Sci.*, **105**, 815

Venables, P. H. and Wing, J. K. (1962). Level of arousal and the subclassification of schizophrenia. *Arch. Gen. Psychiatry*, **7**, 114

Wing, J. K. (1960). The measurement of behaviour in chronic schizophrenia. *Acta Psychiatr. Neurol. Scand.*, **35**, 245

9

Antibodies to wheat proteins in schizophrenia: relationship or coincidence?

W. TH. J. M. HEKKENS, A. J. M. SCHIPPERIJN
and D. L. J. FREED

Preliminary results were presented (Hekkens, 1978) about the level of antibodies to gliadin in sera of patients with schizophrenia. The idea behind the measuring of gliadin antibodies was that if gliadin or its break-down products can affect the brain in schizophrenia (Dohan et al., 1969), then those peptides have to pass more or less intact through the intestinal wall. We knew already that mucosal damage such as occurs in coeliac disease, gives rise to an increased level of antibodies against gliadin in the serum of these patients. If schizophrenia and coeliac disease are associated, and both are a consequence of the passage of gliadin or its break-down products through the intestinal wall, one could expect that in schizophrenic patients on a diet including wheat the gliadin antibody level would be increased also. Our preliminary results indicated that this was true for only a few of the schizophrenic patients studied. This could mean that there are two groups of patients, one with an increased permeability for gliadin and with a high antigliadin titre, the other with a low permeability and having a low titre. This phenomenon is similar to that described in Chapter 13 by Ashkenazi et al., in the reaction of lymphocytes from psychotic patients. They measured a lymphokine-inducing effect of a gliadin fraction toxic to coeliac patients in only some of the schizophrenic and psychotic individuals. We therefore wanted to investigate a larger group of patients and to compare them with non-schizophrenic patients from the same psychiatric hospital living under the same conditions.

125

We determined the normal range for gliadin antibodies from a group of 29 healthy blood-bank donors and found the upper level of normal to be 52 units. Both the non-schizophrenic and the schizophrenic patients had values higher than the normal level (13% and 17% respectively). The difference between the two groups was not significant. In patients with untreated coeliac disease practically all values were above the upper limit of normal. The results are summerized in Figure 1.

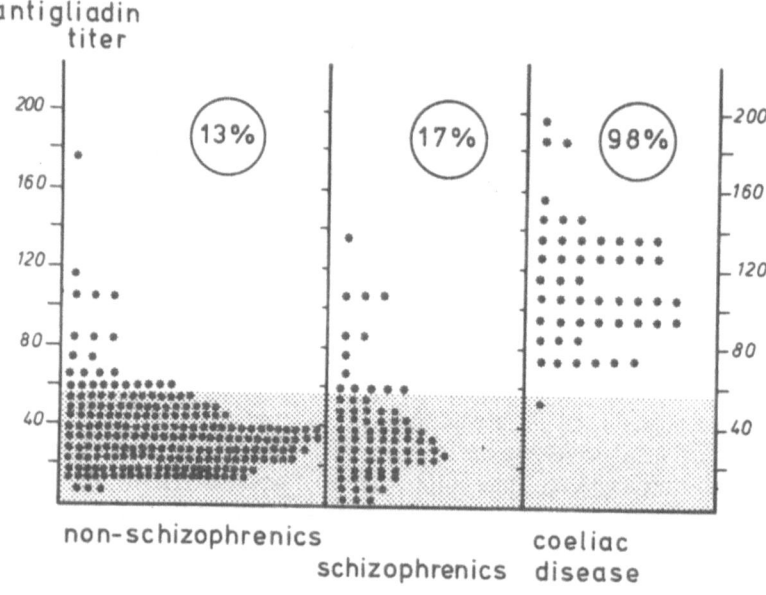

Figure 1 Antibodies against gliadin in normal, non-schizophrenic, schizophrenic and coeliac individuals as determined by the Elisa technique. The normal range is indicated by the stippled area. Cases above normal range given as percentage of each group.

If there are two different groups of patients as Ashkenazi *et al.* suggest, the next question was whether there is any malabsorption indicating intestinal abnormality in the patients with a high gliadin antibody level. Although there was no clinical sign of malabsorption we performed a xylose absorption test in 4 patients (Table 1). If any conclusion can be drawn from these values it is that there is no clearcut demonstrable malabsorption in psychotic patients with a high anti-gliadin titre.

Mascord *et al.* (1978) found an association between mental illness and the number of vegetable foodstuffs against which antibodies were raised. In 20 sera obtained from Manchester (7 normal individuals and 13 schizophrenic patients) the level of antibodies against gliadin and β-lactoglo-

Table 1 Xylose absorption in psychotic patients with an abnormal level of antibodies to gliadin

	Xylose absorption in % of intake (25 g)	Antigliadin level
Schizophrenic		
Patient 1	16	87
Patient 2	18	102
Non-schizophrenic		
Patient 3	11	85
Patient 4	17	106
Normal level	>17	<50

bulin were measured by the Dutch workers. The figures obtained by the Manchester group are related to the *permeability* of the intestinal wall for different proteins; the values found by the Leyden group can be related to the *quantity* of a certain protein that passes the intestinal wall. As can be seen in Figure 2, there is no difference in the range of values between normals and schizophrenics.

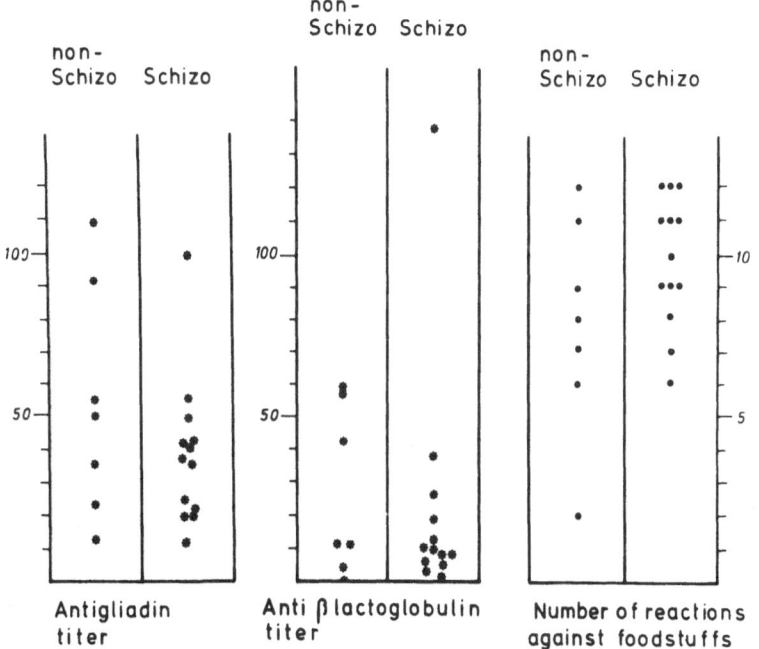

Figure 2 Antibody levels against gliadin and β-lactoglobulin and the number of foodstuffs against which antibodies were raised in normal and schizophrenic individuals

So far it looks as if we are measuring the same phenomenon with different methods. If so, then it was worthwhile to see if the speculation of Freed (see below), that 'normal individuals perceive their foods as varying in their degree of immunogenicity, while those who have the schizophrenic trait are unable to see the difference' also holds true for our method. When we put together the values obtained from Manchester and Leyden (i.e. number of sensitivities *versus* titre of anti-gliadin or anti-β-lactoglobulin) we find a nice correlation for the normal individuals but no correlation for the schizophrenic patients (Figure 3).

From the observations made by the two research groups the following conclusions can be drawn:

(1) With the measurement of antibodies to gliadin no direct correlation between schizophrenia and symptoms of malabsorption as manifest in coeliac disease is found.

(2) In normal individuals there is a correlation between the levels of antibody formation and the number of foodstuffs against which antibodies are found whereas no such correlation is found in schizophrenic patients.

(3) When a normal gut is permeable to dietary antigens it is relatively unselective; breakdown products of milk and wheat are taken up indiscriminately to about the same extent, together with certain other dietary macromolecules. The permeability of the schizophrenic's gut, on the other hand, is more selective, often permitting high titres of antibody against one food but not another. (Alternatively, the selectiveness of the schizophrenic may be a function of his antibody-producing apparatus rather than his gut.)

If the peptide responsible for the primary toxicity in coeliac disease is the same as that causing schizophrenia, it must be small and not readily give rise to antibody formation. In coeliac disease the extra mucosal defect permits also larger breakdown products of gliadin to pass the mucosal layer and give rise to antibody formation. There is no good evidence in our data for a direct relationship between the two diseases.

If the peptide causing mucosal damage in coeliac disease is different from the wheat peptide causing schizophrenia then any relationship between the two diseases is just a coincidence. Although this is not very likely the possibility cannot be excluded until the toxic factor in gliadin has been isolated, characterized and tested in coeliac and schizophrenic patients.

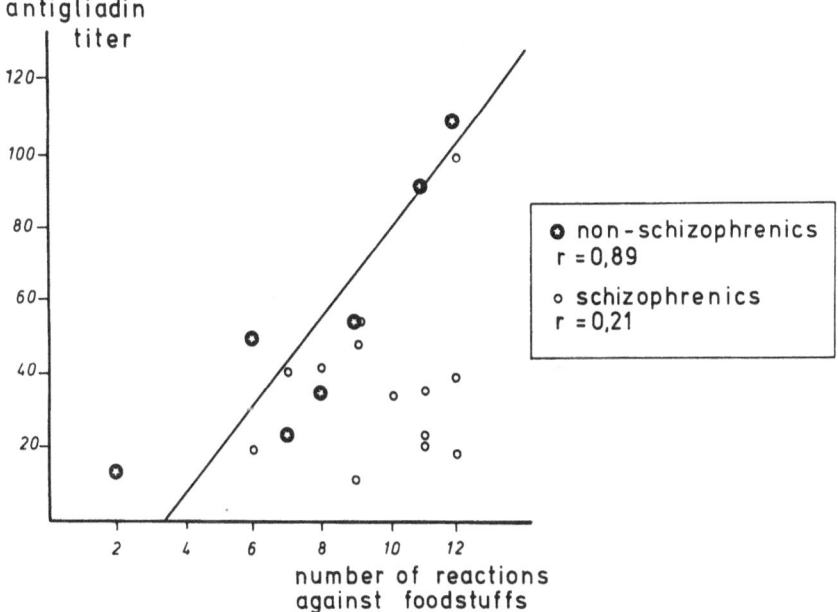

Figure 3A

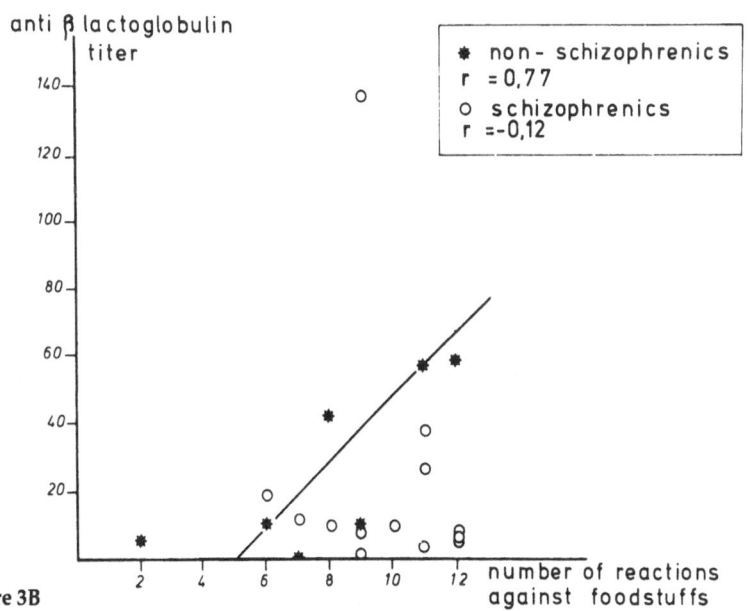

Figure 3B

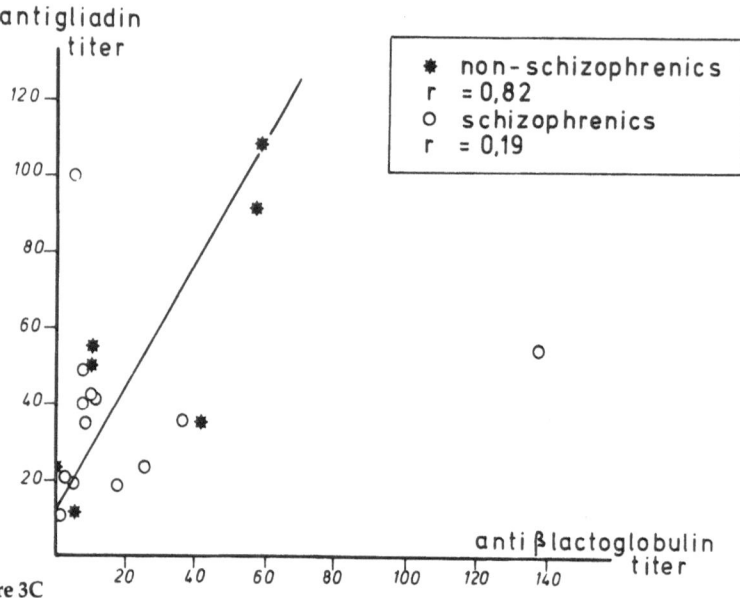

Figure 3C

Figure 3 A, B and C   The correlation between antigliadin level, anti- β-lactoglobulin level and the number of foodstuffs against which antibodies were found in normal (*) and schizophrenic (○) individuals.

Progress Report: March 1979

D. L. J. Freed

Following up an earlier report (Mascord *et al.*, 1978) of an association be-tween schizophrenia and antibodies against vegetable foodstuffs, we have been examining sera of 44 schizophrenic patients residing in Medway Region psychiatric hospitals under the care of Dr B. W. Dur-rant. As controls we have taken sera from 27 normal laboratory personnel who claim to be free of any psychiatric illness (in the 1978 experiment we used as controls unselected hospital patients who may or may not have had concomitant psychiatric illness). We have so far examined all sera for the presence of antibodies to 12 vegetable foodstuffs and 12 animal food-stuffs, using modification of the indirect fluorescent antibody technique (Eterman *et al.*, 1977).

The animal foodstuffs are as follows: beef; ox liver; ox heart; lamb; lamb's liver; lamb's kidney; chicken; chicken liver; pork; bacon; cod; and sardine. Both schizophrenics and normals show reactivity for these sub-strates to some extent varying from 3% positive to 30% positive. For none of these foods is there a significant difference of antibody prevalence between the two groups. Mascord *et al.* (1978) found no difference between schizophrenics and controls with respect to antibody against cow's milk.

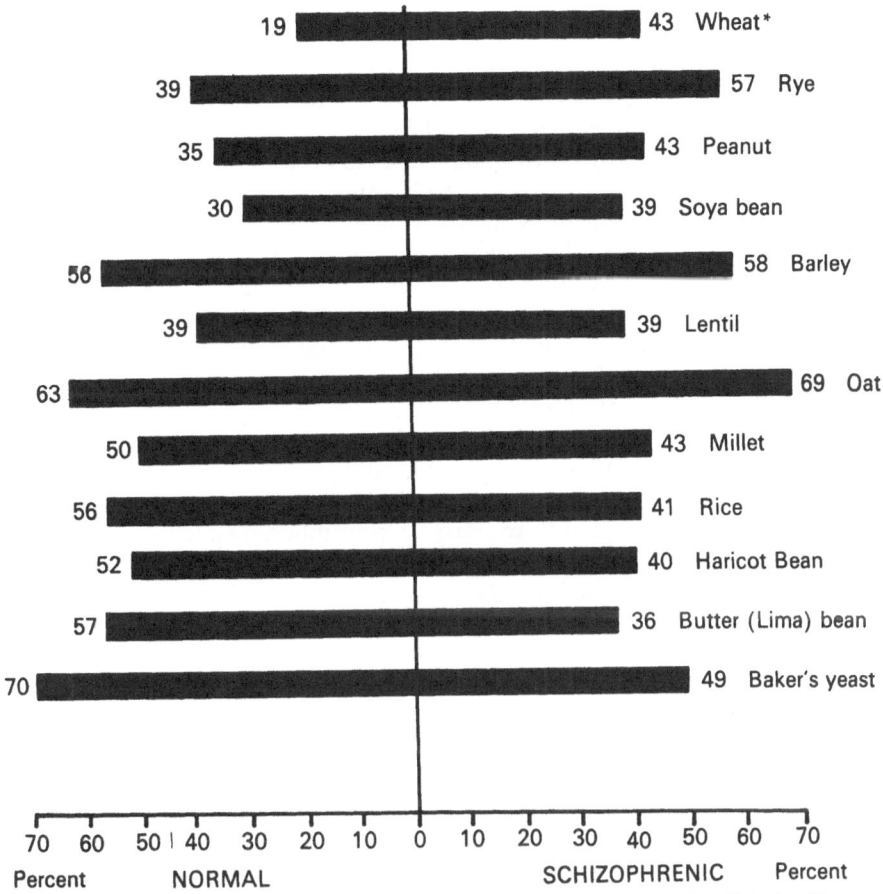

Figure 4 Percentage prevalence of antibodies to 12 vegetable 'seed' foodstuffs in healthy people and hospitalized schizophrenics. The normals show considerable immunological interest in yeast but little in wheat, the other foods lying in between. The schizophrenics, however, are less choosy. *p < 0.05

The vegetable foodstuffs however show a different kind of pattern (see Figure 4). Some evoke antibodies in the majority of normal individuals as well as in some schizophrenics (yeast, oats, barley). The only food that evokes significantly different antibody responses in the two groups is wheat ($\chi = 4.4$; $p < 0.05$); this is not because schizophrenic individuals are more likely than expected to produce the antibody but because normals are *less* likely. Rye shows the same tendency but does not by itself

achieve significance; antibody to wheat and/or rye is however significantly associated with schizophrenia ($\chi^2 = 3.95$; $p < 0.05$). Wheat and rye
are most closely related of all the grass-derived grains, and their gluten is
most damaging to coeliac patients.

In Figure 4 the results have been arranged from top to bottom in
ascending order of normal/schizophrenic ratio. When arranged in this
way a hitherto unsuspected pattern is seen. Among schizophrenics the
distribution of antibodies to the various foodstuffs seems to be fairly uni-
formly distributed between 36% and 69% whereas among the 'normals'
the distribution is skewed from top (19%) to bottom (70%). We may speculate that normal individuals perceive their foods as varying in their
degree of immunogenicity while those who have the schizophrenic trait
are unable to see the difference.

The two studies now done in our laboratory may properly be compared
with each other, as they were different in a number of ways. (i) A different person performed the tests, and since the reading of immunofluorescence is rather subjective it is possible that the two observers had
different criteria in mind for designating a result positive or negative. (ii)
The observer in the first study knew whether the serum he was examining came from the patient group or the control group; his results cannot
therefore be assumed to be unbiased. The second worker was however
issued by a disinterested third party with numbered specimens and did
not know the origin of each serum until her decisions had been written
down. (iii) Although the immunofluorescence method was used by both,
different reagents and different microscopes were used. (iv) The controls
studied were different, as noted above. The first study was therefore less
reliable than the second; however, it would be unlikely that the same
overall conclusion would emerge from both if the interpretation were
spurious.

The first experiment studied six 'seed' foodstuffs: wheat, barley, rice,
soya bean, lentil and haricot bean. The second experiment expanded the
range to include also rye, peanut, oat, millet, butter bean (lima bean) and
baker's yeast. Both observers found a significantly higher prevalence of
antibodies to wheat in the psychiatric group, and both agreed the
absence of any association with antibody to cow's milk. The first observer
also detected a significant excess of anti-lentil antibodies in that group,
and an excess of antibody against haricot bean in the control group ($\chi^2 =$
6.4); neither was confirmed by the second worker (Table 2). It was not
possible to confirm by the second study the tentative conclusion of the
first of an association between mental illness and the *number* of vegetable
foodstuffs against which antibodies were raised.

The two studies do not therefore agree on all points (the disputed foods
being lentil and haricot bean). The difference may be due to methodologi-
cal weakness in the first (or, less likely, the second), or may reflect a genu-

Table 2 Percentage prevalence of antibodies against various foods in psychotic and control groups in two Manchester/Medway studies

	First Study		Second Study	
	Psychotic	Normal	Psychotic	Normal
Wheat	16	2**	43	19*
Lentil	19	2*	39	39 (NS)
Haricot bean	4	23**	40	52 (NS)

* = $p<0.05$ ** = $p<0.025$ NS = not significant

ine discrepancy. If the latter then the difference is presumably between the two control groups, since all of the 'psychiatric' sera came from the same source (Dr B. W. Durrant). This underlines the folly of drawing overenthusiastic conclusions from the work so far reported. Our knowledge of serological reactivity against foods in the population at large is still sparse; furthermore we have no reason to assume that a group of psychiatric patients under the care of one psychiatrist in Medway are representative of psychiatric patients in general. All the same, it is of interest that two separate studies both implicate wheat, thereby supporting the earlier clinical and serological work of Dohan *et al.* (1972).

Acknowledgements

I thank Miss Janet Ditchfield and Ms Phoebe Standart for invaluable technical help, and Sanity and the Schizophrenia Association of Great Britain for funding the present study.

References

Ashkenazi, A. *et al.* (1980). Immunological reaction of psychotic patients to fractions of gluten. Chapter 13, this Volume

Dohan, F. C., Grasberger, J. C., Lowell, F. M., Johnston, H. T. and Arbegast, A. W. (1969). Relapsed schizophrenics: More rapid improvement on a milk and cereal-free diet. *Br. J. Psychiatry*, **115**, 595

Dohan, F. C., Martin, L., Grasberger, J. C., Boehme, D. and Cottrell, J. C. (1972). Antibodies to wheat gliadin in blood of psychiatric patients: possible role of emotional factors. *Biol. Psychiatry*, **5**, 127

Eterman, K. P., Hekkens, W. T. and Pena, A. S. (1977). Wheat grain: a substrate for the demonstration of gluten antibodies in serum of gluten-sensitive patients. *J. Immun. Methods*, **14**, 85

Hekkens, W. Th. J. M. (1978). Antibodies to gliadin in serum of normals, coeliac patients and schizophrenics. In Hemmings, G. and Hemmings, W. A. (eds.) *The Biological Basis of Schizophrenia*, pp. 259–261. (Lancaster: MTP Press)

Mascord, I., Freed, D. and Durrant, B. (1978). Antibodies to foodstuffs in schizophrenia. *Br. Med. J. I*, 1351

10
The effects of hormones
on immune responses

J. A. McINTYRE and W. PAGE FAULK

Attempts to assign biological effects of hormones on immune functions of complex organisms are difficult, because hormones are known to induce numerous changes, many of which are interrelated and simultaneously operational. Furthermore, the effects produced by many hormones are not uniform in all the mammals. Moreover, the immune response involves an intricate balance of many cellular interactions, and our knowledge of the immune system has grown tremendously. Consequently, before reviewing the effects of hormones on such a biologically complicated system, a brief review of the current understanding of normal immune functions will be presented.

Scientists commonly use animal models to provide experimental data about biological systems since information relating directly to human biology is obtainable only by studying normal individuals or, in rare instances, experiments of Nature such as congenital defects. Much of our knowledge of the immune system has come from rodent studies which have been extrapolated to man. In this respect, the mouse has proved to be a good model for studying immune mechanisms in man, because many immunological parameters described for mice have been identified in man. Surprisingly, however, experiments designed to study the effect of hormones (primarily glucocorticoids) on the immune response have uncovered major differences between mouse and man. Indeed, the mouse is classified as steroid sensitive while man is relatively steroid resistant (Table 1). Because of this discrepancy, extrapolation of these experimental data from mouse to man has not been as scientifically beneficial as one would hope. There are, nonetheless, analogies among these studies many of which are substantiated by the observed changes in human

Table 1 Glucocorticosteroid sensitivity in mammals

Sensitive	Resistant
Mouse	Man
Rat	Monkey
Rabbit	Guinea-pig
Hamster	Ferret
	Dog

transplant recipients, who often receive superpharmacological doses of steroids to combat immunological rejection reactions.

Immune responses can be divided into two categories: cellular and humoral (Bellanti, 1978). Cell mediated immunity (CMI) involves immune responses produced by intact cells whereas humoral immunity is hallmarked by the production of antibodies. During the generation of both cellular and humoral immune responses, cooperation and/or communication among cells of many different types must occur before the responses can be completed. As shown in Figure 1, lymphocytes responsible for the two types of immunity are derived from stem cells (Greaves *et al.*, 1973) and they are acted upon by different tissues during development and maturation. Cells which have the potential to produce antibodies are called B cells or bone-marrow derived lymphocytes, because during their development they have been affected by bone-marrow. Alternatively, cells involved in cellular immunity are designated T cells or thymus derived lymphocytes because they are affected by specialized thymus epithelial cells. Frequently, the T and B lymphocytes interact with one another and at times both are dependent upon interaction with another cell, the macrophage, to mount an immune response. An example of these interactions is seen in Figure 2. This intercellular cooperation has been intensely investigated, but the precise nature of the interaction is not yet clear. The diversity of each lymphocyte population has also been the subject of many investigations (Nabholz and Miggiano, 1977). T lymphocytes represent many functionally distinct cells. For example, suppressor T cells are capable of impeding both humoral and cellular immune responses. Others, designated as helper T cells, are required for the successful generation of humoral immune responses to a group of antigens known as thymus dependent antigens. In many instances, T cell subpopulations must interact with each other to mount cellular immune responses.

For purposes of description, the immune response is said to occur in three phases. The first or afferent phase involves the recognition and

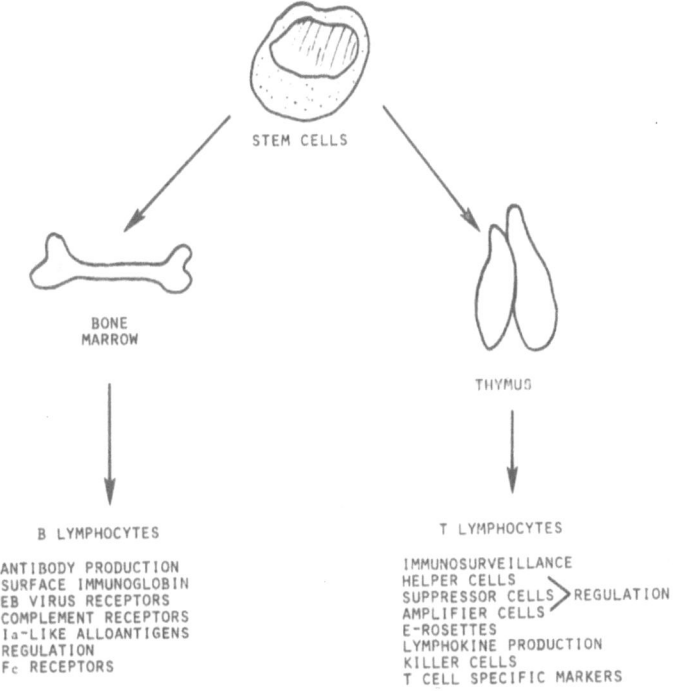

STEM CELLS

BONE
MARROW

THYMUS

B LYMPHOCYTES

ANTIBODY PRODUCTION
SURFACE IMMUNOGLOBIN
EB VIRUS RECEPTORS
COMPLEMENT RECEPTORS
Ia-LIKE ALLOANTIGENS
REGULATION
Fc RECEPTORS

T LYMPHOCYTES

IMMUNOSURVEILLANCE
HELPER CELLS
SUPPRESSOR CELLS REGULATION
AMPLIFIER CELLS
E-ROSETTES
LYMPHOKINE PRODUCTION
KILLER CELLS
T CELL SPECIFIC MARKERS

Figure 1 Lymphoid stem cells migrate either through the thymus or bone marrow to become immunocompetent T and B lymphocytes respectively. Mature cells have several different morphological and functional characteristics

presentation of antigen to the lymphocyte; the second or central phase entails the cellular interactions which lead to proliferation; and the third or efferent phase is represented by the production of antibody molecules or killer T cells. Fortunately, immune responses can be observed *in vitro* using culture systems, thus much of the data pertaining to hormonal effects of immunity have been produced by observing the *in vitro* correlates of *in vivo* immune responses.

Table 2 lists several hormones studied for their effects on the immune system. The percentages represent the frequency that each hormone reviewed for this report appeared in the literature. The most prevalent experimental work has centred around glucocorticoids with thymosin and the sex-related hormones accounting for most of the other studies.

Steroid hormones rarely if ever stimulate antibody production (van Arsdel, 1974) because they are of low molecular weight and are rapidly metabolized. To raise antisera to them for use in radioimmunoassay,

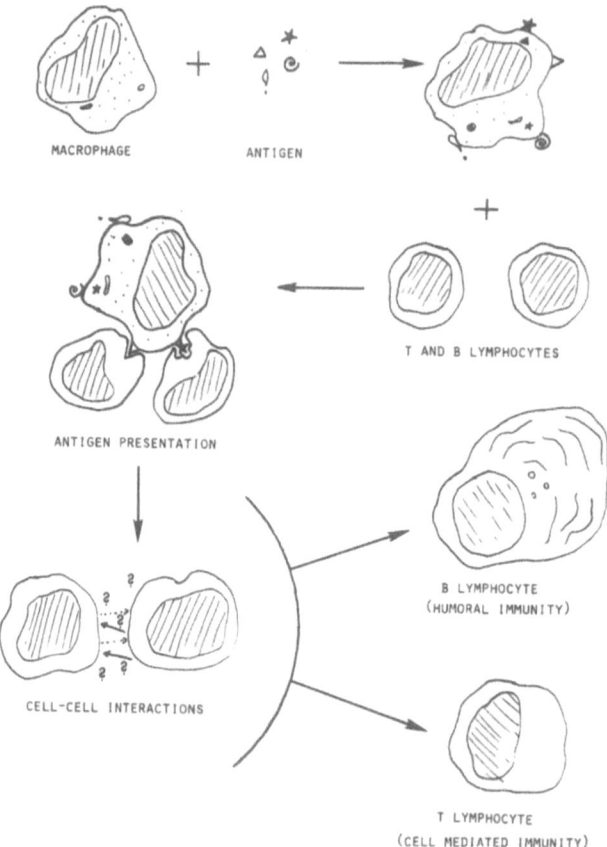

Figure 2 Hypothetical illustration of immune response involving macrophages, T and B lymphocytes. Antigen is 'processed' by macrophages and presented to immunocompetent T and B lymphocytes, which after interacting differentiate, divide and proliferate to produce both humoral and cellular immune responses

these hormones must either be chemically modified or coupled to a protein carrier such as human albumin (Cook *et al.*, 1973). Polypeptide hormones, in contrast, are somewhat different in that they can incite antibody responses; for example, anti-insulin antibodies are present in most persons given insulin (Faulk *et al.*, 1971). Little information is available, however, regarding hormones and their effects on immune responses.

It is reasonable to assume that any endocrine system which influences cell growth will exert its effect on cellular differentiation, proliferation and protein synthesis required for both CMI and humoral immunity.

Table 2 Effect of hormones on the immune response

Glucocorticoids (58%)*	Somatotropins (6%)
Dexamethasone	
Corticosterone	
Hydrocortisone	Gonadotrophins (9%)
Prednisone	
Methylprednisolone	
Thymosin (10%)	Androgens (5%)
Parathyroid hormones (1%)	Oestrogens (9%)

* Relative percentage of experimental data available from literature search

Much of the animal data generated from these studies cannot be extrapolated to other species since many hormonal effects are dependent on the choice of the experimental animal (Claman, 1972). There are however, some similar hormonal effects observed between mouse and man, especially when human cells are exposed to superpharmacological doses of corticosteroids, although it is not clear whether the mechanisms responsible for these effects are the same as would operate if more physiological dosages were used. The fact that receptors for steroids are found in most mammalian tissues is circumstantial but nevertheless good evidence that glucocorticoids probably play an important role as normal physiological regulators (Ballard *et al.*, 1974). However, fundamental knowledge regarding the intracellular biochemistry of the effect of hormones on immunocompetent cells has lagged behind the accumulation of clinical and laboratory observations.

GLUCOCORTICOIDS

Many investigations (Dietrich and Dukor, 1968; Dukor and Dietrich, 1970b; Gisler, 1974; Greenberg and Dimitrov, 1976) have shown that corticosteroids affect phagocytosis when administered during the early or afferent stages of the immune response, thereby interfering with antigen processing and the subsequent induction of immune responses. The mechanism to account for macrophage sensitivity to steroids is speculative; however, there is some evidence to suggest that it may involve a stabilization of lysosomal membranes (Thomas, 1964; Weissman and Thomas, 1964; Greenberg and Dimitrov, 1976), thus preventing the release of enzymes contained in cytoplasmic granules. Support for the membrane stabilization theory may be drawn from studies by Dingle (1963) showing that vitamin A reverses the steroid-induced stability of lysosomal membranes. When vitamin A was given concurrently with cortisone (Cohen and Cohen, 1973) the effect of each was neutralized. It is not known whether these two substances are anticomplimentary or their opposite effects on the immune responses are via entirely different pathways.

Corticosteroids also exhibit varied effects on both cellular and humoral immune responses, which are related to the dosage and/or time of administration. Mice given methylprednisolone (MPS) two days before an antigenic challenge with allogeneic tumour cells showed an increase in the number of cytotoxic T cells (Gerber et al., 1978). This proliferation may be a consequence of steroid destruction of suppressor T cells, thus enabling more killer T cells to be generated.

To achieve maximal stimulatory effects on humoral immunity in vitro it was determined that hydrocortisone (HC) must be added in low doses soon after culture initiation and before exposure to antigen (Sugimoto et al., 1972). High concentrations of HC were inhibitory (Petranyi et al., 1971; Sugimoto et al., 1972; Olson and Schiller, 1978) and were most effective when added before antigen. The effect was not reproducible with either progesterone or deoxycorticosterone (Sugimoto et al., 1972), suggesting that the suppression was due to glucocorticoid activity and not to non-specific steroid toxicity. A decrease in antibody forming cells (AFC) was also noted in vivo when corticosteroids were administered locally to rabbit corneas which had been injected with bovine γ-globulin (BGG) (Hall et al., 1975). Other in vivo studies showed that production of IgG was more sensitive to HC suppression than was synthesis of IgM (Petranyi et al., 1971).

Lymphocytes from steroid-sensitive animals can be divided into subpopulations according to their differential susceptibility. In mice corticosteroids destroy short-lived follicular lymphocytes (Dukor and Dietrich, 1970a), the bone marrow precursors of antibody-forming cells, and lymphocytes located in the thymic cortex (Cohen and Claman, 1971) as well as cortical lymphocytes in other lymphoid organs (Miller and Cole, 1967). Medullary thymocytes and long-lived circulating T cells are much less susceptible to the cytoxic effects of corticosteroid administration. The steroid sensitivity of mouse thymus cells is due to the presence of a hydrocortisone receptor on the lymphocyte membrane. This is present during immaturity but is lost before the lymphocyte migrates into the thymic medulla where it is considered to be an immunocompetent cell. Studies by Cohen and Claman (1971) have shown that HC treatment of mice kills 95% of the thymocytes; however, the remaining 5% in the thymic medulla can still provide 100% of the thymic dependent immune reactivity. These investigators also found that B cells located in the spleen were HC sensitive.

Markham et al. (1978) have shown that corticosteroid immunosuppressive activities are specific for certain T cell subpopulations. Antibody responses to a thymic independent antigen, type III pneumococcal poly-saccharides (SSS) coupled to a thymic dependent antigen, horse ery-throcytes (HRBC) were shown to require interaction between B lym-phocytes and T helper cells. When high doses of HC were given a few hours before priming injections of the thymic-dependent carrier HRBC, the T helper cell activity was abolished. However, the B cell anti-body response to the thymic independent type III-SSS antigen was not; thus, these investigators concluded that HC had no effect on amplifier or suppressor T cells, but rather interfered with either T helper cells or accessory cells such as the macrophage.

Experiments in rats and mice have shown that injection of antigen alone causes significantly measurable increases in blood corticosterone and thyroxin levels (Besedovsky et al., 1975). Thyroxin responses were noted to be biphasic however, in that the initial increase was followed by a significant decrease. In dogs, corticosteroids have little effect on immune responses. In one study (Rosenburg et al., 1975) methylprednis-olone (MPS) was shown to inhibit canine lymphocyte responses to phyto-haemagglutinin (PHA) by 15–50%, but only if MPS was given before addition of PHA. Other dog studies by Sneiderman and Wilson (1975) have shown that corticosteroids inhibit immune haemolysis in vitro, prompting the authors to suggest that steroids may also affect comple-ment metabolism in vivo.

In guinea-pig and man, cortisone treatment results in an initial drop in the circulating peripheral blood lymphocytes (PBL) (Domby and Whit-comb, 1978), and Fauci (1975) has shown that this drop is concomitant with an increased accumulation of PBL in bone marrow. The remaining PBL showed normal responses to most mitogens with the exception of Con A, which was decreased. Bone-marrow lymphocytes, on the con-trary, showed dramatic increases in mitogen responses which were sup-ported by the observation that ^{51}Cr-labelled lymphocytes migrated to bone-marrow after cortisone administration. Attempts to define other actions of HC in guinea-pig by Wahl et al. (1975) have revealed no effect on the ability of macrophages to respond to monocyte chemotactic factor or to the chemotactic fifth component of complement (C5a) in the pres-ence of HC. Likewise, HC does not block interactions between chemo-tactic lymphokines and macrophages, but does inhibit the effects of macrophage inhibition factor (MIF) and macrophage activating factor (MAF) on macrophages.

HC does not interfere with antigen uptake by macrophages as shown by their subsequent ability to activate lymphocytes to produce lymphokines, although it does suppress lymphokine producing cells when present during culture initation. This process is reversible if HC is removed, and the effect is not obtained if the cultures contain serum, presumably because serum proteins such as albumin and transcortin bind and inactivate the steroid.

Although man is steroid resistant, *in vitro* studies with human cells show that if corticosteroid dosages are large enough, most functional capabilities of leukocytes can be suppressed. It is thus important to distinguish between a purely laboratory-related phenomenon versus a truly pharmacological effect produced by corticosteroids when given to patients. It is thought by Boggs *et al.* (1964) that pharmacological concentrations of corticosteroids exert their immunosuppressive effects on lymphoid cells by locally interfering with or altering lymphocyte availability since steroids can also inhibit neutrophil stickiness to inflammatory sites on endothelia (Grant *et al.*, 1962), thus accounting for anti-inflammatory properties. Fauci (1978) has shown that corticosteroids cause neutrophilia both by inducing the premature release of neutrophils from bone marrow and by increasing the half-life of the cell. In addition, certain lymphoid tumour cells have corticosteroid receptors expressed in high density, rendering them susceptible to lysis, and Fauci (1978) has shown that corticosteroid therapy can actually 'shrink' these tumours.

Studies with human cells *in vitro* have shown both dose and time dependent effects of corticosteroids. For example, at 10^{-3} mol/1 HC suppresses antibody responses whereas 10^{-5}-10^{-6} mol/1 enhances them (Fauci *et al.*, 1977), but these effects are dependent on the early addition of steroids to culture. Although corticosteroids cause neutrophilia, absolute counts of monocytes and PBL are depressed, with T cells being more depressed than B cells (Yu *et al.*, 1974). Leukocyte counts return to normal in 24 hours, with lymphocytes recovering more rapidly than monocytes (Yu *et al.*, 1974; Fauci and Dale, 1974). The T cell depression was not thought to be related to an inability to form spontaneous sheep red blood cell rosettes (Fauci and Dale, 1974), as they can do so *in vitro* in the presence of the steroid. Most investigators postulate that the differential decrease in T cells relates to the ability of the steroid to induce changes in surface membranes (Fauci and Dale, 1976), thus causing an aberrant distribution of cells in both the circulatory system and lymphoid compartments (Fauci, 1976; Fan *et al.*, 1978).

Only large corticosteroid dosages can suppress the response of human PBL to the mitogens PHA or pokeweed (PWM) (Fan, *et al.*, 1978), whereas responses to Con A and to antigens such as streptokinase–streptodornase (SKSD) or allogeneic cells are suppressed, even with small steroid doses during the initial 24 hours (Fauci and Dale, 1974; Webel *et al.*, 1974; Cheigh *et al.*, 1975). Reasons for the differential suppression to certain antigens are not known, but this is not due to interference with antigen processing, since addition of macrophages to monocyte-depleted PBL cultures does not restore culture activity (Fauci and Dale, 1974).

Contrary to *in vitro* suppression, Tuchinda *et al.* (1972) have shown augmented responses *in vivo* to the Keyhole limpet haemocyanin (KLH) antigen during prednisone treatment. Also, increased blastogenesis by lymphocytes from renal transplant recipients receiving corticosteroids is thought to represent a non-specific event, unrelated to impending rejection reactions (Pierce *et al.*, 1979). In studies using cortisol concentrations known to exist physiologically in pregnancy, Kasakura (1973) has demonstrated that although pregnant females had lower mixed lymphocyte culture (MLC) responses than non-pregnant women or males, the increased concentration of cortisol associated with pregnancy was not totally responsible for this suppression. Ilfield *et al.* (1977) have demonstrated the autologous MLC reaction to be extremely censitive to corticosteroid suppression, and that this sensitivity is probably indicative of the important role that physiological concentrations of corticosteroids play in modulating T cell autoreactivity. Additional data by Yu *et al.* (1978) have shown that corticosteroid pretreatment of autologous B cells removed their MLC stimulatory potential; however, corticosteroid treated T cells responded normally to untreated autologous B cells.

Recent studies by Rosenburg and Lysz (1978) have shown an inhibitory effect of methylprednisolone (MP) on the generation of human cytotoxic lymphocytes, both by inhibiting MLC generation of cell mediated lymphocytolytic (CML) cells and adversely affecting the ability of killer T cells to lyse ^{51}Cr-labelled target cells after preincubation for three or more hours in the presence of the steroid. Other studies of T cell killing (Fauci, 1975) have proposed that corticosteroids have a protective effect on target cells. Majsky and Abrahamova (1978) have shown a modification of human leukocyte antigens (HLA) on the lymphocytes of patients receiving prednisone treatment.

The effects of corticosteroid on antibody synthesis in humans is variable, but it usually causes a reduction in γ-globulin synthesis (up to 50%) which can continue for as long as 3 months after cessation of treatment (Butler and Rosen, 1973; Baxter and Harris, 1975). Butler (1975) showed that only ongoing antibody synthesis was affected by steroid treatment because antibody responses to KLH were normal despite decreased levels of serum IgG.

The beneficial effects of prednisone suppression of immunity in transplant recipients were shown in a study conducted by Bennett and Barry (1979) who substituted dexamethasone for prednisone in several renal transplant patients. Renal function deteriorated in the dexamethasone treated patients and improved when they were placed back on prednisone. These results were unexpected because dexamethasone competitively blocks prednisone receptors, and it also has a half-life of 4 h versus the 1–2 h half-life calculated for prednisone (Claman, 1972).

New research into the mechanism of corticosteroid action on lymphoid cells has developed slowly. Studies by Munck *et al.* (1972) have examined glucocorticoid-receptor complexes and early events in glucocorticoid activation of rat thymus cells. Although definitive evidence is lacking that similar processes occur in other mammalian cells, there are some data (Baxter and Harris, 1975) to suggest that many of the steps described for rat thymocytes are found in lymphoid cells of other species. According to Munck *et al.* (1972), the earliest detectable event *in vitro* after corticosteroid administration occurs in 15–20 minutes and involves the inhibition of glucose uptake, probably through interference with glucose transport. Cortisol appears to freely penetrate the cell membrane and non-covalently bind to receptors in the cytoplasm of thymus cells. By disrupting the cells in the cold, the presence of these cytoplasmic receptors can be easily demonstrated. Upon warming, the cortisol receptor complex binds to the nucleus. Between the formation of nuclear cortisol receptor complexes and the inhibition of glucose uptake, there are three distinct steps: (1) after 5 minutes, cortisol binding is no longer reversible, and there is an RNA synthesis which is sensitive to actinomycin D; (2) a temperature sensitive step; and (3) a cyclohexamide sensitive step presumably involving protein synthesis. Upon completion of these steps and binding to the nucleus, a newly synthesized protein is thought to appear which is responsible for the inhibition of glucose transport. A similar unmasking of DNA sites by cortisol has been suggested by Ambrose (1970).

THYMIC HORMONES (THYMOSIN)

Unlike the glucocorticoids, the thymic hormone thymosin has a similar biological function in many of the animals studied. Some of the thymic extracts prepared from different mammals have thymosin-like effects on thymectomized animals of other species. Thymosin is purportedly a product of thymic epithelial–reticular cells (Trainin, 1974) which exerts a maturational influence on thymic lymphocytes found in the medullary area of the thymus. Thymosin can provide immunocompetence to neonatally thymectomized adult mouse spleen cells by inducing the production of adenyl cyclase, which in turn raises the intercellular levels of AMP (Kook and Trainin, 1974). Further studies by Trainin (1974) demonstrated that neonatally thymectomized female mice immunologically recovered when they became pregnant, a finding attributed to the production of thymosin by the fetus. Umiel and Trainin (1975) suggest that the target cells for thymosin are the steroid sensitive cortical thymocytes, since corticosteroid resistant cells neither demonstrated enhanced reactivity in the presence of thymosin nor were MLC reactivities enhanced among pooled thymic cells.

Umiel and Trainin (1975) also showed that thymosin exposure was responsible for thymus cells acquiring many T cell characteristics. In studies with immunodepressed hosts, Collins and Morrison (1976) reported that repeated doses of thymosin were able to restore significant levels of delayed type sensitivity (a T cell dependent function) reactions. More recent data from Weksler *et al.* (1978) have prompted these investigators to suggest that a decline in thymic hormone with age may contribute to age associated immune deficiencies, since they could ameliorate these immunodeficiencies by providing their experimental animals with thymosin.

Touraine *et al.* (1975) observed that human bone-marrow cells exposed *in vitro* to extracts of human or calf thymus exhibited the following T cell differentiation patterns: (1) the appearance of antigenic markers; (2) the capacity to form E-rosettes; and (3) the ability to respond to both mitogenic and allogeneic stimuli. Unfortunately, in patients with Swiss type combined immunodeficiency disease (SCID) thymus extract had no effect in producing T cell characteristics, thus providing evidence that the aetiology of this disease is more complex than merely representing a T cell maturation deficiency. The positive influence of thymosin on cell mediated immunological phenomena has been supported by studies with antithymosin serum (White and Goldstein, 1972; Hardy *et al.*, 1968). Contrary to the acceleration of graft rejection in normal mice treated with thymosin, treatment with anti-thymosin serum delayed significantly both first and second set allograft rejection reactions.

GROWTH HORMONE (SOMATOTROPIN)

Growth hormone activity appears to be very closely associated with thymosin activity in that it has been found to specifically bind to thymocytes, whereupon it produces alterations in their mitotic activity and changes in their RNA and protein synthetic profile (Arrenbrecht, 1974; Maor, et al., 1974). In addition, somatotropin (STH) when administered to hypophysectomized rats restored the immune response of the rats to sheep erythrocytes (SRBC) through a mechanism postulated to involve STH stimulation of thymosin production (Pandian and Talwar, 1971; Gisler and Schenkel-Hullinger, 1971). In support of these observations were experiments showing that antibodies to STH when given to rats caused a degeneration of the lymphoid organs which paralleled a decreased ability to synthesize antibody.

SEX-RELATED HORMONES

Early studies of immune responses revealed that females of all species respond to smaller doses of antigen (Kenny and Gray, 1971) and sustain higher antibody titres longer (Batchelor and Chapman, 1965; Cohen and Hamilton, 1976); however, *in vitro* analysis by Kenny and Gray (1971) of individual antibody forming cells (AFC) found no difference between the sexes in the amount of antibody produced per cell.

Oestrogens, like corticosteroids, have biphasic effects on immune responses which are dependent upon the time of their administration relative to antigen exposure. Studies by Thompson *et al.* (1967) showed that oestrogenic hormones impaired the development of stem cells, particularly those with lymphatic potential. Waltman *et al.*, (1971) have shown that oestrogen therapy can also prolong corneal homograft rejection reactions, but in so doing the immune system is depressed, hence the patient is subjected to the opportunistic growth of tumours (Albin *et al.*, 1976). Small doses of oestradiol in mice, according to Kenny *et al.* (1976), when given between 1 and 3.5 days prior to antigen administration, produced a physiological increase in serum oestrogen concentration which remained slightly elevated for many days. While oestrogen levels are raised the number of AFC also increase, an effect independent of phagocytic function and postulated to result from cell division rather than cell differentiation. This view is held because of the observed increased number of mitotic figures in the presence of low hormone concentration. High doses of oestrogens inhibit AFC and even kill thymic cells, thus Feigen *et al.* (1978b) propose that oestradiol directly affects T cell regulatory functions through its ability to suppress DNA synthesis during the early phases of the immune response, i.e. when T helper cell activity is needed. The unique ability of oestradiol to prolong high antibody titres after immune induction is thought to be due to the fact that the B cells, already involved in antibody synthesis, are firmly established; thus the DNA inhibitory properties of oestradiol can affect only suppressor T cells, and by eliminating them a higher rate of antibody synthesis can occur (Feigen *et al.*, 1978a).

That the male hormones (androgens) can cause a decrease in immunological activity was shown in several experiments by Castro (1974a, 1974b) when he observed that orchidectomy in mice produced thymic hypertrophy and accelerated immune rejection reactions. However, these particular effects were applicable only to T cell dependent responses since thymic independent responses (e.g. antibody production to pneumococcal polysaccharide) were unaffected by castration. More recent studies by Fujii *et al.* (1975) showed that low doses of exogenous testosterone injected into mice were biologically inactive, although large doses resulted in a severe depletion of lymphocytes in the thymic independent areas of secondary lymphoid tissues, thus suggesting that testosterone inhibits stem cell proliferation of B cell lines.

PREGNANCY HORMONES

Studies of pregnancy hormones have been difficult and confusing to interpret since it is now known that many of the hormones used were probably not homogeneous. For example, human chorionic gonadotropin (HCG) has been extensively analysed and found to produce very little immunosuppression when used in its chemically pure form (Muchmore and Blaese, 1977). Studies which have previously demonstrated immunosuppressive properties related to HCG, when repeated were able to show that the HCG-suppressive properties were associated with a contaminate (Maes and Chaverie, 1977; Caspary and Hughes, 1977). Consequently, HCG experiments must be interpreted cautiously.

Although cortisol is found in circumstances other than pregnancy, it has been shown to specifically interact with transcortin-like receptors on both syncytiotrophoblast and lymphocytes (Werthamer *et al.*, 1976). Interactions between cortisol and its protein receptor (an α_2-macroglobulin) apparently trigger internalization of complexed cortisol, where an intercellular enzyme cleaves the cortisol–receptor complex leaving a small polypeptide which is reportedly able to inhibit subsequent protein synthesis by the lymphocyte, thus causing a non-specific immunosuppression.

In a series of experiments designed to study the effects of ovine prolactin on PHA-stimulated PBL Karmali *et al.* (1974) demonstrated up to 40% reduction in lymphocyte responses. In this regard, treatment of schizophrenic patients with phenothiazine derivatives is known to elevate prolactin levels (Wiles *et al.*, 1976; Chalmers and Bennie, 1978), but no information is readily available regarding the immune status of these patients.

PARATHYROID HORMONES

In rats, parathyroid hormone (PTH) has been shown to effect immune responses through its ability to modulate extracellular calcium (Swierenga *et al.*, 1976). Calcium is required for DNA synthesis in lectin-induced lymphocyte activation according to Whitfield *et al.* (1976); thus, PTH is necessary for the proliferative phase of immune responses. Parathyroidectomy causes a drop in PTH and a fall of serum calcium levels, and this is thought to be responsible for the decreased antibody synthesis in these animals.

CONCLUSION

In all animals hormones related to emotional stress have been shown to have varying effects on the cells (i.e. T and B lymphocytes and macrophages) participating in immune responses (Kasper, 1974; Gisler, 1974). Moreover, effects upon the complement system have also been described (Kasper, 1974). Certainly a delicate balance exists between hormone interactions. Perhaps the immune responses of individuals undergoing stress-related emotional disorders should receive more consideration in view of the many changes described in this report.

Acknowledgements

Supported in part by grants from the World Health Organization, the Kroc Foundation, Juvenile Diabetes Foundation, Medical Research Council and the East Grinstead Research Trust. We thank Ms Theresa Caldwell and Ms Roxanne Schattle for their excellent secretarial assistance.

References

Ablin, R. J., Bruns, G. R., Guinan, P. D., Alsheik, H. and Bush, I. M. (1976). Hormonal therapy and alteration of lymphocyte proliferation. *J. Lab. Clin. Med.*, **87**, 227

Ambrose, C. T. (1970). The essential role of corticosteroids in the induction of the immune response *in vitro*. In Wolstenholme, G. E. W. and Knight, J. (eds.). *Ciba Found. Study Group Vol. 36*: 100–125.

Arrenbrecht, S. (1974). Specific binding of growth hormone to thymocytes. *Nature (London)*, **252**, 255

van Arsdel, P. P. (1974). Allergy, immunology and hormones. In Williams, R. H. (ed.) *Textbook of Endocrinology* **11**, 970–976

Ballard, P. L., Baxter, J. D., Higgins, S. J., Rousseau, G. G. and Tomkins, G. M. (1974). General presence of glucocorticoid receptors in mammalian tissues. *Endocrinology*, **94**, 998

Batchelor, J. R. and Chapman, B. A. (1965). The influence of sex upon the antibody response to an incompatible tumor. *Immunology*, **9**, 553

Baxter, J. D. and Harris, A. W. (1975). Mechanism of glucocorticoid action: General features, with reference to steroid-mediated immunosuppression. *Transplant. Proc.*, **7**, 55

Bellanti, J. A. (1978). General Immunology. In Bellanti, J. A. (ed.) *Immunology*, Vol. II, p. 69. (Philadelphia: W. B. Saunders)

Bennett, W. M. and Barry, J. M. (1979). Failure of dexamethasone to provide adequate chronic immunosuppression for renal transplantation. *Transplantation*, **27**, 218

Besedovsky, H., Sorkin, E., Keller, M. and Muller, J. (1975). Changes in blood hormone levels during the immune response. *Proc. Soc. Exp. Biol. Med.*, **150**, 466

Boggs, D. R., Athens, J. W., Cartwright, G. E. and Wintrobe, M. M. (1974). The effect of adrenal glucocorticosteroids upon the cellular composition of inflammatory exudates. *Am. J. Pathol.*, **44**, 763

Butler, W. T. (1975). Corticosteroids and immunoglobulin synthesis. *Transplant. Proc.*, **7**, 49

Butler, W. T. and Rosen, R. D. (1973). Effects of corticosteroids on immunity in man I. Decreased serum IgG concentration caused by 3 or 5 days of high doses of methylprednisolone. *J. Clin. Invest.*, **52**, 2629

Caspary, E. A. and Hughes, D. (11977). Experimental allergic encephalomyelitis in the Guinea Pig: Failure to suppress with crude human chorionic gonadotropin. *Science*, **34**, 53

Castro, J. E. (1974a). The hormonal mechanism of immunopotentiation in mice after orchidectomy. *J. Endocrinol.*, **62**, 311

Castro, J. E. (1974b). Orchidectomy and the immune response II. Response of orchidectomized mice to antigens. *Proc. R. Soc. Lond. B*, **185**, 437

Chalmers, R. H. and Bennie, E. H. (1978). The effect of fluphenazine on basal prolactin concentrations. *Psychol. Med.*, **8**, 483

Cheigh, K. H., Stenzel, R. R., Riggio, R. R., Katz, E. B. and Rubin, A. L. (1975). Effects of intravenous methylpredisolone on mixed lymphocyte cultures in normal humans. *Transplant. Proc.*, **7**, 31

Claman, H. N. (1972). Corticosteroids and lymphoid cells. *N. Engl. J. Med.*, **287**, 388

Cohen, B. E. and Cohen, I. K. (1973). Vitamin A: Adjuvant and steroid antagonist in the immune response. *J. Immunol.*, **111**, 1379

Cohen, D. A. and Hamilton, J. B. (1976). Sensitivity to androgen and the immune response: Immunoglobulin levels in two strains of mice, one with high and one with low target organ responses to androgen. *J. Reticuloendothel. Soc.*, **20**, 1

Cohen, J. J. and Claman, H. N. (1971). Thymus-marrow immunocompetence V. Hydrocortisone resistant cells and processes in the hemolytic antibody response of mice. *J. Exp. Med.*, **133**, 1026

Collins, F. M. and Morrison, N. E. (1976). Restoration of delayed hypersensitivity to sheep erythrocytes by thymosin treatment of T-cell depleted mice. *Infect. Immunol.*, **13**, 564

Cook, I. F., Rowe, P. H. and Dean, P. D. G. (1973). Investigations into the immune response to steroid conjugates using corticoids as a model. I. A specific cortosol antibody. *Steroids Lipids Res.*, **4**, 302

Dingle, J. T. (1963). In De Peuck, A. V. S. and Cameron, M. D. (eds.) *Ciba Foundation Symposium on Lysosomes*, p. 384. (Boston: Little, Brown and Company)

Dietrich, F. M. and Dukor, P. (1968). The immune response to heterologous red cells in mice IV. Induction of unresponsiveness to weakly immunogeneic red cells by cyclophospamide and cortisone acetate. *Clin. Exp. Immunol.*, **3**, 783

Domby, W. R. and Whitcomb, M. E. (1978). The effects of corticosteroid administration on the bronchoalveolar cells obtained from Guinea pigs by lung lavage. *Rev. Respir. Dis.*, **117**, 893

Dukor, P. and Dietrich, F. M. (1970a). The immune response to heterologous red cells in mice IV. Effect of cyclophosphamide and cortisone on antigenic competition. *J. Immunol.*, **105**, 118

Dukor, P. and Dietrich, F. M. (1970b). Prevention of cyclophosphamide-induced tolerance to erythrocytes by pretreatment with cortisone. *Proc. Soc. Exp. Med.*, **133**, 280

Fan, P. T., Yu, D. T. Y., Clements, P. J., Fowlston, S., Euman, J. and Bluestone, R. (1978). Effect of corticosteroids on the human immune response; comparison of 1 and 3 day 1 gm pulses of methylprednisolone. *J. Lab. Clin. Med.*, **91**, 627

Fan, P. T., Yu, D. T. Y., Targoff, C. and Bluestone, R. (1978). Effect of corticosteroids on the immune response: Suppression of mitogen-induced lymphocyte proliferation by 'pulse' methylprednisolone. *Transplantation*, **26**, 266

Fauci, A. S. (1975). Mechanisms of corticosteroid action on lymphocyte subpopulations I. Redistribution of circulating T and B lymphocytes to the bone marrow. *Immunology*, **28**, 669

Fauci, A. S. (1976). Glucocorticosteroid therapy: Mechanisms of action and clinical considerations. *Ann. Intern. Med.*, **84**, 304

Fauci, A. S. (1978). Clinical aspects of immunosuppression: use of cytotoxic agents and corticosteroids. In Ballanti, J. (ed.) *Immunology*, Vol. II, p. 740. (Philadelphia: W. B. Saunders)

Fauci, A. S., and Dale, D. C. (1974). The effect of *In Vitro* hydrocortisone on subpopulations of human lymphocytes. *J. Clin. Invest.*, **53**, 240

Fauci, A. S. and Dale, D. C. (1975). The effect of hydrocortisone on the kinetics of normal human lymphocytes. *Blood*, **46**, 235

Fauci, A. S., Pratt, K. R. and Whalen, G. (1977). Activation of human B lymphocytes IV. Regulatory effects of corticosteroids on the triggering signal in the plaque forming cell response of human peripheral blood B lymphocytes to polyclonal activation. *J. Immunol.*, **119**, 598

Faulk, W. P., Karam, J. H. and Fudenberg, H. H. (1971). Human anti-insulin antibodies. *J. Immunol.*, **106**, 1112

Feigen, G. A., Fraser, R. C. and Peterson, N. S. (1978b). Sex hormones and the immune response II. Perturbation of antibody production of Estradiol 17β^1. *Int. Arch. Allergy Appl. Immunol.*, **57**, 488

Feigen, G. A., Fraser, R. C., Peterson, N. S. and Dandliker, W. B. (1978a). Sex hormones and the immune response I. Host factors in the production of penicillin-specific antibodies in the female guinea-pig. *Int. Arch. Allergy Appl. Immunol.*, **57**, 385

Fujii, H., Nawa, Y., Tsuchiya, H., Matsuno, K., Fukumoto, T., Fukuda, S. and Kotani, M. (1975). Effect of a single administration of testosterone on the immune response and lymphoid tissue in mice. *Cell. Immunol.*, **20**, 315

Gerber, M., Andness, D., Pioch, Y., Radel, M. and Serrou, B. (1978). Effect of cyclophosphamide and methylprednisolone on *in vitro* cellular immune responses to allogeneic tumor cells correlation with *in vitro* rejection. *Transplantation*, **26**, 142

Gisler, R. H. (1974). Stress and the hormonal regulation of immune reactivity in mice. *Psychother. Psychosom.*, **23**, 197

Gisler, R. H. and Schenkel-Hulliger, L. (1971). Hormonal regulation of the immune response II. Influence of pituitary and adrenal activity on immune responsiveness *in vitro*. *Cell. Immunol.*, **2**, 646

Grant, L., Palmer, P. and Sanders, A. G. (1962). The effect of heparin on the sticking of white cells to endothelium in inflammation. *J. Pathol. Bacteriol.*, **83**, 127

Greaves, M. F., Owen, J. T. and Raff, M. C. (1973). *T and B Lymphocytes: Their Origin, Properties and Roles in Immune Responses*. (Amsterdam: Excerpta Medica)

Greenberg, C. S. and Dimitrov, N. V. (1976). The effect of hydrocortisone on the immune response of mice treated with Corynebacterium parvum. *Clin. Immunol. Immunopathol.*, **5**, 264

Hall, J. M., Meyer, R. F., Smolin, G. and Okumoto, M. (1975). Effect of pretreatment with local corticosteroids on antibody-forming cells in the eye and draining lymph nodes. *Canad. J. Opthalmol.*, **10**, 487

Hardy, M. A., Quint, J., Goldstein, A. L., State, D. and White, A. (1968). Effect of thymosin and antithymosin serum on allograft survival in mice. *Proc. Natl. Acad. Sci. USA*, **61**, 875

Ilfield, D. N., Krakauer, R. S. and Blaese, R. M. (1977). Suppression of the human autologous mixed lymphocyte reactions by physiologic concentrations of hydrocortisone. *J. Immunol.*, **119**, 428

Karmali, R. A., Lauder, I. and Horrobin, D. F. (1974). Prolactin and the immune response. *Lancet*, **2**, 106

Kasakura, S. (1973). Is cortisol responsible for inhibition of mixed lymphocyte culture (MLC) reactions by pregnancy plasma? *Nature (London)* **246**, 496

Kasper (1974).

Kenny, J. F. and Grey, J. A. (1971). Sex differences in immunologic response: Studies of antibody production by individual spleen cells after stimulus with *Escherichia coli* antigen. *Pediatr. Res.*, **5**, 246

Kenny, J. F., Paugburn, P. C. and Trail, G. (1976). Effect of estradiol on immune competence: *In vivo* and *in vitro* studies. *Infect. Immun.*, **13**, 448

Kook, A. I. and Trainin, N. (1974). Hormone-like activity of a thymus humoral factor on the induction of immune competence in lymphoid cells. *J. Exp. Med.*, **139**, 193

Maes, R. F. and Chaverie, N. (1977). The effect of preparations of human chorionic gonadotropin on lymphocyte stimulation and immune response. *Immunology*, **33**, 351

Maor, D., Englander, T., Eylar, E. and Alexander, P. (1974). Participants of hormone in the early stages of the immune response. *Acta Endocrinol.*, **75**, 205

Markham, R. B., Stashak, P. W., Prescott, B., Amsbaugh, D. F. and Baker, P. J. (1978). Selective sensitivity to hydrocortisone of regulatory functions that determine the magnitude of the antibody response to type III pneumococcal polysaccharide. *J. Immunol.*, **121**, 829

Majsky, A. and Abrahamova, J. (1978). Modification of human leukocyte antigens in patients with malignancies following hormone therapy. *Tissue Antigens*, **11**, 181

Miller, J. J. and Cole, L. J. (1967). Resistance of long-lived lymphocytes and plasma cells in rat lymph nodes to treatment with prednisone, cyclophosphamide, 6-mercaptopurine and actinomycin D. *J. Exp. Med.*, **126**, 109

Muchmore, A. V. and Blaese, R. M. (1977). Immunoregulatory properties of fractions from human pregnancy urine: evidence that human chorionic gonadotropin is not responsible. *J. Immunol.*, **118**, 881

Munck, A., Wira, C., Young, D. A., Mosher, K. M., Hallahan, C. and Bell, P. A. (1972). Glucocorticoid-receptor complexes and the earliest steps in the action of glucocorticoids on thymus cells. *J. Steroid Biochem.*, **3**, 567

Nabholz, M. and Miggiano, V. C. (1977). In Loor, F. and Roelants, G. E. (eds.) *B and T cells in Immune Recognition*. (New York: John Wiley and Sons)

Olson, C. E. and Schiller, E. L. (1978). Strongyloides ratti infections in rats II. Effects of cortisone treatment. *Am. J. Trop. Med. Hyg.*, **27**, 527

Pandian, M. R. and Talwar, G. P. (1971). Effect of growth hormone on the metabolism of thymus and on the immune response against sheep erythrocytes. *J. Exp. Med.*, **134**, 1095

Petranyi, Jr., G., Benczur, M. and Alfoldy, P. (1971). The effect of single large dose hydrocortisone treatment on IgM and IgG antibody production, morphological distribution of antibody producing cells and immunological memory. *Immunology*, **21**, 151

Pierce, G. E., Thomas, J. H., Vessella, R. L., Hermreck, A. S. and Barth, R. F. (1979). Corticosteroids and leukocyte blastogenesis in renal transplantation. *Transplant. Proc.*, **9**, 364

Pierpaoli, W. and Maestroni, G. J. M. (1977). Pharmacological control of the immune response by blockade of the early hormone changes following antigen injection. *Cell. Immunol.*, **31**, 355

Rosenberg, J. C., Colburn, W. A., Brennan, P., Lysz, K., Palutke, M., Stubs, S. S. and Rosenberg, S. A. (1975). *In vitro* effect of methylprednisolone on protein synthesis of activated canine thymus derived lymphocytes. *Transplant. Proc.*, **7**, 547

Rosenberg, J. C. and Lysz, K. (1978). Suppression of human cytotoxic lymphocytes by methylprednisolone. *Transplantation*, **25**, 115

Sneidermann, C. A. and Wilson, J. W. (1975). Effects of corticosteroids on complement and the neutrophilic polymorphonuclear leukocytes. *Transplant. Proc.*, **7**, 41

Solomon, G. F., Amkraut, A. A. and Kasper, P. (1974). Immunity, emotions and stress. *Psychother. Psychosom.*, **23**, 209

Sugimoto, M., Tamura, S., Kurata, T. and Egashira, Y. (1972). Effects of hydrocortisone on the *in vitro* primary immune response of mouse spleen cells to sheep erythrocytes. *Jpn. J. Med. Sci. Biol.*, **25**, 345

Swierenga, S. H. H., MacManus, J. P., Braceland, B. M. and Youdale, T. (1976). Regulation of the primary immune response *in vivo* by parathroid hormone. *J. Immunol.*, **117**, 1608

Thomas, L. (1964). Possible mechanism for the action of cortisone in reactions to tissue injury. In Thomas, L., Uhr, J. and Grant, L. (eds.) *Int. Symp. of Injury, Inflammation & Immunity*, pp. 312–319.

Thompson, J. S., Crawford, M. K., Reilly, R. W. and Severson, C. D. (1967). The effect of estrogenic hormones on immune responses in normal and irradiated mice. *J. Immunol.*, **98**, 331

Touraine, J. L., Touraine, F., Incefy, G. S. and Good, R. A. (1975). Effect of thymic factors on the differentiation of human marrow cells into T-lymphocytes *in vitro* in normals and patients with immunodeficiencies. *Ann. N.Y. Acad. Sci.*, **249**, 335

Trainin, N. (1974). Thymic hormones and the immune response. *Physiol. Rev.*, **54**, 272

Tuchinda, M., Newcomb, R. W. and Devald, B. L. (1972). Effect of predinisolone treatment on the human immune response to keyhole limpet hemocyanin. *Int. Arch Allergy Appl. Immunol.*, **42**, 533

Umiel, T. and Trainin, N. (1975). Increased reactivity of responding cells in mixed leukocyte culture (MLC) reaction by a thymic humoral factor. *Eur. J. Immunol.*, **5**, 85

Wahl, S. M., Altman, L. C. and Rosenstreich, D. L. (1975). Inhibition of *in vitro* lymphokine synthesis by glucocorticosteroids. *J. Immunol.*, **115**, 476

Waltman, S. R., Burde, R. M. and Berrios, J. (1971). Prevention of corneal homograft rejection by estrogens. *Transplantation*, **11**, 196

Webel, M. L., Ritts, R. E., Taswell, H. F., Donadio, J. V. and Woods, J. E. (1974). Cellular immunity after intravenous administration of methylprednisolone. *J. Lab. Clin. Med.*, **83**, 383

Weissman, G. and Thomas, L. (1964). The effects of corticosteroids upon connective tissue and lysosomes. *Recent Prog. Horm. Res.*, **20**, 215

Weksler, M. E., Innes, J. B. and Goldstein, G. (1978). Immunological studies of aging IV. The contribution of thymic involution to the immune deficiencies of aging mice and reversal with thymopoietin. *J. Exp. Med.*, **148**, 996

Werthamer, S., Govindarej, S. and Amaral, L. (1976). Placenta, transcortin, and localized immune response. *J. Clin. Invest.*, **57**, 1000

White, A. and Goldstein, A. L. (1972). Hormonal regulation of host immunity. In Borek, F. (ed.) *Immunogenecity*. (Amsterdam: Elsevier–North-Holland Publishing Co.)

Whitfield, J. F., MacManus, J. P., Rixon, R. H., Boynton, A. L., Youdale, T. and Swierenga, S. (1976). The positive control of cell proliferation by the interplay of calcium ions and cyclic nucleotides; A Review. *In Vitro*, **12**, 1

Wiles, D. H., Kolakowska, T., McNeilly, A. S., Mandelbrote, B. M. and Gelder, M. G. (1976). Clinical significance of plasma chlorpromazine levels. I. Plasma levels of the drug, some of its metabolites and prolactin during acute treatment. *Psychol. Med.*, **6**, (3) 407

Yu, D. T. Y., Clements, P. J., Paulus, H. E., Peter, J. B., Levy, J. and Barnett, E. V. (1974). Human lymphocyte subpopulations – Effect of corticosteroids. *J. Clin. Invest.*, **53**, 565

Yu, D. T. Y., Ramer, S. J. and Clements, P. J. (1978). Effect of methylprednisolone on autologous mixed lymphocyte cultures. *Transplantation*, **25**, 163

11
Binding of chlorpromazine and HLA-A1 antibodies to human lymphocyte membranes

M. DONNER and J. N. MEHRISHI

Investigations over the last decade have clearly shown in mouse and in man that the effect of the neuroleptic drug, chlorpromazine (CPZ), is under the control of the major histocompatibility complexes (MHC), H-2 and HLA, respectively (Kalow, 1966; Füller, 1970). An HLA-A1 related favourable response to treatment with CPZ was observed in 33 chronic schizophrenic patients (Smeraldi and Scorza-Smeraldi, 1976). Treatment of HLA-A1 positive lymphocytes with CPZ *in vitro* decreased the ability of these cells to absorb HLA-A1 antibodies, but not other HLA antibodies directed against antigens of cells bearing the corresponding specificities (Smeraldi and Scorza-Smeraldi, 1976). This led the authors to suggest that HLA-A1 antigens were responsible for the binding of CPZ and the favourable response. β-Adrenergic receptors which bind CPZ are present on lymphocyte plasma membrane. They may well be closely linked to HLA gene products which might influence their interaction with CPZ. An alternative explanation offered was that there is perhaps some analogy between the structures of HLA-A1 antigens and the β-adrenergic receptors. Therefore, HLA-A1 antigens might well act as receptors for CPZ (Smeraldi and Scorza-Smeraldi, 1976). Svejgaard and Ryder (1976) suggested that HLA antigens could interfere in non-immunological receptor–ligand interactions.

Since very little is known at present about CPZ–cell interactions, the basic mechanism of the interference of HLA-A1 antigens remains to be elucidated. Furthermore, it would be of interest to obtain quantitative information about the action of CPZ on T and B cell subpopulations involved in the different steps of immune responses.

Major physico-chemical factors which are believed to govern cell interactions, include the cell surface electrical charge. By the use of the analytical cell/particle electrophoresis, we have determined the anodic electrophoretic mobility (EPM) of cells before and after treatment with clinically relevant, non-toxic concentrations of CPZ. By this means, we have monitored the lymphocyte surface membrane, the binding of CPZ and the role of HLA antigens.

For this study, we have investigated lymphocytes bearing HLA-A1 and A2 antigens, since HLA-A1 patients showed a favourable response to treatment with CPZ, whereas HLA-A2 was associated with a poor response (Smeraldi et al., 1976).

MATERIALS AND METHODS

Blood donors and lymphocyte isolation

Venous blood from normal healthy adult donors on the panel of the Blood Transfusion Service, was drawn between 8 and 9 a.m. The time of day when blood is taken from donors may be relevant when the question of the circadian rhythm needs to be considered. Mononuclear cells were isolated by Ficoll–Hypaque centrifugation and washed twice in MEM medium. In some experiments, cells were immediately resuspended in medium used for CPZ treatment. In other experiments, Ficoll–Hypaque processed cells were separated on the basis of nylon wool adherence.

Cell fractionation on nylon wool columns

Nylon wool separation of Ficoll–Hypaque processed cells was performed as described by Julius et al. (1973). After the recovery of non-adherent cells in the effluent, nylon wool columns were rapidly washed with 100 ml MEM (+ 10% fetal calf serum) and adherent cells were recovered by compressing the nylon wool with a syringe plunger as described (Handwerger and Schwarz, 1974).

HLA-A antibodies treatment

Anti HLA-A1 serum was a gift from Professor H. Festenstein, London, and anti HLA-A2 was obtained from Blood Transfusion Center, Nancy. Nylon wool non-adherent or adherent cells (10×10^6 cells in 0.5 ml) were mixed with 0.5 ml anti HLA-A serum. Cells were incubated for 30 min at 37° C, then washed twice in Dulbecco's medium without Ca^{++} and Mg^{++} ions. One aliquot of cells was investigated for surface electrical charge.

The other aliquot was treated with CPZ and the EPM determined.

Chlorpromazine treatment

Chlorpromazine-HCI (CPZ) powder without any additives was obtained from SPECIA 21, rue Jean Goujon, 75360 Paris Cedex 08.

Experiments on human red cells were carried out to establish the optimal conditions of time of incubation and the non-toxic concentrations of CPZ. Cells at a concentration of 10×10^6 cells/ml were incubated for 20 min at room temperature with CPZ (25×10^{-6} mol/1) in Dulbecco's buffer without Ca^{++} and Mg^{++} ions. It is known that Ca^{++} ions interfere with CPZ binding (Leterrier *et al.*, 1977). Our preliminary experiments showed some reversibility in the action of CPZ when the drug was removed by centrifugation. It was decided to determine the EPM of treated cells without further washing.

Viability of cells and suspending medium

The viability of cells was tested by trypan blue. It was usually 90–95%. It should be emphasized that for these experiments the manipulation of cells took up to two hours. To ensure a high degree of viability of cells and minimize cell death, Dulbecco's medium was used.

Analytical cell electrophoresis

The EPM was determined at 25° C by the use of an electrophoresis apparatus (Cam-Apparatus, Impington, Cambridge, UK) equipped with a chamber of a circular cross section, capacity of 0.8 ml, and reversible silver–silver chloride–potasium chloride (1.0 mol/l) electrodes (Mehrishi, 1972).

The EPM was expressed as 10^{-4} cm^2 s^{-1} V^{-1}. The reliable performance of the apparatus was monitored by determining the EPM of human erythrocytes (in 0.145 mol/l NaCI adjusted to pH 7.2 $\pm$ 0.1 with NaHCO$_3$). Under these conditions, human erythrocytes exhibit a reproducible EPM of $-1.08 \pm 0.03 \times 10^{-4}$ cm^2 s^{-1} V^{-1}.

RESULTS

Table 1 presents the electrokinetic data on Ficoll–Hypaque processed cells bearing HLA-A1 antigens (favourable response to CPZ) or HLA-A2 (poor response to CPZ). CPZ treatment of HLA-A1 cells leads to a significant decrease in the mean EPM. In contrast, under similar conditions, HLA-A2 cells exhibited an unexpected increase (8–18%) in the mean EPM.

Table 1 Normal adult human peripheral blood lymphocytes bearing different HLA antigens. Changes in the anodic electrophoretic mobility (EPM ± S.D.) induced by chlorpromazine

Cell donor and HLA-A specificity	Sex and age of caucasian donors	Blood group	Mean EPM (10^{-4} cm^2 s^{-1} V^{-1} ± S.D.) of Ficoll-processed cells		EPM variations in % (p values)†
			Control cells	CPZ treated cells	
M.C., 1, 19	M	54 yrs	O	-1.16 ± 0.02 (64)*	-1.06 ± 0.03 (84)	-8.6% (<0.01)
M.T., 1, 3	F	35 yrs	AB	-1.10 ± 0.01 (57)	-1.00 ± 0.02 (75)	-9.0% (<0.01)
M.A.L., 1, 26	F	33 yrs	B	-1.13 ± 0.02 (86)	-1.02 ± 0.03 (59)	-9.6% (<0.01)
J.M.J., 2, –	M	49 yrs	O	-1.09 ± 0.03 (65)	-1.18 ± 0.02 (73)	+8.3% (< 0.01)
M.A.H., 2, 11	F	30 yrs	O	-1.03 ± 0.03 (62)	-1.22 ± 0.02 (58)	+18.4% (< 0.005)
G.B., 2, 19	M	51 yrs	O	-1.21 ± 0.01 (77)	-1.32 ± 0.01 (57)	+9.1% (<0.01)

* Numbers of cells examined are given between brackets.
† p values of Student's t test.

Table 2 Nylon wool non-adherent lymphocytes isolated from normal adult human peripheral blood: effect of anti HLA-A1 serum and chlorpromazine (CPZ) on the anodic electrophoretic mobility (EPM ± S.D.)

Group no.	1st treatment of cells	2nd treatment of cells	Experiment no. 1	Experiment no. 2	Experiment no. 3
1	—	—	-1.20 ± 0.03	-1.16 ± 0.03	-1.17 ± 0.03
2	—	CPZ	-1.07 ± 0.02 -11%† ($p < 0.01$)	-1.06 ± 0.02 -9% ($p < 0.01$)	-1.05 ± 0.03 -10% ($p < 0.01$)
3	anti HLA-A1* antibodies	—	-1.18 ± 0.02	-1.13 ± 0.02	-1.15 ± 0.03
4	anti HLA-A1 antibodies	CPZ	-1.13 ± 0.03 -4% N.S.‡	-1.11 ± 0.01 -2% N.S.	-1.11 ± 0.01 -4% N.S.

* 10×10^6 cells/0.5 ml were mixed with 0.5 ml antiserum and incubated 30 min at 37° C., then washed twice in Dulbecco's medium. An aliquot of antiserum treated cells was treated with CPZ (25×10^{-6}mol/l) for 20 min at room temperature and EPMs determined † EPM variations in %: p values of Student's t test: ‡ the differences between control and CPZ treated cells are not significant

Table 3 Nylon wool adherent lymphocytes isolated from normal adult human peripheral blood. Effect of anti HLA-A1 serum and chlorpromazine on EPM (± S.D.)

Group no.	1st treatment of cells	2nd treatment of cells	Experiment no.		
			1	2	3
1	–	–	−0.88 ± 0.02	−0.94 ± 0.01	−0.90 ± 0.02
2	–	CPZ	−0.85 ± 0.03 N.S.†	−0.91 ± 0.02 N.S.	−0.88 ± 0.01 N.S.
3	anti HLA-A1* antibodies	–	−0.86 ± 0.03	−0.92 ± 0.03	−0.91 ± 0.03
4	anti HLA-A1 antibodies	CPZ	−0.87 ± 0.02 N.S.	−0.91 ± 0.02 N.S.	−0.89 ± 0.03 N.S.

* As explained in Table 2: † the differences between control and CPZ treated cells are not significant

In other experiments, we investigated both the action of CPZ on T and B cells showing various functional properties and different EPM and a possible genetic influence associated with HLA-A1 specificity. Ficoll–Hypaque processed cells bearing the corresponding antigens were separated on the basis of nylon wool adherence. Nylon wool non-adherent (T cell enriched) and adherent (B cell enriched) cells were treated with anti HLA-A1 serum, then with CPZ and cells were scored for EPM. To determine exactly the influence of HLA-A1 antibodies, several groups of control cells were included within each experiment: (a) untreated cells; (b) cells treated only with CPZ; and (c) cells treated only with anti HLA-A1 serum. The data are presented in Table 2. CPZ (25×10^{-6} mol/l) significantly decreased the EPM of non-adherent cells (T enriched) by about 9%. In contrast, when cells were previously treated with anti HLA-A1 serum, CPZ treatment induced only a small decrease in EPM (about 4%), which is within experimental error. Regarding the adherent cells, various treatments caused no significant variations in the mean EPM (Table 3).

Preliminary experiments on HLA-A2 cells and anti HLA-A2 serum were performed with an identical experimental schedule. Cells previously treated with anti HLA-A2 serum exhibited a mean EPM of $-1.10 \pm 0.02 \times 10^{-4}$ cm^2 s^{-1} V^{-1}. It was noted that this treatment did not affect the changes induced by CPZ on HLA-A2 cells. CPZ treated cells exhibited a mean EPM of $-1.18 \pm 0.03 \times 10^{-4}$ cm^2 s^{-1} V^{-1} (about 7%), nearly similar to that observed with cells not treated with anti HLA-A2 serum.

DISCUSSION

The present electrokinetic data on CPZ treated lymphocytes bearing HLA-A1 and HLA-A2 antigens raise some interesting questions about the markedly different results induced by CPZ treatment. Modification of the cell surface charge might be due to either a mere binding of positively charged CPZ on the cell surface or an alteration in the cell membrane macromolecular components following cell–CPZ interaction.

Using human erythrocytes from a *single* donor as target cells, Tenforde et al. (1978) observed a 9–10% decrease in the EPM after CPZ treatment. These authors reported that the drug effect on surface charge is independent of the transformation of red cells from the discocyte to the stomatocyte form and concluded that the decrease in the EPM merely reflected the contribution of positively charged CPZ to surface charge density. We have also observed a decrease in the EPM of erythrocytes treated with CPZ in agreement with others (data not included) (Mehrishi, 1979 However, a similar assumption clearly cannot explain a decrease and an increase in the EPM of cells treated with CPZ. Obviously, the phenomenon is more complex. It is quite likely that CPZ induces changes in the EPM which are dependent upon the chemical architecture of the cell surface (gene product?) (Crumpton et al., 1978; Donner and Mehrishi, 1978, 1979).

The alternative mechanism involving a possible alteration in cell membrane conformation appears attractive. This conclusion is reinforced by the results obtained in the study of the interaction of phenothiazine derivatives with synaptic membranes (Leterrier et al., 1977). From spin label and fluorescent label studies, it has been concluded that, at moderate concentrations (between 10^{-4} and 10^{-5} mol/l), CPZ induced modifications of the membrane protein arrangement (Leterrier et al., 1977). CPZ has also been reported to inhibit the activation of lymphocytes by Con A and PHA suggesting an interference with some membrane events (Ferguson et al., 1978). Any subtle changes in the chemical architecture of the cell periphery may be monitored as for lymphoid cells stimulated by mitogens (Wioland et al., 1976).

It is relevant to note that CPZ markedly modified T cell enriched subpopulations but not that of nylon wool adherent cells enriched in B lymphocytes (Tables 2 and 3). Several hypotheses may be advanced to explain these results. First, the number of CPZ binding sites may be greater on T cells than on B cells resulting in a marked alteration of T cell periphery after cell-CPZ interaction. It is not possible to rule out this possibility since (i) it has been established that CPZ binds to β-adrenergic receptors on lymphocyte cell surface and (ii) recent data suggested a striking heterogeneity of the β-adrenergic response between T lymphocytes and a B cell enriched lymphocyte population (Galant et al., 1978). An alternative hypothesis is that the alteration of T and B cell surface may be identical after CPZ treatment, but the nature of the modification in EPM is different, dependent upon striking differences in the topography of the ionizable chemical groups contributing the electrokinetic charge of cells.

Regarding the role of HLA antigens, it is somewhat surprising that the modifications in the EPM varied according to the HLA specificity (a decrease in the EPM of A1 cells, but an increase in that of A2 cells). Sheetz and Singer (1974) have proposed that CPZ induces an expansion of the membrane, which is apparently reflected in the alteration of the electrical properties of cells. We suggest that such an alteration is probably different for cells of various HLA types. We have already reported striking differences in the surface topochemistry of splenic T cells and thymocytes of mice of varying MHC haplotypes (Donner and Mehrishi, 1978, 1979). It is very likely that human T cells bearing different HLA antigens also possess striking differences in surface topochemistry. Numerous studies have shown some analogy between the major histocompatibility complex in mouse (H-2) and man (HLA) (Iványi et al., 1976; Silver and

Hood, 1977; Iványi et al., 1978). We are inclined to the view that the unexpected *increase* in the EPM of cells bearing HLA-A2 antigens following the binding of a positively charged molecule is attributable to an alteration of the cell membrane arrangement after CPZ interaction.

Our physico-chemical approach monitoring the electrokinetic properties of lymphocyte membranes at the single level provides direct and clear evidence for the inhibition of CPZ binding by HLA-A1 antibodies (Table 2). This supports the suggestions of Smeraldi and Scorza-Smeraldi (1976); see also Svejgaard and Ryder (1976).

Clinical relevance of the results

Our EPM data show that the decrease in electron charges/cell is about 1×10^6 (Table 2), comparable to that reported for erythrocytes (Tenforde, 1978). It is quite likely that all the CPZ bound to cells may not affect the electrical double layer of cell surface or may not be detectable for a variety of reasons, such as packing or the orientation of CPZ molecules in the cell periphery as shown for other positively charged molecules (Nevo et al., 1955 Mehrishi, 1972).

It is important to ascertain whether the concentrations of CPZ which induced *in vitro* interesting effects are clinically relevant.

Let us assume that a reduction in the negative surface charge density by one elementary electron charge results from the binding of a single positively charged molecule of CPZ, i.e. 5.6 ng CPZ/10^7 T enriched cells. The therapeutic range of CPZ in the plasma of psychiatric patients appears to be 150–300 ng/ml (toxic range 750–1000 ng/ml) (Ferguson et al., 1978). It would therefore seem that there are enough CPZ molecules in the plasma to lead to the changes in the surface properties of lymphocytes as observed in our experiments. It is reasonable to suggest that the concentrations of CPZ which lead to significant alterations in surface topochemistry are clinically relevant.

Studies on lymphocytes from normal individuals are essential to provide a basis for developing monitoring tests of clinical relevance in schizophrenia, manic depressive psychosis and related disorders. Monitoring lymphocytes in peripheral blood of patients would clearly be of great value (Mehrishi, 1979).

The data encourage further detailed investigations.

Acknowledgements

We thank Dr C. Raffoux (Department of Immunology in Blood Transfusion Center, Nancy) for generous help in arranging blood samples, HLA tissue-typing and HLA-A2 antiserum. We thank Professor H. Festenstein for HLA-A1 antiserum. The technical assistance of Mrs S. Droesch and the secretarial help of J. Bara are acknowledged. J. N. Mehrishi is particularly grateful to Professor I. H. Mills for encouragement and providing the facilities for the continuation of the work.

References

Crumpton, M. J., Snary, D., Walsh, F. S., Barnstable, C. J., Goddfellow, P. N., Jones E. A. and Bodmer, W. F. (1978). Molecular structure of the gene products of the human HLA system: isolation and characterization of HLA-A, -B, -C and Ia antigens. *Proc. R. Soc. London. B*, **202**, 159

Donner, M. and Mehrishi, J. N. (1978). The lymphocyte surface. Differences in the surface chemistry of murine spleen T lymphocytes of varying major histocompatibility haplotypes. *Proc. R. Soc. London. B*, **203**, 201

Donner, M. and Mehrishi, J. N. (1979). The lymphocyte surface. Surface topochemistry of murine thymocytes related to the major histocompatibility complex. *Int. Arch. Allergy Appl. Immunol.*, **59**, 173

Ferguson, R. M., Schmidtke, J. R. and Simmons, R. L. (1978). Effects of psychoactive drugs on *in vitro* lymphocyte activation. In Bergsma, D. and Goldstein, A. L. (eds.) *Neurochemical and Immunologic Components in Schizophrenia*, Vol. XIV, p. 379. (Alan R. Liss, Inc.)

Füller, J. L. (1970) Strain differences in the effect of chlorpromazine and chlordiazepoxide upon active and passive avoidance in mice. *Psychopharmacologia*, **16**, 261

Galant, S. P., Underwood, S. B., Lundak, T. C., Groncy, C. C. and Mouratides, D.I. (1978). Heterogeneity of human lymphocyte subpopulations to pharmacologic stimulation. I. Lymphocyte responsiveness to beta adrenergic agents. *J. Allergy Clin. Immunol.*, **62**, 349

Handwerger, B. S. and Schwartz, R. H. (1974). Separation of murine lymphoid cells using nylon wool columns. Recovery of the B cell-enriched population. *Transplantation*, **18**, 544

Iványi, P., Pavljukova, H. and Ivaskova, E. (1976). H-2/HLA cross reactions. Absorption analysis of cytotoxic anti-human activity in anti H-2 mouse sera. *Transplantation*, **22**, 612

Iványi, P., van den Berg-Loonen, E. M. and de Greeve, P. (1978). Individual mice of one inbred strain produce anti H-2 and anti HLA antibodies of different specificities. *Tissue Antigens*, **12**, 32

Julius, M. H., Simpson, E. and Herzenberg, L. A. (1973). A rapid method for the isolation of functional thymus-derived murine lymphocytes. *Eur. J. Immunol.*, **3**, 645

Kalow, W. (1966). Genetic aspects of drug safety. *Appl. Ther.*, **8**, 44

Leterrier, F., Mendyk, A., Breton, J. and Viret, J. (1977). Membranes biologiques et actions pharmacologiques: effet des phénothiazines. *J. Fr. Biophys. Med. Nucl.*, **1**, 61

Mehrishi, J. N. (1972). Molecular aspects of the mammalian cell surface. In Butler, J. A. V. and Noble, D. (eds.) *Progress in Biophysics and Molecular Biology*, (Oxford: Pergamon Press)

Mehrishi, J. N. (1979). Fc receptors of lymphoid cell membranes. In Hemmings, W. A. (ed.) *Transmission of Proteins Across Living Membranes*, p. 83. (Amsterdam: Elsevier North Holland)

Nevo, A., de Vries, A. and Katchalsky, A. (1955). Interaction of basic polyamino acids with the red blood cells. I. Combination of polylysine with single cells. *Biochim. Biophys. Acta*, **17**, 536

Sheetz, M. P. and Singer, S. J. (1974). Biological membranes as bilayer couples. A molecular mechanism of drug–erythrocyte interaction. *Proc. Natl. Acad. Sci. USA*, **71**, 4457

Silver, J. and Hood, L. (1977). Preliminary amino acid sequences of transplantation antigens. Genetic and evolutionary implications. In H. N. Eisen and R. A. Reisfeld (eds.). *Contemporary Topics in Molecular Immunology*, Vol. V, p. 35. (New York: Plenum Press)

Smeraldi, E. and Scorza-Smeraldi, R. (1976). Interference between anti-HLA antibodies and chlorpromaine. *Nature*, **260**, 532

Smeraldi, E., Bellodi, L., Sachetti, E. and Cazullo, C. L. (1976). The HLA system and the clinical response to treatment with CPZ. *Br. J. Psychiatry*, **129**, 486

Svejgaard, A. and Ryder, L. P. (1976). Interaction of HLA molecules with non-immunological ligands as an explanation of HLA and disease associations. *Lancet*, **2**, 547

Tenforde, T. S., Yee, J. P. and Mel, H. C. (1978). Electrophoretic detection of reversible chlorpromazine-HCl binding at the human erythrocyte surface. *Biochim. Biophys. Acta*, **511**, 152

Wioland, M., Sabolovic, D. and Burg, C. (1972). Electrophoretic mobilities of T and B cells. *Nature (London)*, **237**, 274

Wioland, M., Donner, M. and Neauport-Sautes, C. (1976). Modifications of the thymocyte membrane during redistribution of Con A receptors. *Eur. J. Immunol.*, **6**, 273

12
The possible role of prostaglandin E1 deficiency in the immunological abnormalities seen in schizophrenia

D. F. HORROBIN

The evidence that schizophrenia is associated with low levels of prosta-glandin (PG) E1 has been given in detail in Chapter 1. The problem seems to relate to a low PGE1/dopamine ratio and to low levels of 1 series PGs with normal or elevated levels of 2 series PGs. The purpose of this chapter is to demonstrate that a low PGE1 level could be the cause of the immu-nological deficits in schizophrenia. These deficits have been described in other chapters in this book. They can be oversimplified and summarized in the statement that there seems to be evidence, from both *in vitro* studies and clinical observations, of defective T lymphocyte function and excess B lymphocyte function. The T lymphocytes are particularly con-cerned with cellular immunity and resistance to viral infections. The B lymphocytes are concerned with humoral immunity and produce anti-bodies to antigens, usually foreign ones, but also 'self'-antigens in dis-ordered autoimmune states. There are two sub-groups of T lymphocytes, the 'helper' cells which cooperate with B lymphocytes in the production of a strong and specific antibody response to foreign antigens, and the 'suppressor' cells. The suppressor cells control overactive B lymphocytes and prevent them from producing too wide a range of inappropriate anti-body responses to both 'self'-antigens and to commonly encountered antigens in the air, in the food and in contact with the skin. It is currently believed that many hyperallergic individuals have deficient T suppressor cell function with resulting excessive and inappropriate B lymphocyte mediated antibody responses. Evidence presented in other papers strongly suggests that many schizophrenics have immune systems which behave in this sort of hyperallergic manner.

PGE1 AND T LYMPHOCYTES

The evidence that PGE1 is a regulator of T lymphocyte function has recently been reviewed in detail (Horrobin et al., 1979). The thymus which is essential for the development of T lymphocyte function contains substantial amounts of PGE1 (Bergstrom and Samuelsson, 1965; Karim et al., 1967). Zinc (Brummerstedt et al., 1977; Golden et al., 1978), prolactin and the precursor of PGE1, dihomo-gammalinolenic acid (DGLA) (Singh and Owen, 1976) can all stimulate thymus growth. Cortisol and lithium (Perez-Cruet and Dancey, 1977) both of which inhibit PGE1 synthesis (Manku et al., 1979) cause thymus atrophy. The effects of thymic hormone on T lymphocytes can be imitated by PGE1 (Bach and Bach, 1974). PGE1 activates T lymphocyte function in NZB/NZW mice (Zurier et al., 1977a, 1977b). These animals have a disease which is remarkably similar to human systemic lupus erythematosus (SLE), a disease which is frequently accompanied by a schizophrenia-like psychosis. The immunological abnormalities in these animals are characterized by defective T cell and overactive B cell function. The T cells are activated, the overactive B cells are suppressed, and life span is substantially prolonged by PGE1 treatment. There is therefore strong evidence that PGE1 is able to activate T lymphocytes and inhibit B lymphocyte function.

PGE1 DEFICIENCY AND IMMUNOLOGICAL DEFECTS IN SCHIZOPHRENICS

If there is a PGE1 deficit in schizophrenia, then schizophrenics should have reduced numbers of T lymphocytes and increased numbers of B lymphocytes, a prediction which has been precisely fulfilled by Russian workers. They might also be expected to be unable to respond to viral and possibly tubercular infections completely normally. It is possible that the high rates of tuberculosis in schizophrenics in pre-vaccination and chemotherapy days, which were undoubtedly in part due to nutritional problems, may have also been in part due to inherent immunological deficits. The recently reported evidence of viral infection in the cerebrospinal fluid of some schizophrenics is also compatible with a disordered function of T lymphocytes (see Chapter 2, for detailed discussion).

The evidence that *at least some* schizophrenics have overactive B cells and respond badly to a wide variety of normally encountered antigens is now substantial. The *cause* of this hyperallergic state may be a primary deficit of PGE1 formation. A *consequence* of the state will be an exaggeration of the already low ratio of 1 series PGs to 2 series PGs. This is because in immune responses the production of 2 series PGs from arachidonic acid often seems to be substantially increased. If it is the ratio between the 1 and 2 series which matters one would therefore expect the mental state of schizophrenics to deteriorate following exposure to an antigen to which they are susceptible.

Two recent discoveries suggest further mechanisms whereby 'food allergies' may modify immunological status in schizophrenics. Zioudrou *et al.* (1979) have demonstrated that peptides with opiate-like properties (exorphins) are products of partial digestion of a variety of proteins, particularly α-casein of milk and various cereal proteins especially from wheat. These exorphins, if they have properties similar to the opiates, may be able to inhibit PGE1 synthesis (Horrobin *et al.*, Chapter 1). In normal individuals this may not be particularly important but in schizophrenics who already for some reason have a partially depressed PGE1 level, the exorphin may be sufficient to push the schizophrenic 'over the edge' leading to severe psychiatric and immunological abnormalities.

Cholecystokinin (CK) is a peptide hormone released from the gut, particularly in response to a fatty meal. This too has been shown to have opiate-like properties (Schiller *et al.*, 1978). Again in normal people this probably does not matter but in schizophrenics it may be the last straw. This could be a partial explanation of why some schizophrenics respond badly to fatty meals.

THERAPEUTIC CONSEQUENCES

If the concepts proposed in this chapter and Chapter 1 are correct, then restoration of normal PGE1 synthesis should normalize both the psychiatric and immunological status in schizophrenics. If the immunological status becomes normal and the B cell hyperactivity is suppressed, then schizophrenics should cease to develop allergic responses to common food and airborne antigens although this would probably not prevent them reacting badly to exorphin-generating foods. The nightmare of trying to avoid an almost unending list of allergens would thus be by-passed. Proposed methods of elevating PGE1 biosynthesis are outlined in Chapter 1.

References

Bach, M. A. and Bach, J. F. (1974). Effects of prostaglandins and indomethacin on rosette forming lymphocytes: interactions with thymic hormone. In Robinson, H. J. and Vane, J. R. (eds.) *Prostaglandin Synthetase Inhibitors*, pp 24–248. (New York: Raven Press)

Bergstrom, S. and Samuelsson, B. (1965). Prostaglandins. *Annu. Rev. Biochem.*, **34**, 101

Brummerstedt, E., Basse, A., Flagstad, T. and Andresen, E. (1977). Animal model of human disease. Acrodermatitis enteropathica, zinc malabsorption. *Am. J. Pathol.*, **87**, 725

Golden, M. H. N., Golden, B., Harland, P. S. E. G. and Jackson, A. A. (1978). Zinc and immunocompetence in protein-energy malnutrition. *Lancet*, **2**, 1226

Horrobin, D. F., Manku, M. S., Oka, M., Morgan, R. O., Cunnane, S. C., Ally, A. I., Ghayur, T., Schweitzer, M. and Karmali, R. A. (1979). The nutritional regulation of T lymphocyte function. *Med. Hypotheses*, **5**, 969

Karim, S. M. M., Sandler, M. and Williams, E. D. (1967). Distribution of prostaglandins in human tissues. *Br. J. Pharmacol.*, **31**, 340

Manku, M. S., Horrobin, D.F., Karmazyn, M. and Cunnane, S. C. (1979). Prolactin and zinc effects on rat vascular reactivity: possible relationship to dihomo-gammalinolenic acid and to prostaglandin synthesis. *Endocrinology*, **104**, 774

Perez-Cruet, J. and Dancey, J. T. (1977). Thymus gland involution induced by lithium chloride. *Experientia*, **33**, 646

Schiller, P. W., Lipton, A., Horrobin, D. F. and Bodansky, M. (1978). Unsulfated C-terminal 7-peptide of cholecystokinin: a new ligand of the opiate receptor. *Biochem. Biophys. Res. Commun.*, **85**, 1332

Singh, U. and Owen, J. J. T. (1976). Studies on the maturation of thymus stem cells. The effects of catecholamines, hitamine and peptide hormones on the expression of T cell allo-antigens. *Eur. J. Immunol.*, **6**, 59

Tyrrell, D. A. J., Parry, R. P., Crow, T. J., Johnstone, E. and Ferrier, I. N. (1979). Possible virus in schizophrenia and some neurological disorders. *Lancet*, **1**, 839

Zioudrou, C., Streaty, R. A. and Klee, W. A. (1979). Opioid peptides derived from food proteins: the exorphins. *J. Biol. Chem.*, **254**, 2446

Zurier, R. B., Sayadoff, D. M., Torrey, S. B. and Rothfield, N. F. (1977a). Prostaglandin E treatment in NZB/NZW mice. *Arthritis and Rheumatism*, **20**, 723

Zurier, R. B., Damjanov, I., Sayadoff, D. M. and Rothfield, N. F. (1977b). Prostaglandin E1 treatment of NZB/NZW mice. II Prevention of glomerulonephritis. *Arthritis and Rheumatism*, **20**, 1449

13
Immunological reaction of psychotic patients to fractions of gluten

A. ASHKENAZI, D. KRASILOWSKY, S. LEVIN, D. IDAR,
M. KALIAN, A. OR, Y. GINAT and B. HALPERIN

INTRODUCTION

Production of leucocyte migration inhibition factor (LIF) by peripheral blood lymphocytes in response to challenge with gluten fractions was studied in hospitalized schizophrenics and psychotics as compared with normal individuals and children and adolescents with biopsy proven coeliac disease. The schizophrenic and psychotic patients were found to be sub-divided into two groups, one responding in the LIF test like coeliac patients and the other like the normal controls. The psychotic and schizophrenic patients did not show any evidence of malabsorption. It is speculated that in certain psychotic individuals, gluten may be involved in biological processes in the brain.

Coeliac disease due to gluten sensitivity has been associated with dermatitis herpetiformis and other diseases (Scott and Losowsky, 1975). The association of gluten ingestion with schizophrenia was reported by Dohan (1966) as statistical data, and a hypothesis was presented; Dohan (1969) considered the possible association of coeliac disease with schizophrenia and Dohan et al. (1969) reported the good effect of milk- and cereal-free diet on relapsed schizophrenics. There is controversy over the subject, and improvement of the patients' condition was considered by Baker (1973) to be caused by improving the absorption of the phenothiazine drugs given to all patients kept on gluten-free diet. In 1976, Singh and Kay confirmed the good effect of gluten-free diet on schizophrenics, as well as the deleterious effect of gluten reintroduction. A *Lancet* editorial (1976) summarized the available literature on the subject with the statement that 'at present it is very difficult to relate gluten sensitivity to schizophrenia. In the absence of further information, any suggestions that gluten sensitivity is aetiologically related to schizophrenia remain speculative'. To try and answer this important question we decided to examine the response of the peripheral blood lymphocytes (PBL) of schizophrenics to stimulation with fractions of gluten. We have shown that lymphocytes of patients with gluten-sensitive coeliac disease respond to *in vitro* stimulation by subfractions of gluten (B2 and B3), by producing increased amounts of leucocyte migration inhibition factor (LIF) (Ashkenazi *et al.*, 1978). In our hands this is a discriminatory test for gluten sensitivity. We also compared the response of PBL from normal individuals with that of a group of children and adolescents with coeliac disease confirmed by biopsy.

MATERIALS AND METHODS

Twenty one hospitalized patients diagnosed as having schizophrenia, 15 male and 6 female, and who had been sick for 6 months to 20 years, comprised the schizophrenic group. Ten patients, 7 male and 3 female, with psychotic illness other than schizophrenia, comprised the psychotic group. Amongst the schizophrenic group were 13 chronic cases – nine chronic schizophrenic patients, three chronic paranoid and one chronic hebephrenic patient. The mean age for the group was 31 years. The eight patients in the acute schizophrenic group included five with acute paranoic schizophrenia and one each with hebephrenic, affective and atypical schizophrenia. The mean age of this group was 27 years.

The group with other than schizophrenic psychoses (10 patients) consisted of two patients with involution psychosis, two with paranoic psychosis, one with senile paranoia, one with senile depression, one with psychotic reaction and three with psychotic reaction in oligophrenia. The mean age of this group was 44 years. All diagnoses were made clinically by experienced psychiatrists and confirmed by the use of the checklist for the diagnosis of schizophrenia as recommended by Astrachan *et al.*, (1972).

The group of 34 normal controls was made up of normal hospital personnel, and children and adults admitted to a general hospital for elective surgery. The group of 55 coeliac patients included in this study was recently described by Ashkenazi *et al.* (1978). Informed consent was obtained for blood examination after the procedure was fully explained to the psychotic patients and their guardians, as well as to the normal controls and coeliac patients. The B2 and B3 fractions of gluten for the *in vitro* assay were prepared as previously described. The LIF (leucocyte-migration-inhibition factor) test was performed by mixing 1×10^6 peripheral blood lymphocytes (PBL) with 3×10^6 polymorphonuclear (PMN) leucocytes in an agarose droplet in Petri dishes. This was incubated overnight in the presence of either phytohaemagglutinin (PHA) as a positive control, or B2 or B3 fractions plus a negative control without antigen. Inhibition of the migration of the PMN leucocytes by the LIF was measured; migration inhibition above 15% was considered as positive indicating sensitized lymphocytes.

In 10 schizophrenic patients and 5 psychotic patients blood xylose was determined 1 h after ingestion of 0.5 g xylose per kg as a 5% solution. In 12 schizophrenic and 3 psychotic patients serum folate levels were examined by radio-immunoassay (Mincey, 1978). In 13 schizophrenic and 6 psychotic patients serum B12 levels were examined by radio-immunoassay. This was done in order to detect any biological evidence of malabsorption or subclinical coeliac disease.

The diet consumed by the patients was examined by the hospital dietician and was found to be varied and containing the recommended food components including gluten. No patient in this study had digestive disturbances nor were there eating problems.

RESULTS

The results of the LIF test in schizophrenic and psychotic patients is presented in Figure 1. It can be seen that the lymphocytes from the psychotic and schizophrenic patient groups, responded less well to stimulation by PHA, a universal mitogen, which therefore caused less inhibition of migration of leucocytes (mean $21.3\% \pm 8.35$ and $22.35\% \pm 11.9$ respectively) than in the controls ($33\% \pm 13$); $t = 3.56$, $p < 0.003$. Three patients had no LIF production to PHA whatsoever, a finding seen in some immune deficiency states.

By comparing the response of the psychotic patients (Table 1) to the response of the controls it appears that the whole group showed migration inhibition of $14.45\% \pm 8.56\%$ as compared to $4\% \pm 5\%$ in the controls; ($t = 6.074$ and the difference was highly significant, $p < 0.0005$). Comparing the psychotic group ($14.45\% \pm 8.56\%$) to the coeliac group ($24\% \pm 6\%$, $t = 6.055$) again the difference was highly significant ($p < 0.0005$). From these results it appears that the group of psychotic patients is intermediate between the normal controls and the coeliac patients.

In our laboratory 15% or greater is considered a positive LIF response to gluten. We divided the psychotic patients into two groups: (a) positive

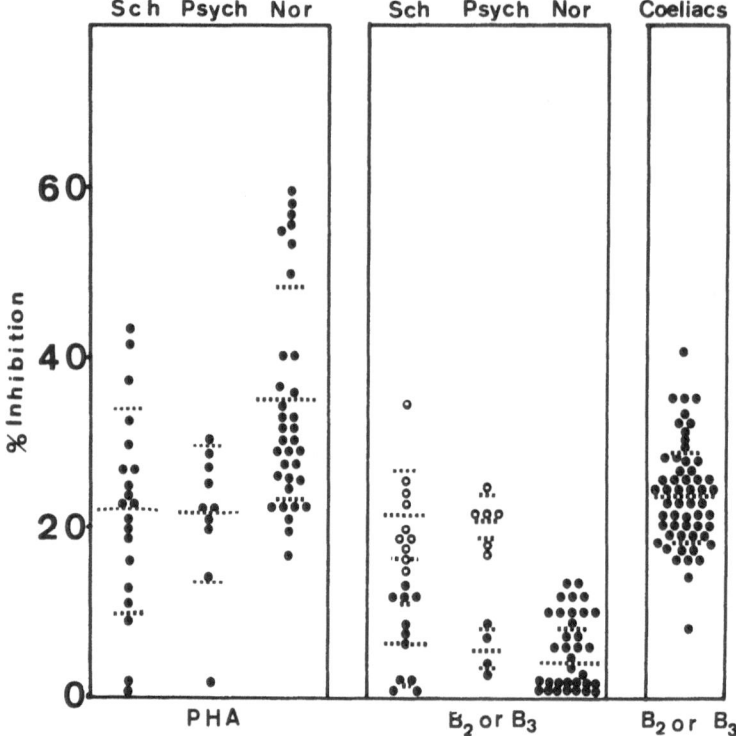

Figure 1   LIF production by lymphocytes after stimulation by PHA and B2 or B3 fractions of gluten. The response of the schizophrenic and psychotic patients to B2 or B3 is divided into responders (>15% inhibition – ○) and non-responders (<15% inhibition – ●). Mean ± SD is indicated

'responders' and (b) negative 'non-responders'. The 'responders' resemble the coeliac patients and the 'non-responders', the normal controls. Analysis of the two groups can be observed in Figure 1 and Tables 2 and 3.

Table 1   LIF response (% inhibition) to fractions of gluten by psychotic patients, coeliac patients and controls

	Normal controls		Psychotic patients (responders and non-responders)		Coeliac patients
N	34		31		55
Mean	4		14.45		24
SD	5		8.56		6
		$t = 6.074$		$t = 6.055$	
		$p < 0.0005$		$p < 0.0005$	

Table 2 Clinical and biochemical parameters in psychotic patients with positive LIF response to gluten

	Age (years)	Sex	LIF (% inhibition)	Blood xylose (mg%)	Serum folate (ng/ml)	Diagnosis
S.K.	20	m	18	—	—	CPS
L.S.	19	m	17	—	—	PS
T.G.	29	m	15	—	—	PS
T.S.	16	m	23	—	—	CS
E.B.	40	f	24	55	9.5	CS
S.R.	31	f	35	—	5.5	PS
N M.	29	m	20	26	3	CS
C.Z.	28	m	26	31.2	8	CS
M.O.	19	f	19	—	—	CS
M.M.	26	f	19	—	—	AS
A.G.	31	f	17	36	6	IP
Z.J.	77	m	25	38	6	DS
R.N.	19	m	22	33.6	—	PP
H.H.	24	m	18	30	—	PS, MD
Z.J.	36	m	22	28	6.4	PP
H.D.	23	m	22	—	—	P, MD
n	16		16	8	7	
mean	29.18		21.4	34.7	6.34	
SD	14.38		4.8	9.1	2.0	
t^*	0.348		5.052	0.198	0.495	
p	0.4		< 0.0005	0.45	0.3	

t^* – comparison with the respective group of non-responders (Table 3); CPS – chronic paranoid schizophrenia; PS – paranoid schizophrenia; CS – chronic schizophrenia; AS – atypical schizophrenia; IP – involutional psychotics; DS – depressive state; PP – paranoid psychotics; PS – psychotic state; MD – mental deficiency; P – psychotic

In Tables 2 and 3 a summary of some clinical and biochemical parameters in all the psychotic patients are summarized and analysed statistically. No statistically significant differences were found between the schizophrenic patients and the non-schizophrenic patients. The mean age of responders was 29.1 ± 14.38 years, non-responders 34.33 ± 15.31 years; $t = 0.348$, $p = 0.4$ (non-significant difference). Five of the 16 responders were female, compared with four females out of 15 non-responders.

It has already been shown that the LIF response of the psychotic patients is significantly higher than that found in normal individuals. Of

Table 3 Clinical and biochemical parameters in psychotic patients with negative LIF response to gluten

	Age (years)	Sex	LIF (% inhibition)	Blood xylose (mg %)	Serum folate (ng/ml)	Diagnosis
K.J.	29	m	12	27	3.5	CS
P.A.	35	m	13	39.6	16	SAS
L.S.	28	m	9	39	4	CS
S.N.	32	f	12	28	9	PS
D.J.	37	m	2	—	—	CS
A.M.	19	m	7	—	—	PS
G.J.	20	m	0	—	—	HS
B.N.	28	m	8	40	2.7	CS
O.D.	27	m	12	—	3.5	PS
A.A.	58	m	0	49.2	6.3	ES
D.M.	21	f	8	62.5	14	PS
M.A.	32	m	3	—	—	IP
R.T.	46	f	9	—	—	IP
A.E.	27	m	7	—	—	PS
M.Z.	76	f	4	—	—	PSP
n	15		15	7	8	
mean	34.33		7.06	40.75	7.37	
SD	15.31		4.38	12.25	5.15	
t^{**}	0.348		5.052	0.198	0.495	
p	0.4		< 0.0005	0.45	0.3	

t^{**} – comparison with the respective group of responders (Table 2); SAS – schizo-affective schizophrenia; HS – hebefrenic schizophrenia; ES – exacerbation of schizophrenia; PSP – paranoid senile psychosis. See Table 2 for other abbreviations.

interest is the fact that the LIF response in the non-responders group is also higher than the response in the normal controls, but the difference is not significant. Blood xylose examined in 8/16 responders (mean 34.7 mg% ± 9.1 mg%) was not different from that found in 7/15 non-responders examined (mean 40.75 mg% ± 12.25 mg%; $t = 0.198$, $p = 0.45$). All patients examined had normal levels (> 22 mg%).

There was no difference in serum folate levels in 7/16 responders examined (mean 6.34 ng/ml ± 2 ng/ml) and in 8/15 non-responders tested (mean 7.37 ng/ml ± 5.15 ng/ml); $t = 0.495$, $p = 0.3$.

The serum B12 in 19 patients examined was within normal limits, i.e. higher than 300 pgm/ml.

DISCUSSION

The connection between wheat gluten and schizophrenia has been suspected since the end of the Second World War (Dohan, 1966). From that time until now two groups of investigators, Dohan and colleagues (1969) and the group of Singh and Kay (1976), have published studies trying to elucidate the connection between wheat ingestion and schizophrenia. Others have raised objections to this possible relationship (Baker, 1973; Lancet editorial, 1976).

The results show that the response of lymphocytes from 10 out of 21 schizophrenic patients and 6 out of 10 psychotic patients to stimulation with subfractions of gluten was similar to that obtained with the lymphocytes from coeliac patients. On the other hand, unlike in coeliac patients, the psychotic and schizophrenic patients did not show any evidence of malabsorption or impairment of xylose absorption, or significant impairment of folate absorption. B12 levels were also normal. This reflects the good nutritional status of this group of patients. It is therefore possible that not only does gluten react with and damage the intestinal mucosa in coeliac patients, but in certain susceptible individuals, gluten may interfere with normal biological processes in the brain. Recently Klee *et al.* (1978) reported on the presence of endorphin-like and opioid-antagonist polypeptides in wheat gluten. These polypeptides, after absorption from the gastro-intestinal tract of susceptible individuals can act on the brain and cause psychotic symptoms. Our findings show that 50% of psychotic and schizophrenic patients examined apparently absorb the polypeptides leading to sensitization of their lymphocytes to gluten polypeptides. The response of LIF positive and negative psychotic and schizophrenic patients to withdrawal of gluten from their diet is presently under investigation.

References

Ashkenazi, A., Idar, D., Handzel, Z. T. Ofarim, M. Levin, S. (1978). An *in-vitro* immunological assay for the diagnosis of coeliac disease. *Lancet*, **1**, 627
Astrachan, B. M., Harrow, M., Adler, D. *et al.*, (1972). A checklist for the diagnosis of schizophrenia. *Br. J. Psychiatry*, **121**, 529
Baker, G. A. (1973). Effects of Nutrition on Schizophrenia. *Am. J. Psychiatry*, **130**, 1401
Dohan, F. C. (1966). Cereals and schizophrenia, data and hypothesis. *Acta Psychiatr. Scand.*, **42**, 125
Dohan, F. C. (1969). Is coeliac disease a clue to the pathogenesis of schizophrenia? *Ment. Hyg.*, **53**, 525
Dohan, F. C., Grasberger, J. C., Lowell, F. M., Johnston, H. T., Arbegast, A. W. (1969). Relapsed schizophrenics: More rapid improvement on a milk and cereal-free diet. *Br. J. Psychiatry*, **115**, 595
Editorial (1976). Gluten and schizophrenia. *Lancet*, **1**, 844
Klee, M. A., Ziondrou, C., Streaty, R. A. (1978). Exorphins – Peptides with opioid activity

isolated from wheat gluten, and their possible role in the etiology of schizophrenia. In Usdia, E. (ed.) *Endorphins in Mental Health Research*, (London: Macmillan)

Mincey, E. K., Wilcox, E., Morrison, R. T. (1974). Estimation of serum and red cell folate by a simple radiometric technique, in radio-immuno-assay and related procedures in medicine. *Proceedings of symposium*, Istanbul, 10–14 Sept. 1973. Vol. II, pp. 205–220. (Vienna: International Atomic Energy Agency)

Scott, B. B. and Losowsky, M. S. (1975). Coeliac disease: A cause of various associated diseases? *Lancet*, **2**, 956

Singh, M. M. and Kay, S. R. (1976). Wheat gluten as a pathogenic factor in schizophrenia. *Science*, **191**, 401

Section 3:
ADDICTION

14
β-endorphin and endoloxone: messengers of the autonomic nervous system for the conservation or expenditure of bodily resources and energy in anticipation of famine or feast

D. L. MARGULES

SUMMARY

Two new divisions of the autonomic nervous system are postulated that direct the conservation or expenditure of bodily resources (water, CO_2, Na^+, Ca^{++}, heat, fuels) and energy and coordinate these movements with the degree of anticipated nutrient shortage or excess in the environment. One division (the endorphinergic division) conveys the message of expected shortage and stimulates the organism to build up stores for an impending famine in the following manner: almost all forms of excretion cease and retention occurs of water, CO_2, Na^+, Ca^{++}, heat, and fuels; many energy expending activities cease as do urges toward activity; food, water, and salt appetites and intakes increase and overeating produces obesity and oedema. Pre-famine feeding is associated with hyperinsulinaemia because its purpose is to build the stores necessary to survive famine. The endorphinergic system accomplishes these preparations, in part, by a release of β-endorphin and adrenocorticotrophic hormone (ACTH) from the pituitary gland. β-Endorphin, a morphine-like peptide induces a state of lethargy, passivity and skeletal muscle relaxation. In this state, an attenuation occurs of the arousal capacity of many of the classical stimuli for the activation of the sympathetic nervous system including pain, cold, asphyxiation, oxygen lack and the emotions of fear and rage. This serves to conserve energy and to prevent wasteful expenditures. β-Endorphin also reduces overall energy expenditures by the reduction of thyrotrophin release, the lowering of the set point for body temperature and the elevation of the set point for carbon dioxide tension in the blood. Drops in body temperature, respiration rate, cardiovascular output, sympathetic tone, and thyroid hormone release, reduce the energy production and oxygen consumption in almost every tissue in the body. β-Endorphin also acts in conjunction with glucagon, and insulin, whose release it stimulates, to conserve and extract and store every remaining bit of nutrient, water and minerals in the body. This occurs in various ways, including the inhibition of excretion in many organs. Sphincters for defecation, urination and bile release are tightly contracted. Simultaneously, propulsive peristalsis is inhibited and instead the gastrointestinal contents are stirred and mixed in place within the small intestine and large intestine. β-Endorphin stimulates the release of antidiuretic hormone which acts on the kidney to conserve water. β-Endorphin also acts to inhibit the release of the gonadotrophic hormones thus reducing the sexual urges. The actions of β-endorphin are supported by ACTH release which stimulates the adrenal cortex to release the mineralocorticoids and glucocorticoid hormones. These hormones further conserve sodium and carbohydrates and reduce the rate of their utilization. Finally β-endorphin appears to have appetite and thirst stimulating abilities. Hibernation is an extreme form of the results of preparations implemented by endorphinergic division of the autonomic nervous system. Hibernation represents an almost perfect adaptation to seasonal food shortages. The other new division of the autonomic nervous system (the endoloxonergic division) antagonizes all of the actions of the endorphinergic division. Its actions are mimicked by opioid antagonists such as naloxone. It conveys a message of an expected environmental surplus and it allows the organism to release internal stores by the excretion of water, CO_2, Na^+, Ca^{++}, heat and nutrients from the body. It increases energy expenditures and it stimulates activities that use up energy rapidly. It inhibits food appetite, water appetite and salt appetite. These events are compatible with an expected surplus of nutrients in the environment (feast). This system produces a type of shivering and related movements known as 'wet dog shakes' that resemble a convulsant condition. These shakes and related movements are heat-generating devices that can rapidly produce an elevation in body temperature necessary for example, to arouse an animal rapidly from hibernation. Small doses of naloxone increase the heart rate and respiration rate of hibernating hamsters and arouse them prematurely from the hibernating state. The endoloxone (endogenous naloxone) system intensifies the arousal capacity of many of the classical stimuli for activation of the sympathetic nervous system including pain, cold, asphyxiation, oxygen lack and the emotions of fear or rage. The pituitary hormones that integrate the activation of the antistarvation system and mediate its various functions are unknown. There is evidence however, that calcitonin and/or certain fragments of ACTH such as CIP (ACTH-38) and α- as well as β-melanocyte stimulating hormones (MSH) have endoloxonergic activity. Calcitonin stimulates the urinary excretion of Na^+Cl^-, Ca^{++} and other ions, and causes body weight loss. The MSH hormones produce an increase in excreted urine volume and sodium concentration and CIP inhibits the ACTH induced cortical steroid release. Other endoloxone-like actions may be discovered for these peptides and/or peptides derived or related to the calcitonin, CIP and/or MSH sequences. These actions include the stimulation of thyrotrophin, the raising of body temperature set point, the stimulation of respiration, the increase of cardiovascular output and the increase of sympathetic tone. Endoloxone activity produces excretion from many other sources including lacrimation, vomiting, diarrhoea, urination, sweating, release of bile and other digestive secretions, sweat and ejaculation. ACTH release is inhibited and mineralocorticoid activity decreases. Drops in aldosterone allow sodium to be released in the urine. Drops in glucocorticoid release allow carbohydrate utilization to be stimulated. There is an increase in sympathetic tone all over the body along with painful contractions of skeletal muscles that resemble convulsions.

INTRODUCTION

The feeding pattern of mammals evolved long before the current era of plentiful food and energy. In those early millenia, species survived which could take advantage of infrequent feasts in order to store enough calories to survive the long intervening periods of famine. As a result, many mammals, including humans, acquired the capacity to eat one half to all of their daily basal calorie requirements in a single 10-minute meal (Owen et al., 1979). If given the opportunity, many people tend toward overeating and gorging themselves. They store the extra nutrient in adipose tissue. This tissue is kept plump so that it can yield back enough calories to provide the ability to survive the inevitable famine. Today in affluent nations obesity is quite common and it represents a preparation for the famine that never comes.

Major physiological systems control the inflow and outflow of nutrients in response to feast or famine. These systems involve smooth muscle and glands that operate automatically and are not under voluntary control. They are a part of the autonomic nervous system that controls the energy metabolism and the conservation of nutrients and integrates these with many bodily reactions including respiration, body temperature, metabolic rate, and others, which will be discussed below. In order to account for these widespread and relatively rapid preparations the existence of two new divisions of the autonomic nervous system is postulated. This is necessary because the pattern of bodily changes involved in feast and famine cannot be produced by any pattern of known parasympathetic or sympathetic nervous system actions.

Homeostasis, or the oscillation around a set point, maintains the constancy of the milieu interne. This concept has dominated thinking and research on feeding, drinking and salt appetite and on the autonomic nervous system for many years (Cannon, 1929). Many of the physiological reactions that assure constancy of the milieu interne involve the activation of the sympathetic nervous system. This system preserves homeostasis particularly during a crisis that requires a massive muscular exertion (fight or flight), such as an immediate threat to the organism's life (Cannon, 1929). Under some threats, however, such as food shortage and starvation, the animal may not benefit from the fight or flight response. A starving organism cannot afford a massive expenditure of calories and energy in a futile attempt to defend a high homeostatic set point. It is better off modifying its set points for homeostasis, reducing energy expenditures, conserving bodily resources and waiting out the famine.

Species vary as to their ability to lower metabolic rate, body temperature and respiratory quotient, but many animals, including humans, retain the ability to lower these values substantially in response to a prolonged fast (Owen et al., 1979). The lowering of these set points during starvation involves an inhibition of the sympathetic nervous system (Brodie et al., 1965). Until recently no mechanism has been known to accomplish this. This paper presents the theory that the anti-sympathetic actions associated with starvation are accomplished by the activation of the endogenous morphine-like system or the endophinergic system. The endophinergic system provides a variety of additional benefits to the starving organism that help conserve energy and bodily resources. The set point for some important required substances is modified, such as for nutrients, water and CO_2 tension in the blood. Some of these changed set points are maintained for relatively long periods, but eventually all of them are restored, sometimes quite violently by an antagonist system that has a naloxone-like action. In this chapter, the concept of homeostasis is extended from a fixed set point notion to a shifted set point theory. A better word that describes such regulation around radically different set points is 'heterostasis'. Two new divisions of the autonomic nervous system are postulated for implementation of these shifts in set points. Finally, an integrated and widespread physiological role is proposed for the body's morphine-like and naloxone-like naturally occurring peptides and their receptors.

Food shortages stand among a group of critical environmental events that shape the course of biological evolution. In the course of evolution, organisms have evolved many major physiological adaptations that had survival value during periods of food shortage. Hibernation, estivation and migration, dramatic examples of such adaptations, involve major physiological changes with widespread and influential effects at many levels of organization throughout all the tissues and organs of the body (Mrosovsky, 1971). Often, when food shortage is seasonal, animals anticipate their famine by the accumulation of extra calories either on their bodies as adipose tissue or in their nest as hoarded foods. Very little is known about the physiological or chemical nature of adaptive changes in preparation for food shortages. Moreover, no one has considered the possibility that an integrated and influential system may exist for the orderly organization and control of the various adaptive reactions to anticipated food shortages. A large body of information can be incorporated by such a theory from the literature of several unrelated and somewhat neglected disciplines: hibernation; the pharmacology of the opioids, morphine, β-endorphin and enkephalin; the biochemistry of starvation; and the physiology of the autonomic nervous system. Also included are certain areas in endocrinology common to all of these disciplines.

A highly integrated system is called into action prior to and during the early phase of a seasonal food shortage. Energy expenditures are reduced, the excretion of nutrients (sodium, water and intestinal contents) is inhibited, and feeding and drinking behaviours are stimulated. This system maximizes the inflow of calories into storage sites and minimizes the outflow. Thus glycogen and triglycerides are built up to provide a large reservoir of stored supplies. It also conserves energy in many other ways. In general it acts to inhibit sympathetic nervous system reactions at many places simultaneously. It is not simply a widespread parasympathetic activity, for this system does not promote digestive secretions, nor does it enhance excretion. Its actions fit into no known configuration of sympathetic or parasympathetic activity. This system may be a previously unrecognized modulator of autonomic nervous system activity that produces a unique series of reactions. It may be best to identify this pattern in individual organs. For the purpose of this paper this set of actions will be called 'endorphinergic' and the system as the 'endorphinergic system'.

Stimuli that ordinarily activate the sympathetic nervous system such as pain, exposure to cold, asphyxiation, oxygen lack, and strong emotions (rage and fear) lose a part of their ability to do so when the endorphinergic system is active. The adaptive significance here relates to the fact that a starving individual cannot afford a massive expenditure of its dwindling caloric resources; it must conserve energy in all but the most dangerous situations.

CHEMICAL BASIS OF THE ENDORPHINERGIC RESPONSE

The morphine-like substances which occur naturally in the body, including β-endorphin and enkephalin, provide the chemical basis for the antisympathetic reaction. These substances act as hormonal and synaptic transmitter messages that attenuate arousal properties of various stimuli and conserve energy. Nowhere is this more clearly evident than from the analgesic actions of morphine (Goodman and Gilman, 1975), β-endorphin (Tseng et al., 1976) and enkephalin (Akil et al., 1976). This attenuation of the reactivity to pain should be viewed as a small part of a broad adaptation to food shortage, mediated by the endogenous opioid substances. The message serves to conserve energy in all but the most painful situations.

Pain is not the only sensation attenuated by morphine and morphine-like bodily peptides. These substances lower the set point for body temperature, substantially (Tseng et al., 1976; Ferre et al., 1978). In other words, they prevent the occurrence of a heat-generating sympathetic response. This allows the body temperature of homeostatic animals to reach levels lower than normal. Larger drops in body temperature occur during hibernation. Small drops in body temperature that occur in non-hibernators may be an adaptive response to starvation that reduces metabolism and conserves fuel. Morphine also raises the set point of the respiratory centre to carbon dioxide tension (PCO_2), thus depressing respiration (Moss and Friedman, 1978). All phases of respiration are depressed including rate of breathing, minute volume and tidal exchange (Goodman and Gilman, 1975). This makes an oxygen lack less likely to arouse a compensatory sympathetic reaction. It also contributes to a lower metabolic rate and the conservation of energy and water (lost as expired water vapour). Finally morphine and β-endorphin reduce emotional reactivity (rage and fear) and produce apathy, lessened physical activity, skeletal muscle relaxation, lethargy, drowsiness and passivity (Goodman and Gilman, 1975).

In summary, the effects of all of the classical stimuli for sympathetic arousal are attenuated by morphine including pain, exposure to cold, asphyxiation, oxygen lack and strong emotions. The whole constellation is consistent with an adaptive reaction to food shortage that helps the organism conserve heat, energy, fuel, water and sodium, and calcium, and to reduce substantially the possibility of a wasteful expenditure of energy or massive muscular exertion. The receptors that mediate these actions are located mainly in the organs of the peritoneal cavity and are affected during starvation by β-endorphin released primarily from the pituitary. We have preliminary evidence in collaboration with Dr Candace Pert and Dr James Flynn that starvation induces a large increase in pituitary immunoreactive β-endorphin content, 10 times the level of non-starved controls.

FREE FATTY ACID, GLUCOSE AND INSULIN REQUIREMENTS DURING STARVATION

Three mechanisms produce the release of stored metabolic fuels. These are called into action in an orderly sequence depending upon the intensity of the caloric demands of the body. Ordinary or low demand between meals is satisfied by the release of free fatty acids from the adipose tissue. The mechanism involves neuronal norepinephrine produced at first by sympathetic neural messages (Brodie *et al.*, 1965). As deprivation continues and demand rises, free fatty acids continue to be released into the blood but neuronal norepinephrine declines and some other substance takes over. This has been demonstrated in experiments that show starvation-induced increases in free fatty acids are not affected by noradrenergic blockage or by chemical sympathectomy (Goodman and Knobil, 1959; Brodie and Maickel, 1963; Stern and Maickel, 1963; Maickel *et al.*, 1977). The substance which takes over the job of stimulation of free fatty acid release has not been identified. Morphine stimulates the release of free fatty acids (Borison *et al.*, 1962; Feldberg and Shaligram, 1972) and this raises the possibility that β-endorphin or enkephalin may be the unidentified stimulant for the starvation-induced increase in free fatty acid. However, we have found that naltrexone does not effect the rate of body weight loss of obese or lean mice during starvation. This suggests that opioid receptors are not involved in the lipolytic events necessary for survival during starvation. Other non-opioid hormones which may contribute to lipolysis include α- and β-melanocyte stimulating hormones, glucagon, secretin, ACTH, arginine, vasopressin and epinephrine.

Free fatty acids are used as fuel for muscle and liver but not for the brain, particularly early in starvation (Cahill, 1976). At that time the brain is still an obligatory glucose-dependent organ very vulnerable to a glucose shortage. The glucose supply to the brain is assured by the glycogen stores in liver and muscle. These stores are made available mainly by the action of glucagon released from the pancreas and epinephrine released from the adrenal medulla. Both hormones release glucose from the liver but only epinephrine releases glucose from the muscle (Cahill, 1976). During starvation the release of epinephrine probably occurs without a concomitant sympathetic nervous system arousal.

Morphine stimulates the epinephrine-induced increase in blood plasma glucose (Borison et al., 1962; Feldberg and Shaligram, 1972). This raises the possibility that β-endorphin and/or enkephalin may contribute to the stimulation of epinephrine release. In any case, the neural pathway that activates the adrenal medulla does not stimulate any other part of the sympathetic nervous system. In order to ensure that mobilized glucose reaches the brain and the brain alone, it is necessary to reduce or abolish insulin activity, otherwise glucose bound for the brain will be taken up by other body organs before it reaches the central nervous system. The food deprived individual accomplishes this by the reduction of the release of insulin and by the reduction of the sensitivity of the insulin receptor. These events are implemented as starvation continues and liver glycogen, which is a small reservoir, nears depletion. This requires a shift into the hormonal state known as gluconeogenesis, which produces amino acids by the hydrolysis of proteins. Some of these amino acids are converted to glucose in the liver from the gluconeogenic amino acids such as glutamic and aspartic acid, alanine, arginine, asparagine, cysteine, glutamine, and glycine. Thus, the glucose supply of the brain is extended (Cahill, 1976).

GLUCONEOGENESIS

Two hormonal systems promote gluconeogenesis. One is the glucagon system of the endocrine pancreas, the other is the pituitary ACTH–adrenal cortex axis. Neither of these systems require sympathetic neural activation and their output is not blocked by chemical sympathectomy. The glucagon system in the pancreas is activated by morphine or β-endorphin (Ipp et al., 1978). Whenever β-endorphin is released from the pituitary there is a concomitant release of ACTH (Guillemin et al., 1977). This suggests that the endogenous opioid substances may participate in the activation of gluconeogenesis by the stimulation of glucagon release and by the concomitant release of ACTH.

During this more intensive stage of food deprivation the body is sacrificing protein to make glucose. This glucose primarily must go to the brain and it is essential to maintain the reduced sensitivity of the insulin receptors. This is accomplished by the anterior pituitary, which produces a substance that reduces the sensitivity of the insulin receptor. Removal of the pituitary (hypophysectomy) reduces the ability of animals to maintain their blood glucose levels in the fasted condition. They can not release glucose from storage sites in the liver. At the same time, hypophysectomized animals show a striking increase in their sensitivity to insulin. The effect is powerful enough to ameliorate pancreatic diabetes (the Houssay effect).

The pituitary substance (or substances) responsible for the decrease of sensitivity to insulin and for the fasting-induced release of glucose from the liver appears to be related to ACTH. In fact, ACTH itself contributes to the adaptation to starvation by stimulation of the release of the adrenal cortical hormones, particularly the glucocorticoids. These hormones stimulate gluconeogenesis, restore the glycogen content of the liver, reduce the sensitivity of the insulin receptors, and discourage the utilization of glucose already in cells. The glucocorticoids are the hormones par excellence for the production, conservation and protection of the brain's glucose supply. It is not surprising that removal of the adrenal gland is fatal within a week or two. Death can be prevented by replacement therapy with the adrenal cortical hormones or by the administration of large amounts of the sodium ion. There is no satisfactory explanation for the ability of sodium to replace the adrenal glands. Perhaps it is related to the ability of sodium to favour the binding of endoloxone (Pert and Snyder, 1974). Animals without adrenal glands have an increased sensitivity to insulin and they fail to maintain their blood glucose levels when food is withheld. A large part of the effects produced by hypophysectomy may be due to the loss of adrenal cortical hormones and the consequent loss of glucose and sodium.

However, this is not the whole story of the role of the pituitary in the defence of the brain's glucose and sodium supply. The β-endorphin released from the pituitary appears to contribute substantially to the gluconeogenesis via its stimulatory action on pancreatic glucagon (Ipp et al., 1978). I have already mentioned the numerous anti-sympathetic actions present during starvation. The release of β-endorphin from the pituitary would strengthen these actions all over the body. Occupation of opioid receptors increases blood glucose via the stimulation of the epinephrine-induced breakdown of glycogen in the liver, and β-endorphin release would enhance such stimulation. The possibility exists that β-endorphin or a related pituitary peptide mediates the reduction in insulin receptor sensitivity. Finally a non-opioid related peptide may be involved in the starvation induced release of free fatty acids from adipose tissue.

The degree of glucose need probably influences the extent of the mobilization of stored calories as follows: mild needs can be met by glucagon release alone, which mobilizes liver stores; moderate needs require the addition of epinephine which mobilizes both liver and muscle stores; severe needs require the involvement of the pituitary ACTH and β-endorphin systems. Amino acids necessary for gluconeogenesis are not called for in mild deprivation, but they are needed for example after an overnight fast (Cahill, 1976). Glucagon alone may provide for this type of gluconeogenesis. Continuation of the gluconeogenesis leads to its reinforcement by the pituitary ACTH and β-endorphin systems. Finally, the need for fatty acids appears to be met at first by means of sympathetic induced release of norepinephrine and later from some non-sympathetic substance.

CONSERVATORY ACTIONS OF β-ENDORPHIN

Morphine and the naturally occurring opioid polypeptides have many actions consistent with the hypothesis that they serve to help the organism adapt to food shortage. The powerful effect of opioid substances on the gastro-intestinal tract is well known; they decrease the propulsive contractions of the stomach, small intestine and large intestine and increase the contractions that stir and mix the gastro-intestinal contents (Daniel, 1968). In the small intestine this type of movement helps to extract every remaining nutrient and in the large intestine it aids in the extraction of every remaining bit of water. To insure that these stirring and mixing movements do not result in excretion, the anal sphincter is tightly contracted by a direct action of the opioid substances. Moreover, morphine produces an inattention to the normal sensory stimuli for the defecation reflex by an action on the central nervous system. This reduces the chances of overcoming the contraction by means of a command from the brain (Goodman and Gilman, 1975).

A starving individual cannot afford the expenditure of energy needed to seek water. Moreover, he needs to have built up water stores in his body in order to be able to hydrolyse emergency fuel available from muscle and other protein sources. β-Endorphin and morphine act to conserve water by the stimulation of the release of antidiuretic hormone (ADH), which acts on the kidneys to reduce the urinary output of water (Tseng et al., 1978; Wenick, 1979). In addition, urine retention is increased in the bladder by contraction of the ureters and the increase in vesical sphincter tone (Goodman and Gilman, 1975). Water is also conserved by an opioid induced reduction of the following digestive secretions: saliva; hydrochloric acid; bile; and the exocrine secretions of the pancreas and small intestine (Goodman and Gilman, 1975; Konturek et al., 1978).

It is possible that some of these effects of opioid substances are mediated in part via opioid pepticles released with glucagon. This mixture is known to reduce the volume of gastric juice and its acid concentration. This mixture also reduces the propulsive motility of the gastro-intestinal tract and eliminates pancreatic juice. The loss of these secretions not only provides water but also a source of amino acid made available by the hydrolysis of the digestive enzymes and gastro-intestinal hormones. The amino acids obtained by this hydrolysis are converted into glucose by gluconeogenesis in the liver. The digestive juices are the first protein sources to be sacrificed during starvation. Water also is conserved by a reduction of water vapour lost in respiration. All of these water retaining responses may contribute to the peculiar famine oedema that occurs frequently during starvation particularly in men and children (kwashiorkor) (Gopalan and Gopalan, 1975; Wenick, 1979).

Opioids save energy by the reduction of thyroid hormone release (Goodman and Gilman, 1975). This reduces the energy production and oxygen consumption of almost all the other tissue in the body. Opioids accomplish this decrease by decreasing the release of pituitary thyrotrophin (TSH). The decrease in body temperature set point is a consequence of the lowered thyroid hormone release and reduced calorigenesis. Stress also decreases the release of TSH. It is tempting to suggest that stress may cause its decrease in TSH, partly by the release of pituitary ACTH and β endorphin.

Starvation not only decreases tri-iodothyronine (T_3) levels in the serum but also increases serum levels of reverse T_3, an inactive form of T_3 (Vagenakis et al., 1975). Cardiovascular output is decreased by the opioids (Florez and Mediavilla, 1977). β-Endorphin reduces arterial blood pressure and produces a decrease in vascular sympathetic tone. These changes are compatible with the decrease in respiration and the reduction of energy production and oxygen consumption in the bodily tissue. β-Endorphin produces a marked sedation and reduction in muscular activity including motivational weakness and apathy. These behavioural changes are seen during the later stages of starvation (Gopalan and Gopalan, 1975). It is tempting to speculate that β-endorphin contributes to the apathetic and passive condition of the starved.

Just as the starving individual cannot afford to expend energy in the search for water, he also cannot afford this expenditure in the search for sexual gratification. Starving individuals have no libido (Gopalan and Gopalan, 1975). β-Endorphin or enkephalin may be responsible for the marked reduction in libido seen during starvation. The administration of opioids reduces the pituitary gonadotropins, particularly follicle stimulating hormone (FSH) but also luteinizing hormone (LH) (Brun et al., 1977; Blank et al., 1979). Such administration also inhibits copulatory behaviour (Quarantotti et al., 1978). As a result of the loss of pituitary gonadotropins the gonadal hormone output is reduced. The loss of gonadal hormones is responsible for the loss of libido.

It is of interest that TSH, LH and FSH are all glycosylated hormones and require a carbohydrate content as part of their structure. During starvation carbohydrates are in short supply and there may not be enough carbohydrate available for the proper glycosylation of these hormones. If obesity is a sign of sustained preparation for famine, this could explain why it is often accompanied by low thyroid and gonadal function. (See

Margules, 1978, for discussion.)

β-Endorphin stimulates feeding behaviour when administered intraventricularly or directly into the brain. Pituitary and blood levels of β-endorphin were found by Margules *et al.* (1978) to be elevated substantially in genetically obese mice (*ob/ob*) and rats (*fa/fa*). The obesity of these rodents may be due to an elevated set point for body adipose stores brought about by the high opioid levels. These animals show many of the other signs of elevated opioid levels including lethargy, hypothermia and constipation. This raises the possibility that the cause of their obesity is a false message of starvation, that induces overeating.

The actions of naloxone (Maikel *et al.*, 1977) and naltrexone (Demetrios and Renault, 1966) are consistent with the idea of an endogenous opioid that stimulates feeding, drinking and weight gain. In direct support of this idea, small doses of naloxone abolish overeating in genetically obese rodents (*fa/fa* and *ob/ob*) without affecting the feeding of the lean littermate controls (Margules *et al.*, 1978). On the other hand the message may not be a false message, but rather a message of imminent starvation. Such a message occurs prior to the prolonged fast of hibernation, migration and estivation, and contributes substantially to the adipose stores that are accumulated prior to the fast. This raises another possibility that has not received attention in the literature. β-Endorphin release may contribute to the naturally occurring obesity of hibernating or migrating animals. Moreover, the actions of β-endorphin and the metabolic changes are in the same direction as the hibernating state including the lowering of the body temperature set point, the reduction of respiration and cardiovascular output. Similarly the opioid induced retention of urine and faeces can be viewed as a means of prevention of the freezing of the animal in his own waste products during hibernation.

The hibernating animal is also going through a period of starvation and requires many of the same metabolic and hormonal changes required in a non-hibernating starvation state. We have preliminary data demonstrating that small doses of naloxone reverse the hibernation state and shift it substantially toward arousal. This suggests that hibernation is maintained by the release of an endogenous opioid such as β-endorphin.

SEIZURES AS HEAT GENERATING DEVICES

The hibernator is capable of a rapid rise in body temperature and a reversal of the starvation state in all of its various manifestations. Very little is known about this reversal. It does seem to involve a convulsant-like state, markedly increased heart rate and respiration. Extremely high doses of morphine, systematically administered, produce convulsions. Direct injections of 5 µg of β-endorphin into the lateral ventricle of the rat brain produce electrical evidence of typical epileptic seizures in the limbic system (Henriksen *et al.*, 1978). These paradoxical seizures and epileptic activity may be viewed as heat generating reactions which help to raise body temperature quickly. These reactions may play a physiological role in the termination of hibernation and the restoration of normal body temperature.

We have preliminary evidence that naloxone (0.2 mg/kg s.c.) arouses hamsters from deep hibernation. These reactions are opposite in direction to the primary actions of the opioids. They bring to mind the well known withdrawal symptoms that occur either after the abrupt cessation of chronic opioid activity or after the administration of an opioid antagonist, such as naloxone. Other withdrawal reactions in addition to convulsions include: diarrhoea; exaggerated respiratory response to CO_2; elevation in heart rate and blood pressure; pilomotor erection; muscle spasms; spontaneous ejaculation and orgasm; anorexia; and increased body temperature (Goodman and Gilman, 1975). It should be noted that these responses counteract all of the aspects of the endorphinergic induced changes.

TOLERANCE, PHYSICAL DEPENDENCE AND WITHDRAWAL REACTIONS

The phenomena of tolerance, physical dependence and withdrawal reactions occur with all opioid substances including the naturally occurring opioid peptides (Teng *et al.*, 1976; Wei and Loh, 1976). Tolerance develops most rapidly with the more or less continuous administration of opioids. With intermittent administration it is possible to avoid the development of tolerance for an indefinite period (Goodman and Gilman, 1975). Starvation calls for a continual release of opioid substances as long as the food shortage lasts. Such a release produces the development of tolerance. Thus the system would have to put out more opioids in order to maintain the same degree of functional output.

The adaptive significance of this strategy is clear when the individual happens to be hibernating. Tolerance would represent a latent induction of the antagonistic system that will eventually be required to reverse the hibernation state. The required reversal involves a violent upheaval in order to achieve the metabolic requirements. Often at the end of a hibernation state caloric reverses are low. Thus it makes sense to begin the preparations for the induction of the anti-hibernation reaction before the time of the required arousal. This is another type of anticipatory preparation that is analogous to the pre-hibernation obesity. Such anticipatory responses seem to be a major feature of these systems. Non-hibernating mammals may have developed advantageous ways for the use of these anticipatory systems without the loss of consciousness. These involve the accumulation of calories either in the body or hoarded in the nest.

ANATOMICAL BASIS FOR THE ENDORPHINERGIC SYSTEM

β-Endorphin is produced by the following cells: all cells of the intermediate pituitary lobe; scattered cells of the anterior pituitary lobe; all the gastrin-producing cells of the stomach (G cells); certain neuronal cells in the arcuate nucleus of the hypothalamus and in other portions of the brain. Enkephalin is produced in a variety of brain cells and in neuronal cells in the smooth muscle of the small intestine and vas deferens. Thus a variety of cells are capable of producing these substances both in the periphery and in the brain. The major set of cells from the point of view of the quantity produced is the intermediate lobe of the pituitary. This provides a hormonal basis for the widespread anti-sympathetic effects of this system.

Receptors for β-endorphin exist in the stomach, intestinal tract, liver, pancreas, kidney, heart, lungs, spleen, skeletal muscle and brain, as determined by the capacity of those tissues to take up and retain $[^{125}I]$ β-endorphin after it has been injected intravenously (Reilly et al., 1968). Thus, all of the organ systems participating in the many adaptive changes discussed above seem to have receptors for the opioid substances. These appear to be on neuronal cells that control motor or endocrine output. It is unclear if any sensory elements exist in the periphery which are sensitive to endorphin or endoloxone.

AN EXPLANATION OF PIGMENT CHANGES DURING STARVATION

Profuse infiltrations of brown pigment occur in the posterior portion of the pituitary of starving humans (Wenick, 1979). In addition the skin is covered with a dirty brown pigment that concentrates around the neck, rump, sides of the torso and on the back of the arms and the thighs (Gopalan and Krishnaswarmy, 1975). These pigment changes can be explained by the present theory. Increases in β-endorphin are accompanied by increases in α-melanocyte stimulating hormone by virtue of a common precursor shared by both hormones. This precursor, pro-opiocortin contains other hormones as well, including ACTH and CLIP. It appears that all of the hormones derived from pro-opiocortin are in excess in genetically obese mice, including α-melanocyte stimulating hormone (Beevar et al., 1977; Rossier et al., 1979). Thus, if this is also the case in starvation, α-melanocyte stimulating hormone may be responsible for the darkening of the skin and pituitary. This is the first chemical explanation of the pigment changes during starvation.

THE ENDOLOXONERGIC SYSTEM

The evidence for the existence of an endogenous substance with naloxone-like activity is not as strong as the evidence for the endorphinergic system. The firm establishment of such a system is hindered by the lack of the identification of endogenous substance with naloxone-like activity. Nevertheless, it is clear that an intact pituitary is necessary in order for naloxone to exert the pain augmenting action of reducing the escape latency of mice on the hot plate (Gopalan and Krishnaswarmy, 1975). This suggests that the pituitary contains a hyperalgesic factor and that naloxone acts to release this substance. Of the known pituitary substances, three seem to have actions particularly compatible with the release of nutrients from the body, which is a cardinal characteristic of the endoloxonergic state.

Calcitonin enhances the urinary excretion of water and various ions in young animals (Rasmussen, 1974). It also inhibits feeding behaviour and produces body weight losses (Rasmussen, 1974). Recently, in collaboration with Dr Cary W. Cooper, we have found elevated calcitonin levels in the pituitary and thyroid glands but not in the blood of genetically obese rats (fa/fa) (Margules, Flynn, Walker and Cooper, 1979). This work represents the first quantitative determination of calcitonin-like immunoactivity in the pituitary gland. There is a good chance that a substance with calcitonin-like immunoreactivity participates in the suppression of overeating in middle-aged rats. The capacity to release substances with calcitonin-like immune reactivity into the blood is found in the Fisher 344 rat, one of the few rodents to remain lean throughout its entire lifespan. The fa/fa rat seems to lack this capacity.

Another candidate for an endoloxonergic substance is the group of melanocyte stimulating hormones (MSH). These hormones increase substantially the concentration of sodium in the urine at doses as low as 5 ng in trained, fasted, water-loaded rats (Orias and McCann, 1972). They also produce yawning (an expulsion of CO_2), one of the signs of morphine withdrawal.

The other possible pituitary substance with naloxonergic activities is corticotropin-inhibiting peptide (CIP) (ACTH 7–38) which has been shown to inhibit ACTH-stimulated corticosterone production in isolated rat adrenal cells. A reduced corticosterone level encourages the utilization of carbohydrates, inhibits the formation of glucose from tissue protein and inhibits the deposition of glycogen in the liver. These events are compatible with an expected surplus of nutrients in the environment (feast). It is possible that there are a series of endoloxone hormones that reinforce each other in the preparations for arousal from hibernation and for feasting, just as β-endorphin and ACTH reinforce each other in the preparation for famine.

EMOTIONAL STATES AS SIGNS OF ENDORPHINERGIC OR ENDOLOXONERGIC ACTIVITY

The ability to tolerate comfortably a series of repeated exhalations without the need for inhalation occurs during periods of laughter. During this time the carbon dioxide tension in the blood must be increasing. At the same time a laughing individual must be in an analgesic state, for otherwise he would not be able to tolerate the discomfort of a continual series of exhalations. If a laughing individual released β-endorphin this would account for all the phenomena involved, including the depression in respiratory rate, the analgesic state and the ability to tolerate higher tensions of carbon dioxide in the blood. Laughter may be a sign of a build up of endorphinergic activity and an inflow of carbon dioxide into the body. Its hedonistic aspects can be attributed to endorphinergic activity rather than simple anoxia.

Yawning is an early sign of the withdrawal syndrome in opioid addicted individuals. It indicates the beginning of a process meant to return carbon dioxide tension levels in the blood to lower levels. The yawn is a prolonged exhalation that blows carbon dioxide out of the body. It is an indication that endoloxonergic activity is building up. Often yawning is associated with the uncomfortable state of being bored. Yawning is not as efficient in expelling CO_2 as hyperventilation, which occurs during the arousal from hibernation.

Crying is almost always caused by a sharp increase in pain. It is an indication of strong endoloxonergic activity. Crying is more common in infants and children than in adults. Calcitonin loses its ability to lower blood calcium in adults. It is tempting to speculate that the greater tendency of infants and children to pain and crying is due to their increased sensitivity to calcitonin (growing pains?). Thus calcitonin may be a major endoloxonergic hormone of the childhood years. Whenever endoloxonergic activity increases there is an outflow of fluids and other substances from the body. Thus, sharp stimuli which induce pain may release endoloxone, a substance that increases pain sensitivity and reactivity, increases sympathetic tone and precipitates a withdrawal syndrome. The release of tears may be a sign of an endoloxone induced withdrawal state.

A big smile opens the lips and teeth which guard the gastrointestinal system and this is preparation for an inflow. Smaller smiles only open the lips and not the teeth. Nevertheless a smile prepares for an expected inflow and can be classified on the endorphinergic side rather than on the endoloxonergic side. Smiles sometimes precede laughing which might be a stronger indication of endorphinergic activation.

Stretching is an extremely important activity necessary for optimal exposure of receptors to the endoloxone and endorphin hormones. During sexual activity it is necessary to both engorge the gonads with blood and to repeatedly stretch or rub them in order to reach orgasm. Sensory neurons that feed back the message of orgasm to the brain require the release of pituitary substance, the absorption of this hormone in the gonads, (which is facilitated by engorgement) and the exposure of the receptors to the agonist (which requires stretching of the gonadal tissue). Sexual pleasure involves endoloxone in order to build up to orgasm and to ejaculate. After orgasm endorphin is necessary in order to relax afterwards. Weaker orgasm-like sensations can also be produced by stretching of the bladder and rectum and this helps to explain some of the pleasurable relief of urination and defecation. Stretching the stomach can convey pleasurable sensations of fullness or uncomfortable sensations of nausea. In both cases exposure to the endogenous peptide (endorphin or endoloxone) may contribute to these sensations. Stretching striated muscles produces pleasure as in massage. Stretching probably also is involved in laughing as the air forced against the tissue of the lung stretches it. Stretch receptor physiology in smooth muscles has been severely neglected probably because these receptors are difficult to isolate and record from.

Gonadal hormones such as oestrogen and testosterone facilitate sexual activities, and to the extent that these are energy consuming they are endoloxonergic. The hormones of the pituitary and hypothalamus related to gonadal function may be the major endoloxonergic hormones of adolescence and young adulthood. In support of this connection, withdrawal from morphine, a major endoloxonergic upheaval, produces spontaneous ejaculation and orgasm.

Acknowledgements

This work was supported by grant No. BNS 77–22630, from the National Science Foundation.

References

Akil, H., Madden, R. P., and Barchas, J. D. (1976). Opiates and endogenous opioid peptides. In Kosterlitz, H. (ed.) *Opiates and Endogenous Peptides*. p.63 (Amsterdam: North-Holland)

Beevar, S., Beloff-Chain, A., Donaldson, A. L. and Edwardson, J. A. (1977). Stress-induced increase in endogenous opiate peptides – concurrent analgesia and its partial reversal by nolotone. *J. Physiol.*, **275**, 550

Blank, M. S., Panerai, A. E. and Friesen, H. G. (1979). Opioid peptides modulate luteinizing hormone secretion during sexual maturation. *Science*, **203**, 1129

Borison, H. L., Fishbaum, B. R., Bende, N. K. and McCarthy, L. E. (1962). Morphine-induced hyperglycemia in the cat. *J. Pharmacol. Exp. Ther.*, **138**, 229

Brodie, B. B. and Maickel, R. P. (1963). Role of the sympathetic nervous system in drug induced fatty liver. *Ann. N.Y. Acad. Sci.*, **104**, 1049

Brodie, B. B., Maickel, R. P. and Stern, D. N. (1965). Autonomic nervous system and adipose tissue. In *Handbook of Physiology, Adipose Tissue*, Section 5, pp. 583–600. (Washington, D.C.: American Physiological Society.)

Brun, J. F., van Vugt, D., Marshall, S. and Meites, J. (1977). Effects of naloxone, morphine and methionine encephalin on serum prolactin, lutenizing hormone, follicle stimulating hormone, thyroid stimulating hormone, and growth hormone. *Life Sci.*, **21**, 461

Cahill, Jr., G. F. (1976). Starvation in man. *Clin. Endocrinol. Metab.*, **5**, 397

Cannon, W. B. (1929). *Bodily Changes in Pain, Hunger, Fear, and Rage*, 2nd Edn. (New York: Appleton)

Daniel, E. E. (1968). Pharmacology of the gastrointestinal tract. In *Handbook of Physiology*, Section 6, Volume 4, pp. 2267–2324. (Washington, D.C.: American Physiological Society)

Demetrios, J. and Renault, P. (1966). *Narcotic Antagonist: Naltrexone Progress Report*. NIDA Research Monograph 9. Available from the National Technical Information Service, Springfield, Va. 22161, order no. PB255833

Feldberg, W. and Shaligram, S. V. (1972). The hyperglycaemic effect of morphine. *Br. J. Pharmacol.*, **46**, 602

Ferre, S., Reina, R. A., Santagostino, A., Scoto, G. M. and Spadaro, C. (1978). Effects of met-encephalin on body temperature of normal and morphine tolerant rats. *Psychopharmacology*, **58**, 277

Florez, J. and Mediavilla, A. (1977). Respiratory and cardiovascular effects of *meta*-enkephalen applied to the ventral surface of the brain stem. *Brain Res.*, **138**, 585

Freed, W. J., Perlow, M. J., Carman, J. S. and Wyatt, R. J. (1978). *Calcitonin and Feeding*. Abstract 528, *Soc. Neurosci.*, **4,**

Goodman, H. M. and Knobil, E. (1959). Effect of adrenergic blocking agents on fatty and mobilization during fasting. *Proc. Soc. Exp. Biol. Med.*, **102**, 493

Goodman, L. S. and Gilman, A. (1975). *The Pharmacological Basis of Therapeutics*. (New York: Macmillan Publishing Company)

Gopalan, C. and Krishnaswarmy, K. (1975). Famine oedema. *Prog. Food Nutri. Sci.*, **1**, 207

Grivert, P., Baizman, E. R. and Goldstein, A. (1978). Naloxone response of hypophysectomized and adrenalectomized mice. *Life Sci.*, **23**, 723

Guillemin, R., Vargo, T., Rossier, J., Minick, S., Ling, N., Rivier, S., Vale, W. and Bloom, F. (1977). *Science*, **197**, 1367

Henriksen, S. J., Bloom, F. E., McCoy, F., Ling, N. and Guillemin, R. (1978). β-Endorphin induces non-convulsive limbic seizures. *Proc. Natl. Acad. Sci.*, **75**, 5221

Holaday, J. W. and Faden, A. I. (1978). Naloxone reversal of endotoxin hypotension suggests role of endorphens in shock. *Nature (London)*, **275**, 450

Ipp, E., Dobbs, R. and Unger, R. H. (1978). Morphine and β-endorphin influence the secretion of the endocrine pancreas. *Nature (London)*, **276**, 190

Konturek, S. J., Tasler, Aeszkowski, M., Jaworeb, J., Cov, D. H. and Schally, A. V. (1978). Inhibition of pancreatic secretion by enkephalin and morphine in dogs. *Gastroenterology*, **74**, 851

Stetoemetrias, J. and Renault, P. (1966). *Narcotic Antagonists: Naltrexone Progress Report*. NIDA Research Monograph 9. Available from the National Technical Information Service, Springfield, Va. 22161, order no. PB 255833

Maickel, R. P., Braude, M. C. and Zabik, J. E. (1977). The effects of various narcotic agonists and antagonists on deprivation-induced fluid consumption. *Neuropharmacology*, **16**, 863

Maickel, R. P. and Brodie, B. B. (1963). Interaction of drugs with the pituitary adrenocortical system in the production of the fatty liver. *Ann. N.Y. Acad. Sci.*, **104**, 1059

Margules, D. L. (1978). Molecular theory of obesity sterility and other behavioural and endocrine problems in genetically obese mice (*ob/ob*). *Neurosci. Bio. Behav. Rev.*, **2**, 231

Margules, D. L., Flynn, J. J., Walker, J. and Cooper, C. W. (1979). Elevation of calcitonin immunoreactivity in the pituitary and thyroid glands of genetically obese rats (*fa/fa*). *Res. Bull.*, **4**, 589

Margules, D. L., Moisset, B., Lewis, M. J., Shibuya, H. and Pert, C. B. (1978). β-Endorphin is associated with overeating in genetically obese mice (*ob/ob*) and rats (*fa/fa*). *Science*, **202**, 988

Moss, I. R. and Friedman, E. (1978). k -endorphin: effects on respiratory regulation. *Life Sci.*, **23**, 1271

Mrosovsky, N. (1971). *Hibernation and the Hypothalamus.* (New York: Appleton-Century-Crofts)

Orias, R. and McCann, S. M. (1972). Natriuresis induced by α- and β-melanocyte stimulating hormone (MSH) in rats. *Endocrinology*, **90**, 700

Owen, O. E., Reichard Jr., G. A., Patel, M. S. and Boden, G. (1979). Energy metabolism in feasting and fasting. In Klacko, D. M., Anderson, R. R. and Heimberg, M. (eds.) *Hormones and Energy Metabolism.* (New York: Plenum Press).

Pert, C. B. and Snyder, S. H. (1974). Operate receptor binding agonists and antagonists affected differently by sodium. *Mol. Pharmacol.*, **10**, 868

Quarantotti, B. P., Corda, M. G., Paglielli, E., Biggio, G. and Gessa, G. L. (1978). Inhibition of copulatory behaviour in male rats by D-ALA²-Met-enhephalinamide. *Life Sci.*, **23**, 673

Rasmussen, H. (1974). Parathyroid hormone, calcitonin and the calciferols. In Williams, R. H. (ed.) *Textbook of Endocrinology.* (Philadelphia: W. B. Saunders)

Reilly, M. A., Kline, N. I. and Smith, A. A. (1978). Uptake of 125 by mouse tissue after intravenous injection of [¹²⁵I] β-endorphin. *Fed. Proc.*, **37**, 237

Rossier, J., Rodgers, J., Hibasaki, T., Guillemin, R. and Bloom, F. E. (1979). Opiod peptides and α-melanocyte-stimulating hormone in genetically obese (*ob/ob*) mice during development. *Proc. Natl. Acad. Sci. USA*, **76**, 2077

Stern, D. and Maickel, R. P. (1963). Studies in starvation induced hypermobilization of free fatty acids. *Life Sci.*, **2**, 872

Tseng, L., Loh, H. H. and Li, C. H. (1976). Human β-endorphin: development of tolerance and behavioural activity in rats. *Biochem. Biophys. Res. Commun.*, **74**, 390

Tseng, L. F., Loh, H. H. and Li, C. H. (1978). β-Endorphin: antidiurectic effects in rats. *Int. J. Protein Res.*, **12**, 173

Vagenakis, A. G., Burger, A., Portray, G. I., Rudolph, M., O'Brian, J. T., Azizi, F., Arky, R. A., Nicod, P., Ongbar, S. H. and Braverman, L. E. (1975). Diversion of peripheral thyroxine metabolism from activating to inactivating pathways during complete fasting. *J. Clin. Endocrinol. Metab.*, **41**, 191

Wei, E. and Loh, H. (1976). Physical dependence on opiate-like peptides. *Science*, **193**, 1262

Wenick, M. (ed.) (1979). *Hunger Disease: Studies by the Jewish Physicians in the Warsaw ghetto.* (New York: John Wiley and Sons)

15
The pharmacology of tobacco smoking in relation to schizophrenia

G. H. HALL

The smoking of tobacco in its various forms has persisted for centuries and continues today in spite of the tremendous publicity given to its adverse effects. The reasons why people smoke are varied and complex. Sociological, psychological and pharmacological factors all play an important role in the development and maintenance of the smoking habit. It is now generally accepted that many smokers who inhale are smoking for and become dependent on the nicotine content of tobacco smoke. Studies in both experimental animals and man during the last decade have contributed to a better understanding of the effects of nicotine and tobacco smoke on the central nervous system and to the establishing of a pharmacological basis for the tobacco smoking habit (Armitage, Hall and Morrison, 1968; Hall, 1970; Hall and Morrison, 1973; Ashton et al., 1978; Hall, Francis and Morrison, 1978).

In a recent survey carried out by the Schizophrenia Association of Great Britain, approximately 50% of those who responded indicated an addiction to smoking, possibly reflecting a dependence on nicotine. Whilst the sample was relatively small and the results therefore difficult to place in perspective with regard to the smoking population as a whole, it is nevertheless of interest to consider briefly the data obtained. 43% of those schizophrenics who were smokers indicated that they smoked thirty or more cigarettes per day. The number of cigarettes smoked also appeared with some individuals to be related to the particular stage of the illness and the amount of tension or agitation experienced.

Studies in both experimental animals and human subjects have demonstrated that nicotine and tobacco smoking can produce dose-related stimulant and depressant effects on the brain (Armitage, Hall and Sellers, 1969; Ashton *et al.*, 1978). A consideration of the pharmacology of tobacco smoking in relation to schizophrenia may therefore provide a further understanding of the pharmacological and biochemical mechanisms which play a role in the onset and recurrence of the disease process. In this context, effects on the central nervous system of tobacco smoke and more particularly of nicotine will be considered, with the emphasis on effects on chemical neurotransmitter and related systems. In addition, attention will be directed to a possible relationship between tobacco smoking, stress and schizophrenia.

NEUROTRANSMITTERS AND NEUROMODULATORS

Acetylcholine

In 1944, Cohen *et al.* reported on the striking amelioration of one patient's schizophrenic illness following the administration of acetylcholine. The study involved the administration of convulsant doses of acetylcholine to a group of eleven schizophrenic patients, eight of whom showed no general therapeutic benefit. In one patient there was slight, and in another moderate improvement. The condition of a third patient underwent a dramatic remission. However, it was concluded that the therapeutic results did not justify the continued use of acetylcholine as a form of treatment in schizophrenia, since the margin of safety of the drug appeared to be extremely slight. More recently, there have been a number of pharmacological and metabolic investigations focussed on the possible role of cholinergic mechanisms in schizophrenia and these have been reviewed by Davis *et al.* (1978). Some studies have indicated that increasing central cholinergic activity may improve schizophrenic symptoms. For example, exacerbation of the symptoms of schizophrenia by the intravenous administration of the dopamine agonist methylphenidate was shown to be reversed by injection of physostigmine. However, in contrast, other studies have shown that intravenous physostigmine does not improve schizophrenic symptoms.

Dale (1914) when studying the actions of certain esters of choline including acetylcholine, concluded that 'two distinct types of action can be detected – a "muscarine" action, paralysed by atropine, and a "nicotine" action, paralysed by excess of nicotine'. Thus many of the central and peripheral actions of acetylcholine can be mimicked by nicotine, in that nicotine can act on specific cholinoceptive structures or receptor sites at which acetylcholine would normally act to produce a nicotinic effect.

Some central actions of nicotine are potentiated by physostigmine, indicating an involvement of acetylcholine in the response, and nicotine has also been shown to release acetylcholine from the central nervous system. Nicotine injected into a lateral ventricle of the brain of conscious or anaesthetized cats causes a twitching of the ears, salivation, respiratory changes and a fall in blood pressure sometimes accompanied by a decrease in heart rate. Physostigmine injected intravenously, or neostigmine injected into a lateral ventricle, potentiated the ear response and fall in blood pressure produced by intraventricular nicotine (Armitage and Hall, 1967). The involvement of acetylcholine in the nicotine response was further confirmed by demonstrating inhibition of the response by the acetylcholine synthesis inhibitor hemicholinium, followed by restoration of the response with choline. The effects of small amounts of nicotine on electrocortical activity and cortical acetylcholine release were studied in anaesthetized cats (Armitage, Hall and Sellers, 1969). The most common effect of nicotine given intravenously, in a dose of 2 μg/kg every 30 s for 20 min, was to cause desynchronization of the electrocorticogram, indicating cortical activation, and an increase in the release of cortical acetylcholine. A larger dose given less frequently (4 μg/kg every min for 20 min) caused in some experiments an increase and in others a decrease in cortical activity. Such changes were accompanied respectively by an increase or decrease in cortical acetylcholine output. The amounts of nicotine that affected the electrocorticogram and modified acetylcholine release were similar to those absorbed by the cigarette smoker who inhales.

Catecholamines

Noradrenaline

In 1971, Stein and Wise postulated that the fundamental symptoms of schizophrenia were due to a dysfunction of central noradrenergic pathways. Their hypothesis was based on a concept of schizophrenia in which disturbance of affect was thought to occur as a consequence of a deficiency in the 'pleasure resources' of the schizophrenic subject. They demonstrated that reward and goal-oriented behaviour, which are disturbed in schizophrenia, are the function of a dorsal noradrenergic pathway which orginates in the locus coeruleus and innervates the cerebral cortex and hippocampus. They further demonstrated that dopamine-β-hydroxylase was significantly reduced in the central nervous system of schizophrenic patients and that this enzyme deficit was particularly pronounced in the diencephalon and hippocampus (Wise and Stein, 1973).

Seevers (1968) has proposed that cigarette smoking induces psychological dependence as a consequence of the stimulant action of nicotine on brain reward systems. If nicotine increases directly, or indirectly, the excitability of reward systems, it should be possible to demonstrate that nicotine can (a) facilitate the rewarding effects of electrical stimulation of the hypothalamus and (b) cause release of noradrenaline at central synapses associated with reward mechanisms. Nicotine has been shown to have a facilitatory effect on self-stimulation (Wanner and Battig, 1968), and thus indirectly on pleasure-seeking behaviour. It has been suggested that nicotine, by acting on a central cholinergic receptor, may indirectly cause release of noradrenaline which, in turn, produces the facilitatory effect on self-stimulation (Pradhan and Bowling, 1971). Similarly, nicotine like acetylcholine causes a release of noradrenaline from the hypothalamus (Hall and Turner, 1972). Cigarette smoke introduced into the lungs and nicotine injected intravenously, or perfused through the hypothalamic region of the third cerebral ventricle, increased the efflux of [^{3}H]-noradrenaline into the perfusate collected from the cerebroventricular system of the anaesthetized cat (Hall and Turner, 1972).

Nicotine has also been shown to cause changes in the output of [^{3}H]-noradrenaline from perfused rat hypothalamic slices (Hall and Turner, 1972) and Balfour (1973, 1978) has demonstrated an increase in the release and a decrease in retention of [^{3}H] noradrenaline by synaptosomes prepared from rat hypothalumus. Experimental evidence is therefore available which may provide a link for the suggestion that some schizophrenic subjects appear to be heavy smokers and this may be as a consequence of an action of nicotine on brain reward systems, possibly mediated by the release of noradrenaline at central synapses.

Dopamine

It is now generally accepted that dopamine plays a key role in mental function, although Carlsson (1978) rightly draws our attention to the fact that whereas a primary disturbance in dopaminergic function in schizophrenia cannot be ruled out, the intimate relationship between dopaminergic and other systems must be emphasized and the possible involvement of other transmitters cannot be disregarded. Systemic injection of nicotine in rats causes a decrease followed by an increase in the firing rate of nigrostriatal dopaminergic neurons. However, applied directly to the cell by micro-iontophoresis, only an increase in cell firing occurred without the transient initial depression (Lichtensteiger et al., 1976). In contrast, physostigmine injected systemically elicited an increase in the firing rate of zona compacta neurons followed by a prolonged decrease. Lichtensteiger et al., (1976) have suggested that the effects of nicotine suggest the existence of a cholinergic input to nigral dopaminergic neurons and that the biphasic effect of nicotine may indicate a complex local circuitry consisting of stimulatory as well as inhibitory cholinergic mechanisms. Systemic administration of nicotine was also shown to cause a significant rise in homovanillic acid in the caudate nucleus.

Treatment of animals with nicotine causes a marked lowering of prolactin and growth hormone levels in the rat (Lichtensteiger et al., 1978). The effect of nicotine on prolactin secretion appeared to have been mediated by tuberoinfundibular dopamine neurones, since it was completely reversed by pimozide. In contrast, this dopamine blocking agent did not affect the reduction of serum growth hormone by nicotine.

Prostaglandins

Recently, evidence has been presented which suggests a possible link between schizophrenia and a disturbance in prostaglandin metabolism in the central nervous system. Feldberg (1976) has postulated that schizophrenia may be associated with increased prostaglandin synthesis in certain parts of the brain. This hypothesis was based on the findings that (i) catalepsy, which is the nearest equivalent in animals to human catatonia, develops in cats when prostaglandin E_1 is injected into the cerebral ventricles and when during endotoxin or lipid A fever the prostaglandin E_2 level in cisternal cerebrospinal fluid rises to high levels; however, when fever and the prostaglandin level was brought down by non-steroidal antipyretics which inhibit prostaglandin synthesis, catalepsy disappeared as well and (ii) febrile episodes are a genuine syndrome of schizophrenia.

In contrast, Horrobin (1977, 1979) has suggested that schizophrenia may be a prostaglandin deficiency disease. This proposal was based on the prolactin and therefore prostaglandin stimulating properties of antischizophrenic drugs, on the resistance to pain, inflammation, and inflammatory diseases shown by schizophrenics and on the occurrence of schizophrenic-like psychoses in individuals treated with drugs which have prostaglandin antagonist actions. Nicotine and tobacco smoke have not yet been shown to have an action on prostaglandins within the brain. However, using the perfused isolated heart of the rabbit, Wennalm (1978) demonstrated that nicotine increased the outflow of a prostaglandin-like material, probably by an action dissociated from its noradrenaline liberating properties. The exposure of rats to tobacco smoke has been shown to cause a decrease in the metabolism of prostaglandin E_2 in the lungs (Bahkle et al., 1979). If nicotine and tobacco smoke can modify prostaglandin metabolism in peripheral tissues, then the possibility exists that they could exert similar actions within the brain.

In suggesting that schizophrenia may be associated with increased prostaglandin synthesis in certain parts of the brain, Feldberg (1976) cited evidence from the literature which demonstrates that an elevated body temperature may be a syndrome of schizophrenia. It is therefore of interest to consider that nicotine injected into or perfused through the cerebral ventricles, or directly into specific regions of the hypothalamus of rat (Lomax and Kirkpatrick, 1969; Knox and Lomax, 1972), cat (Hall, 1972) and rhesus monkey (Hall and Myers, 1971, 1972) can cause changes in body temperature. In the cat and monkey, depending on the route and site of injection, the most common effect of nicotine was to produce a fall in body temperature, similar responses being obtained with an acetylcholine–physostigmine mixture and with noradrenaline. It is not the intention to suggest that if the smoking of tobacco appears to be particularly important for some schizophrenics, then this is due to the fact that they are smoking to obtain nicotine in order to counter an elevated body temperature possibly accompanying a psychotic episode or state. Simply, it may indicate that if the mechanisms responsible for the psychosis and febrile episode result from an imbalance of the same chemical substance within the brain, particularly neurotransmitters, then the fact that nicotine can reduce body temperature, possibly by release of noradrenaline, may suggest some disturbance of noradrenergic systems in schizophrenia.

STRESS

Studies of the environmental circumstances which may contribute to the development of the smoking habit suggest that nicotine, in the medium of tobacco smoke, may help to alleviate the effects of stress mediated by psychological or physical discomfort. Smokers do appear to smoke, or to smoke more, when exposed to an emotionally stressful situation (Kissen, 1960), and from the available evidence it seems that such a situation can contribute not only to the beginning of the smoking habit, but also to its continuation and to the number of cigarettes consumed.

It is thus of interest that Hartmann (1976) has put forward the theory that in schizophrenia there may be some form of basic deficit producing a vulnerability to stress. Hartmann suggests that a deficient functioning of brain noradrenaline systems may underline the deficit, which could be in the area of feedback processing. He further postulates that the basic deficit, which is probably genetic, producing susceptibility to schizophrenia could be at the dopamine-β hydroxylase step and suggests that this could explain the acute sensitivity of schizophrenics to stress, since at times of stress noradrenaline would be reduced and synthesis of dopamine but not of noradrenaline would be increased. If this theory is accepted, the ability of nicotine to cause release of noradrenaline within the brain may account for the fact that not only do supposedly normal subjects appear to react to stressful situations by increasing their nicotine intake, but also in schizophrenics the number of cigarettes smoked appears to relate, at least for some individuals, to the amount of tension or agitation experienced.

In 1973, Hall and Morrison presented new evidence for a relationship between tobacco smoking, nicotine dependence and stress. This followed from an attempt to find an animal model for a stressful situation in which habitual smokers might feel the need to smoke and become dependent on nicotine. It was shown that dependence on nicotine could be demonstrated in animals following prolonged administration of the drug (Hall and Morrison, 1973; Hall, Francis and Morrison, 1978). In these experiments, it was necessary to choose a situation in which measurable and adaptive behaviour could be evoked, thus enabling the effects of nicotine and its withdrawal to be studied. A shock avoidance schedule was chosen (Sidman, 1953), because any disruption of lever pressing behaviour resulting from the withdrawl of nicotine would be readily detectable as an increase in the number of shocks received. Whilst rats can be trained to avoid programmed electric shocks by pressing a lever, this type of behaviour is difficult to learn and the situation is stressful (Weiss, 1971). The greatest stress is produced by avoidance shedules in which there are no signals preceding the delivery of shock or following an effective response.

Rats which had received nicotine during training pressed the lever more often and took fewer shocks than their saline trained partners. When saline was substituted for nicotine, the number of shocks received by the nicotine trained rats increased to such an extent that most took more shocks than did their saline trained partners. The nicotine trained rats had thus become dependent on nicotine for a successful performance and in its absence they coped less effectively with the situation than did rats which had never experienced the drug.

A second series of experiments was performed to study the effects of withdrawing nicotine in a less stressful situation, using a feedback or 'safety' signal to indicate a correct response. This safety signal reduces the stressful effects of an avoidance situation (Weiss, 1971). In this situation, there was no disruption of behaviour following substitution of saline for nicotine, as indicated by the number of shocks received. However, when the safety signal was discontinued, and saline substituted for nicotine, the performance of the nicotine trained rats deteriorated. Thus rats which had learned under the influence of nicotine to avoid an electric shock in the absence of any feedback signal had become dependent on nicotine for an effective performance. The presence of the safety signal reduced this dependence, probably by reducing the degree of stress to which the animal was exposed. The stressful effects of unsignalled avoidance schedules and a reduced level of stress in signalled avoidance schedules are well documented (see Hall and Morrison, 1973).

The possibility that tobacco smoking may alleviate stress as a result of an action of nicotine on pituitary–adrenocortical function has been suggested by Hall, Francis and Morrison (1978). Nicotine injected into or perfused through the cerebral ventricles of anaesthetized cats and rats caused a fall in plasma corticosteroid levels. However, in contrast, nicotine administered systemically can cause a rise in circulating plasma corticosteroid concentrations, possibly due to direct stimulation of the adrenal cortex (Rubin and Warner, 1975). In individuals having an inadequate response to stress, cigarette smoking may therefore enhance their ability to cope with stressful situations by augmenting steroid output, or may alleviate a stress response by reducing activity in the pituitary–adrenocortical system.

Thus the ability of nicotine to modify a stress response may be one of the reasons why the normal population and also schizophrenic subjects indulge in the tobacco smoking habit.

References

Armitage, A. K and Hall, G. H. (1967). Further evidence relating to the mode of action of nicotine in the central nervous system. *Nature (London)*, **214**, 977

Armitage, A. K., Hall, G. H. and Morrison, C. F. (1968). Pharmacological basis for the tobacco smoking habit. *Nature, (London)*, **217**, 331

Armitage, A. K., Hall, G. H. and Sellers, C. M. (1969). Effects of nicotine on electrocortical activity and acetylcholine release from the cat cerebral cortex. *Br. J. Pharmacol.*, **35**, 152

Ashton, H., Millman, J. E., Rawlins, M. D., Telford, R. and Thompson, J. W. (1978). The use of event related slow potentials of the brain in the analysis of effects of cigarette smoking and nicotine in humans. In Battig, K. (ed.) *Behavioural Effects of Nicotine*, pp. 26–37. (Basel: Karger)

Bahkle Y. S., Hartiala, J., Toivonen, H. and Votila, P. (1979). Effects of cigarette smoke on the metabolism of vasoactive hormones in rat isolated lung. *Br. J. Pharmacol.*, **65**, 495

Balfour, D. J. K. (1973). Effects of nicotine on the uptake and retention of noradrenaline and 5-hydroxytryptamine by rat brain homogenates. *Eur. J. Pharmacol.*, **23**, 19

Balfour, D. J. K. (1978). Biochemical approach to the study of nicotine dependence in rats. In Battig, K. (ed.) *Behavioural Effects of Nicotine*, pp. 83–93. (Basel: Karger)

Carlsson, A. (1978). Antipsychotic drugs, neurotransmitters and schizophrenia. *Am. J. Psychiatry*, **135**, 164

Cohen, L. H., Thale, T. and Tissenbaum, M. J. (1944). Acetylcholine treatment of schizophrenia. *Arch. Neurol. Psychiatry*, **51**, 171

Dale, H. H. (1914), The action of certain esters and ethers of choline and their relation to muscarine. *J. Pharmacol. Exp. Ther.* **6**, 147

Davis, K. L., Berger, P. A., Hollister, L. E. and Barchas, J. D. (1978). Cholinergic involvement in mental disorders. *Life Sci.*, **22**, 1865

Feldberg, W. (1976). Possible assocation of schizophrenia with a disturbance in prostaglandin metabolism: a physiological hypothesis. *Psychol. Med*, **6**, 359

Hall, G. H. (1970). Effects of nicotine and tobacco smoke on the electrical activity of the cerebral cortex and olfactory bulb. *Br. J. Pharmacol.*, **38**, 271

Hall, G. H. (1972). Changes in body temperature produced by cholinomimetic substances injected into the cerebral ventricles of unanaesthetized cats. *Br. J. Pharmacol.*, **44**, 634

Hall, G. H., Francis, R. L. and Morrison, C. F. (1978). Nicotine dependence, avoidance behaviour and pituitary-adrenocortical function. In Battig, K. (ed.) *Behavioural Effects of Nicotine*, pp. 94–107. (Basel: Karger)

Hall, G. H. and Morrison, C. F. (1973). New evidence for a relationship between tobacco smoking, nicotine dependence and stress. *Nature (London)*, **243**, 199

Hall, G. H. and Myers, R. D. (1971). Hypothermia produced by nicotine perfused through the cerebral ventricles of the unanaesthetized monkey. *Neuropharmacology*, **10**, 391

Hall, G. H. and Myers, R. D. (1972). Temperature changes produced by nicotine injected into the hypothalamus of the conscious monkey. *Brain Res.*, **37**, 241

Hall, G. H. and Turner, D. M. (1972). Effects of nicotine on the release of ^{3}H-noradrenaline from the hypothalamus. *Biochem. Pharmacol.*, **21**, 1829

Hartmann, E. (1976). Schizophrenia: a theory. *Psychopharmacology*, **49**, 1

Horrobin, D. F. (1977). Schizophrenia as a prostaglandin deficiency disease. *Lancet*, **1**, 936

Horrobin, D. F. (1979). Possible role of prostaglandin deficiency in schizophrenia: Relevance for the dopamine, opioid and pineal deficiency concepts of the disease. (This volume)

Kissen, D. M. (1960). Psycho-social factors in cigarette smoking motivation. *Med. Offr.*, **104**, 365

Knox, G. V. and Lomax, P. (1972). The effect of nicotine on thermosensitive units in the rostral hypothalamus. *Proc. West. Pharmacol. Soc.*, **15**, 179

Lichtensteiger, W., Felix, D., Lienhart, R. and Hefti, F. (1976). A quantitative correlation between single unit activity and fluorescence intensity of dopamine nerones in zona compacta of substantia nigra as demonstrated under the influence of nicotine and physostigmine. *Brain Res.*, **117**, 85

Lichtensteiger, W., Richards, J. G. and Kopp, H. G. (1978). Changes in the distribution of non-neuronal elements in rat median eminence and in anterior pituitary hormone secretion after activation of tuberoinfundibular dopamine neurones by brain stimulation or nicotine. *Brain Res.*, **157**, 73

Lomax, P. and Kirkpatrick, W. E. (1969). Cholinergic transmission in the thermoregulatory centers. (Abstract) *4th International Congress of Pharmacolgy*, p. 223. (Basel: Schwabe)

Pradhan, S. N. and Bowling, C. (1971). Effects of nicotine on self-stimulation in rats. *J. Pharmacol. Exp. Ther.*, **176**, 229

Rubin, R. P. and Warner, W. (1975). Nicotine-induced stimulation of steroidogenesis in adrenocortical cells of the cat. *Br. J. Pharmacol.*, **53**, 357

Seevers, M. H. (1968). Psychopharmacological elements of drug dependence. *J. Am. Med. Assoc.*, **206**, 1263

Sidman, M. (1953). Avoidance conditioning with brief shock and no exteroceptive warning signal. *Science*, **118**, 157

Stein, L. and Wise, D. (1971). Possible etiology of schizophrenia: Progressive damage to the noradrenergic reward system by 6-hydroxydopamine. *Science*, **171**, 1032

Wanner, H. V. and Battig, K. (1968). Die Wirkung von Nicotin und Amphetamin auf die subkortikale Selbstreizung der Ratte. *Z. Prav. Med.*, **13**, 101

Weiss, J. M. (1971). Effects of coping behaviour with and without a feedback signal on stress pathology in rats. *J. Comp. Physiol. Psychol.*, **77**, 22

Wennalm, A. (1978). Effects of nicotine on cardiac prostaglandin and platelet thromboxane synthesis. *Br. J. Pharmacol.*, **64**, 559

Wise, C. D. and Stein, L. (1973). Dopamine beta-hydroxylase deficits in the brain of schizophrenic patients. *Science*, **181**, 344

16
Alcoholism and schizophrenia: A basic science approach

J. M. LITTLETON

In this chapter I do not intend to draw any inferences as to a connection between alcoholism and schizophrenia. I feel that would not be justified by the evidence available. I do intend to draw some parallels between the condition of alcoholism and that of schizophrenia, and then to illustrate the direction in which research on alcoholism is now proceeding. I will also make some speculations as to whether a similar approach is possible in schizophrenia research, and whether this might be rewarding. The position I have taken, as suggested by the title, is that of a basic experimental scientist working in research. It is too soon to say that the approach to alcoholism which I will outline will have any relevance to the clinical treatment of alcoholism and similar constraints apply to all of my comments about schizophrenia.

PROBLEMS POSED BY RESEARCH INTO ALCOHOLISM AND SCHIZOPHRENIA

The first problem which confronts the research worker is one of definition, and here the parallels between alcoholism and schizophrenia are immediately apparent. Both are clinical conditions whose definition is vague and open to different interpretations. However, both have central characteristics on which most workers are agreed; alcoholism must have alcohol intake as the causative agent; schizophrenics should show evidence of hallucinations in one or more of the senses; and so on. After the establishment of these main signs, agreement ends; even when lip service is paid to some international definition interpretation between centres can vary widely. In the case of alcoholism there has recently been a move away from this largely indefinable term to consider the alcoholic in the quantifiable terms of his (or her) alcohol tolerance and alcohol dependence (Edwards and Gross, 1976). Quantifiable and precise terms are also needed in schizophrenia research, particularly if any correlation is to be obtained between a quantifiable postulated cause of the disease and the severity of the disease itself.

Implicit in my treatment to date has been the conviction that both alcoholism and schizophrenia can be regarded as disease states. In both cases the concept of a 'disease' has not been universally accepted, and it is only relatively recently that a majority of workers would accept a primarily biological basis for either condition. The concept of a 'disease' implies a physical or chemical cause and this is much more easy to defend in the case of alcoholism. Here the cause is obvious; it is alcohol. And yet the enormously varied presentation of alcoholism has been used to bring into question whether alcohol intake is *the* most important cause of the illness. This argument seems to me to ignore a fundamental point in medicine that all illness is the end result of an interaction between the causative agent, the host and the environment. When one considers the enormous variation in human response which the same acute dose of alcohol may produce in different individuals, it does not seem at all surprising that chronic excessive intake should also affect people in different ways.

Similar arguments have been used for schizophrenia. Its presentations vary so widely that it is hard to imagine that one causative agent is involved and it is suggested that, if it is a disease at all, then many different causes are responsible. I do not necessarily share this view. Schizophrenia can be regarded as a disease entity in that patients so diagnosed do share some characteristic signs. The simplest solution is that some basic defect is produced in all schizophrenics and that this is manifest in different ways depending on the individual afflicted (host), and his or her circumstances (environment).

A disease, whether its cause be physical, microbiological or chemical, should be capable of being produced in other animals which share the peculiar aspect of man's physiology or biochemistry affected by the causative agent. In many cases, including alcoholism and schizophrenia, this has been particularly difficult to achieve. It is only about 10 years since viable animal models of alcohol dependence were achieved for use with laboratory animals (for review, see Friedman and Lester, 1977) and this has meant great advances in our ability to study this condition. Before this development many workers had despaired of ever achieving an animal model which reproduced so many of the psychological and physical aspects of alcoholism, and the acceptance of such models is still far from universal. In the case of schizophrenia the situation is far more difficult; animal models based on acute administration of an hallucinogenic drug or chronic administration of amphetamines have been used, but there is of course no way of knowing precisely whether the perceptual and psychological changes they produce in an animal can be equated with those experienced by the schizophrenic. In any event just because the final outcome of drug administration bears a resemblance to a disease, this does not necessarily mean that the mechanism of drug action bears any relationship to the cause of the disease.

Many other problems are posed by work into alcoholism and schizophrenia, and these can largely be attributed to difficulties inherent in clinical research into disease processes affecting the central nervous system. I refer to the difficulties in comparing results between individuals, obtaining viable material from human brain, obtaining material before treatment has been instituted and so on. All are problems met in both conditions, but the difference is that animal models for alcohol dependence now exist, and this has helped researchers focus on areas where useful clinical results in man may be sought. With the exception of focusing of attention on the dopamine and serotonin systems, partially attributable to knowledge gained from the pharmacology of hallucinogenic drugs on animals, such a situation does not yet obtain in schizophrenia research.

SOME BROAD SIMILARITIES BETWEEN ALCOHOLISM AND SCHIZOPHRENIA

Many of the *apparent* similarities between alcoholism and schizophrenia are products of the problems inherent in their investigation and have been discussed, albeit indirectly, in the last section. However, some similarities may provide evidence of a more fundamental relationship and these will now be treated briefly.

First alcoholism can itself be associated with a psychosis which mimics some aspects of schizophrenia. Delirium tremens, now generally acknowledged as a manifestation of the syndrome of withdrawal or partial withdrawal of alcohol, often includes hallucinations of the visual or tactile senses. Whether this drug withdrawal state can give any clues to the aetiology of schizophrenia is doubtful, but there is little doubt that some aspects of the end result are superficially similar (but see Alpert and Silvers (1970) for distinguishing characteristics).

The role of heredity in schizophrenia is a much advanced argument for the biochemical disease concept of the condition. In general terms it seems that liability to schizophrenia involves some genetic component, but that this is not as strong as that seen in many other inherited diseases. Much the same comments can be made of alcoholism (e.g. see Shields,

1977). The alcoholic seems to have some genetic predisposition, either to becoming addicted to the drug, or to its doing him or her particular physical or psychological harm. This need not imply that the causes of schizophrenia and alcoholism are genetically transmitted, as has often been argued, but simply that the contribution of host susceptibility to the causative agent is influenced by genetic complement.

There are as many theories of the basic mechanism of production of alcoholism as there are of schizophrenia, and this probably reflects the problems inherent in their study, as well as the unsatisfactory nature of all hypotheses advanced to date! A catalogue of some of the areas where hypotheses of alcoholism coincide with those of schizophrenia may be salutary. References are given only for alcoholism; those for schizophrenia will be found elsewhere in this book. Much work on alcoholism suggests involvement of the monoamine neurotransmitters in the brain (e.g. Tabakoff, 1977) and, like schizophrenia, alterations in dopamine receptor sensitivity have been suggested to play a role in alcohol tolerance (e.g. Hoffman & Tabakoff, 1977). Alcoholism has also been associated with peptide neurotransmitters (see Blum *et al.*, 1977) and a link between alcohol, amines and opiate-like peptides has been suggested by the possibility that tetrahydroisoquinoline compounds with morphine-like effects may be formed during chronic ethanol administration (e.g. Hirst *et al.*, 1977). It is interesting to see that isoquinolines have now been implicated in the altered dopamine receptor function thought to occur in schizophrenia (see Abell, Chapter 6). Alcoholism, like schizophrenia, has been suggested to be associated with food allergies (Ulett *et al.*, 1974) although how these could *produce* the central nervous system condition I have never fully understood. The effects of environment, age, stress and hormonal changes have all been proposed as important in the genesis of alcoholism and schizophrenia, and it seems very likely that there is truth in these generalizations, although such observations do not necessarily take us any closer to the cause of the conditions.

One aspect of both conditions, which has impressed me, but which may well be disputed by others, is the wide variety of disorders (or absence of disorders) associated with the conditions. For example, schizophrenics have been reported to show disorders in their platelet function (see Chapters 1, 6 and 13) as have alcoholics (Haut and Cowan, 1974). Schizophrenics have lower incidence of inflammatory disease; moderate intake of alcohol may protect against coronary heart disease (Barboriak *et al.*, 1979). Numerous other examples can be cited where research workers have claimed differences in this or that peripheral response between control subjects and patients with schizophrenia or alcoholism. In the case of alcoholics the reason is not difficult to find; alcohol itself is a very non-specific drug. Given in sufficient quantities it will affect the cell membrane of every cell in the body (see below). It is unsurprising therefore, that many tissues are affected by chronic administration of alcohol, and that alcoholics show dysfunction of many organs. If the same is true of schizophrenics, and here there is dispute, then schizophrenia should perhaps be viewed as a widespread disorder which affects many tissues, but which has its most noticeable effect, like alcohol, on the central nervous system.

One approach to alcohol research, which has recently begun to bear fruit, is to investigate the effects of chronic administration of the drug, not only on cells of the mammalian central nervous system, but also on cells of other organisms and on peripheral mammalian cells. Schizophrenia research has not yet exhausted the possibilities of looking at cells from the peripheral tissues of schizophrenics for disorders which may mirror the changes in the brain. From my position of relative ignorance, a likely candidate for investigation as a neuronal model in this respect might be the blood platelet. The ubiquity of reported differences between normal subjects and schizophrenics suggests that some fundamental response of the cell might be altered, and that areas such as membrane function, responses of membrane-bound enzymes and the release of intracellular components would be interesting areas to consider. In this respect Professor Horrobin's hypothesis (Chapter 1) suggesting a widespread defect in prostaglandin E_1 metabolism seems to me to be along the right lines, but at the moment too narrow a hypothesis, and with far too little direct evidence to support the edifice he has erected.

This brief consideration of hypothetical mechanisms for alcoholism and schizophrenia leads me to the conclusion that neither have been approached in a very coherent manner by the groups of research workers concerned. This is much more excusable in the case of schizophrenia, where lack of knowledge of the causative agent and inability to use animals for research are grave setbacks. In the case of current alcohol research I believe the climate is changing and that a basic understanding of the mechanism of action of the drug and of the responses which bring about tolerance and dependence in the mammal exposed to ethanol is now close to being achieved. This has been aided by what I call 'a basic science approach' and I make no excuses for my bias toward this line of research and the results obtained from it. Time alone will tell whether it has any more validity than its predecessors.

BASIC CONSIDERATIONS OF ALCOHOLISM

Alcoholism implies social, psychological or physical harm from chronic excessive intake of ethanol; as discussed previously it is a vague concept, and in many respects it is not applicable to the animal experiments which I shall mainly consider. I shall deal primarily with the effects of acute administration of ethanol, the development of tolerance to these acute effects and the development of physical dependence when administration is continued.

Acute administration of alcohol to laboratory animals, or man, in doses which produce brain ethanol concentrations of about 0.5–1.0 $mg\,g^{-1}$ tissue is associated initially with excitement. If the concentration continues to rise, general signs of central nervous system depression supervene, associated with motor non-coordination at 2–3 $mg\,g^{-1}$ and stupor, coma and death at concentrations in excess of these. Responses vary somewhat between individuals based on previous history of exposure to alcohol, the circumstances under which the alcohol is given, and other factors of which comparatively little is known. This pattern of gradually increasing central depression seems to be common to most species, and the tissue levels of ethanol required to achieve each response do not vary markedly between individuals, strains or species.

On prolonged or repeated administration of alcohol all organisms seem capable of developing relatively normal function at higher and higher doses of the drug. This is explained in two ways. The organism may come to be able to excrete the drug more rapidly, preventing tissue concentrations from rising as high as in the 'naive' animal and eliminating the ethanol more rapidly. This is often referred to as 'dispositional' or 'metabolic' tolerance. Another kind of tolerance is referred to as 'functional' tolerance; in this state, the animal functions relatively normally despite higher and higher concentrations of ethanol in the central nervous system. This may be a function of the ability of the neurons themselves to adapt to the presence of ethanol and it is therefore often called 'cellular' tolerance.

If prolonged and heavy administration of ethanol is continued, to man and many other mammals, a state of physical dependence is induced. This is not well understood, but if ethanol is now removed from the animal concerned, it undergoes an ethanol withdrawal syndrome. In most animals this includes signs of intense excitation, followed by prostration in which severe convulsions may occur. In man hallucinations are also frequently reported. A high mortality can be associated with the untreated physical withdrawal syndrome (see Victor, 1970).

In my view the majority if not all the effects of ethanol just described can be explained by a simple interaction with the mammalian cell membrane.

ACUTE EFFECTS OF ETHANOL ON CELL MEMBRANES

Alcohols and anaesthetics, besides being central nervous system depressants, also have physical properties in common. One of the properties which correlates best with depressant activity within the homologous series of alcohols is their lipid solubility. There is considerable evidence (see Seeman, 1972) that the depressant properties of alcohols and anaesthetics are related to their ability to enter the lipids of cell membranes, and to expand and increase the fluid nature of these. In the brain one might predict that this increased 'fluidity' of synaptic membranes might initially cause excitation as more transmitter is released from presynaptic membranes, but be followed by depression at higher concentrations of ethanol, as postsynaptic receptor systems are disrupted and the normal mechanisms of transmitter release ultimately inhibited.

Until relatively recently there was no direct evidence that ethanol had any effect on the membranes of the mammalian synapse in concentrations associated with intoxication rather than anaesthesia. Indeed the lipid solubility of ethanol is low, making some workers reluctant to accept that it could act in the same general way as other alcohols. However, Chin and Goldstein (1977a) have now shown that ethanol can indeed increase the fluidity of synaptic membranes of brain, as well as cell membranes from other tissues, at concentrations similar to those found in intoxicated animals *in vivo*. The low lipid solubility of ethanol however probably makes a difference as to how far toward the centre of the membrane the alcohol can penetrate. A diagram showing how the situation may appear at the molecular level is shown in Figure 1.

The acute effects of ethanol on the mammal may therefore result from a purely physical effect on the lipids in the region of the water/lipid interface at the surfaces of synaptic membranes in the brain. This could produce the variety of changes in neurotransmitter metabolism, release and receptor sensitivity that have been reported after ethanol administration, since all membrane functions including those of membrane proteins, such as receptors and enzymes, are influenced by the fluidity of the surrounding lipid (for review see Farias *et al.*, 1975).

As yet we do not know the depth to which ethanol molecules can penetrate the membrane, although investigation of this is technically possible. It seems likely that the lipids which would be most influenced by ethanol include the phospholipid head groups, the proximal parts of their fatty acid side chains, and the molecules of cholesterol which are interpolated into mammalian membranes in various amounts (see Figure 2). It is these membrane lipids which should be most affected by ethanol. As to the effect of ethanol on membrane protein function our knowledge is as yet very imperfect. We can speculate however, that proteins which rest on the membrane, or which have active sites close to the lipid/water interface, will be those most affected. Since these proteins and lipids are probably those most affected by ethanol it is logical to look at them from the point of view of deciding which cell-membrane components might alter in order to overcome the continued physical presence of ethanol, i.e.

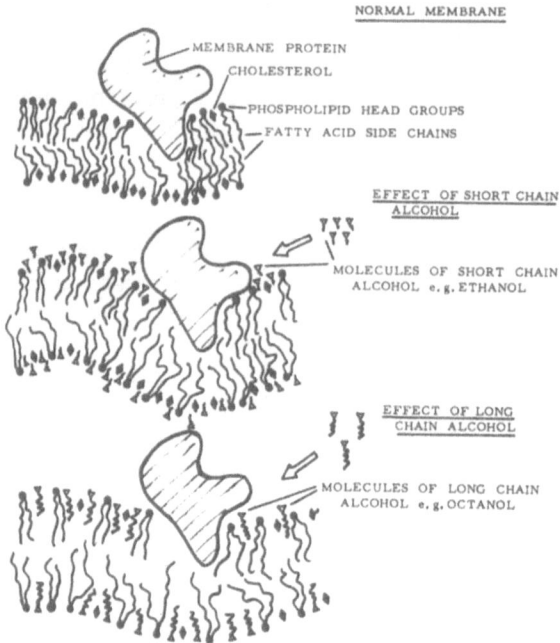

Figure 1 Normally mammalian cell membranes are thought to exist as a relatively fluid lipid bilayer of phospholipids and cholesterol. Alcohols can enter this bilayer and expand and increase its fluid nature. In the case of the relatively lipid-insoluble shortchain alcohols, such as ethanol, this effect is relatively confined to the water–lipid interfaces, but more lipid-soluble alcohols can interpolate their longer hydrocarbon chains deeper into the bilayer and produce more widespread fluidization

to produce cellular tolerance. I shall concentrate on alteration in lipids, but there is no doubt that changes in protein configuration, and other membrane properties could also be associated with ethanol tolerance.

Alcohol tolerance at the level of the synaptic membrane

Before we can consider how a neuronal cell might respond to an agent (ethanol) which makes the surfaces of its cell membranes more fluid, we need to know a little of the biophysics of membranes in general. The fluidity of lipids is partly influenced by their unsaturation. Margarines which contain vegetable oils are more fluid, and "spread straight from the fridge", because they contain polyunsaturated fatty acids, whereas butter is relatively hard because it contains saturated fats. The same principle is true of mammalian cell membranes, the phospholipids, which usually represent the major lipid component of the membrane, have a head group, which may vary in nature, and two fatty acid side chains. The degree of unsaturation of the fatty acid side chains influences the overall fluidity of the membrane. The molecular organization is shown in Figure 2.

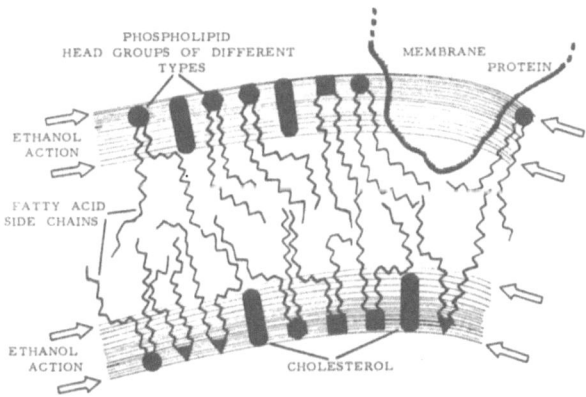

Figure 2 The sphere of influence of ethanol at the surface of the membrane probably does not extend further than the parts of the fatty acid side chains proximal to the phospholipid headgroups. This includes in addition, cholesterol molecules and possibly some active sites of membrane associated proteins

However, it is not only the unsaturation of fatty acids which influences the fluidity in the region of the membrane surfaces; cholesterol and the phospholipid head groups also have important functions here. Cholesterol molecules in the membrane tend to rigidify it at the surface, but this may allow the fatty acid chains even more freedom of movement in the centre of the membrane. We can perhaps say that the presence of cholesterol makes the outside of the membrane less fluid and the inside more fluid. The same may be true of alterations in the headgroups of membrane phospholipids, for example an increase in ethanolamine headgroups at the expense of choline headgroups may rigidify the exterior surface of the membrane (e.g. Michaelson *et al.*, 1974). Much of this theoretical treatment, and more besides, is given in reviews by Cronan and Gelmann (1975) and Bretscher and Raff (1975).

Now it should be clear that, in order to overcome the effects of a fluidizing agent, like ethanol, at the membrane surface, mammalian synaptic membranes have a variety of possible solutions. The neurone could alter its degree of membrane fatty acid unsaturation, the phospholipid headgroups or the cholesterol content. First, we should consider whether there is any evidence that synaptic membranes do indeed alter their physical response to ethanol after its prolonged administration, and then consider which mechanism is most likely.

It was Chin and Goldstein (1977a) who first showed the physical effect of ethanol in low concentrations on mammalian synaptic membranes and it was the same authors (1977b) who subsequently showed tolerance to this effect *at the level of the membrane*. They took synaptic, and red blood cell membranes, from mice which they had made tolerant to ethanol, and demonstrated that these membranes *in vitro* were now resistant to the physical fluidizing effects of ethanol. The membranes must have changed their composition in some way to have become 'less fluidizable' by alcohol. Another group (Johnson *et al.*, 1979) have taken the findings a stage further by preparing artificial membranes from the lipids *only* of mouse synapses, and shown that the change responsible for *in vitro* ethanol tolerance resides in the membrane lipids.

The evidence so far strongly suggests that mammalian synaptic membranes do alter their lipid composition, and that this alteration is associated with physical resistance to ethanol at the level of the membrane, and perhaps with functional tolerance to ethanol at the level of the intact animal. The next question is obviously 'What is the specific alteration responsible for ethanol resistance and tolerance?'; but this is not such an easy question as it first appears. We have shown (Littleton and John, 1977) that a small reduction in the unsaturation of synaptic membrane phospholipid fatty acids is associated with ethanol tolerance. This change is not confined to synaptic membranes, as some tissues in the periphery are affected in a similar way (Littleton, John and Grieve, 1979) and it appears to share some genetic features with the development of ethanol tolerance (see Littleton, 1979a). However, the altered fluidity of the membrane produced by ethanol is probably restricted to the surface, whereas the fatty acid side-chains penetrate deep into the interior (see Figure 2). At first sight it seems doubtful that a reduction in fatty acid side-chain unsaturation could prevent ethanol induced membrane fluidization. In fact the changes reported in ethanol tolerant animals are in the most unsturated fatty acids, those with 4 and 6 double bonds, and these do have double bonds in the areas of the membrane relatively close to the surface. It may therefore be that such a change could underlie ethanol resistance but direct evidence is needed.

The other major lipid of mammalian membranes is cholesterol, and this has been reported to increase in synaptic membranes in association with ethanol tolerance (Chin *et al.*, 1979). Cholesterol rigidifies the outside of the membrane, and so this change would be expected to overcome the effects of ethanol at the membrane surface. However, such direct evidence as exists suggests that a simple increase in membrane cholesterol *content* is not sufficient to account for ethanol tolerance (see later).

Both ourselves (unpublished) and Loh's group in San Francisco (Johnson *et al.*, 1979) have looked for differences in phospholipid head groups in ethanol-tolerant mice without great success. We now believe we may have found a reduction in the relative proportion of phosphatidyl choline (i.e. phospholipids with a choline head group) in a purified synaptic membrane fraction from brains of ethanol tolerant rats but it is as yet too soon to be certain of the significance of this finding.

Direct evidence for the involvement of membrane lipids in alcohol tolerance has been investigated in two ways. Loh's group has investigated the effect of alteration in membrane lipid composition *in vitro* on physical resistance to ethanol; we have altered membrane composition *in vivo* and studied ethanol tolerance in the intact animal. So far these complementary approaches agree very well. Johnson *et al.* (1979) demonstrated resistance to ethanol *in vitro* of the lipids from synaptic membranes of ethanol tolerant mice. They then removed the cholesterol from the membranes and found that the resistance disappeared. Without cholesterol, lipid membranes from ethanol tolerant mice were as much affected by ethanol as were controls. At this stage the evidence clearly suggests that the increased cholesterol content of membranes previously reported by Chin *et al.*, (1978) is responsible for ethanol resistance. However Johnson *et al.*, (1979) then replaced pure cholesterol in the membranes to exactly the same extent; i.e. 'tolerant' and 'control' membranes now had exactly the same cholesterol:phospholipid molar ratio. Ethanol resistance *in vivo* returned to the membranes from the ethanol tolerant mice. This result supports two conclusions: (i) that cholesterol has to be *present* in the membrane to a certain extent before the membrane can demonstrate physical resistance to ethanol; and (ii) that the change in lipid composition of the membrane which is primarily responsible for this resistance is in the phospholipid fraction.

We have been carrying out very similar experiments in intact mice. First, we attempted to produce mice with low amounts of cholesterol in their synaptic membranes by giving a drug which inhibits cholesterol synthesis early in development (Grieve *et al.*, 1979). This prevented the development of tolerance to ethanol by these mice, without altering their initial sensitivity to ethanol. In other words the reduction in membrane cholesterol which we produced did not alter the physical effect of ethanol, but it did prevent the animals making an appropriate response to the continued presence of ethanol. This is exactly what would be predicted from the *in vitro* work of Loh's group (Johnson *et al.*, 1979).

Alteration of brain membrane phospholipid composition has also been attempted by us (Littleton, John and Jones, 1980). We maintained pregnant female mice on a diet high in saturated fat and then continued to feed their offspring the same diet throughout their lives. Preliminary findings (unpublished) show a small reduction in the polyunsaturated fatty acids of synaptic membrane phospholipids of the offspring. These mice were significantly resistant to the central depressant effects of ethanol, and their ability to develop tolerance was unimpaired. If we inhibited cholesterol synthesis in addition to giving these animals the saturated fat diet, we abolished the ethanol resistance, and prevented the subsequent development of tolerance. We interpret these results as meaning that a small change in fatty acid composition, so that the most polyunsaturated fatty acids of membrane phospholipids are reduced, can confer resistance to the depressant effects of ethanol, but only when cholesterol is also present in the membrane. Such an alteration could underlie the development of tolerance to ethanol. The concept is illustrated in Figure 3.

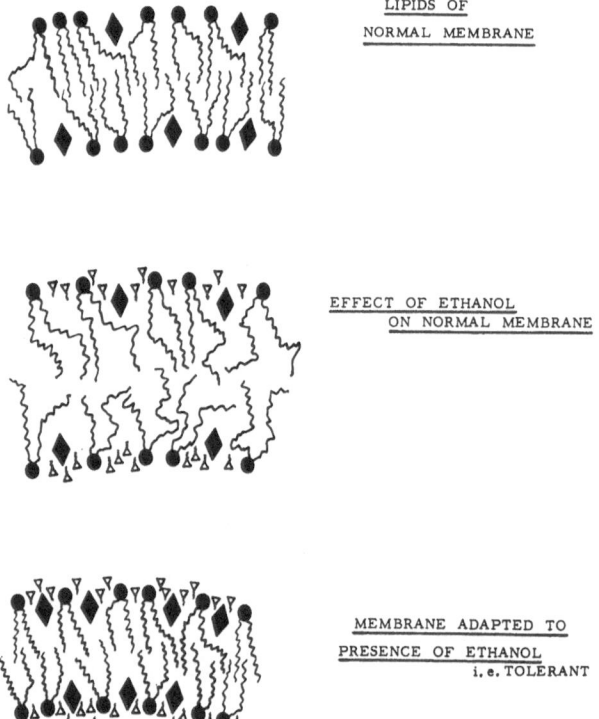

LIPIDS OF
NORMAL MEMBRANE

EFFECT OF ETHANOL
ON NORMAL MEMBRANE

MEMBRANE ADAPTED TO
PRESENCE OF ETHANOL
i. e. TOLERANT

Figure 3 The membrane bilayer and its proposed response to ethanol. Ethanol causes separation and fluidization of the lipid molecules at the membrane surface. The cell responds by reducing the degree of fatty acid unsaturation near the surface and perhaps by an alteration in the phospholipid headgroups. There is an incidental increase in the cholesterol content of the membrane. Without the presence of an optimum amount of cholesterol in the membrane the alteration in phospholipid compostion is an ineffective response to ethanol

There now seems good evidence that an ability of central neurons to alter their membrane lipid composition underlies some of the mechanisms by which mammals develop tolerance to the drug. This basis for tolerance seems to be under genetic control, and may be age related as well as possibly subject to dietary and pharmacological manipulation (see Littleton, 1979a). This level of understanding and the implications which follow from it has been achieved by the application of basic science techniques to the problem in a relatively logical progression of experiments by several groups of workers.

RELATIONSHIP BETWEEN TOLERANCE AND DEPENDENCE

As yet the concepts described above have not been fully integrated into research on physical dependence on ethanol. Most of the changes described above are probably associated with both ethanol physical dependence and tolerance, but their possible role in producing the physical withdrawal syndrome has not yet been investigated. Some general comments about the relationship between tolerance and physical dependence would not however be out of place.

All current theories which relate drug tolerance to physical dependence are variations on the homeostatic hypothesis of Himmelsbach (for review, see Mendelson, 1971). Hill and Bangham (1975) have discussed membrane adaptation to depressant drugs in relation to this homeostatic theory and central depressant drug dependency. The general hypothesis suggests that, as tolerance develops, some change in neuronal metabolism occurs to overcome the effects of the drug. In our theory this change would be altered membrane lipid composition, accounting for development of tolerance to ethanol. When the drug is removed from a dependent individual, the state of altered neuronal metabolism is exposed; it is no longer appropriate as an adaptive mechanism since the drug is no longer present, but it does still produce a functional alteration in the brain. This functional alteration is considered to underlie the withdrawal syndrome.

This simple theory is very attractive, and it adequately explains the almost universal association between functional tolerance and physical dependence. It does not explain however, why functional tolerance should *precede* physical dependence during chronic administration of a drug (see Littleton, 1979a, b). Presumably, at an early stage, the tolerant animal is able to undergo ethanol removal without a functional change, whereas, at a later stage, removal of the drug from the tolerant and dependent animal does result in a functional change. Clearly there is a further effect, rather than just the development of functional tolerance, which happens to the animal in order to render it physically dependent on ethanol.

We have presented evidence in the past, based on genetic differences between mice, that it is the speed of adaption to and from the drug that determines the severity of the withdrawal syndrome (Grieve *et al.*, 1979). Thus mice which have a very slow rate of development of cellular tolerance to ethanol, and presumably also have a slow rate of 'readaptation' from the drug, have a very severe and prolonged ethanol withdrawal syndrome. This has led to the hypothesis (Littleton, 1979b) that the proposed further effect which converts functional tolerance to physical dependence is a breakdown of the capacity for rapid neuronal adaptation; considered here to be related to altered membrane lipid composition. We have just obtained evidence (as yet unpublished) that mice do indeed appear to lose the capacity for rapid adaptation (to ethanol) when they become physically dependent, but we cannot yet say whether this is due to an inability to alter synaptic membrane phospholipid composition. If it is, then an understanding of the biochemical basis of ethanol tolerance and dependence seems very close.

This hypothesis is shown in Figure 4. Stated as simply as possible it suggests that:

(a) Cellular tolerance to ethanol is produced by an alteration in synaptic membrane phospholipid composition, which renders the synapse resistant to the physical effects of ethanol.

(b) When ethanol is removed from a tolerant, but not physically dependent, animal the altered synaptic membrane phospholipid composition rapidly reverts to normal, and is associated with no overt functional change.

(c) At some stage after prolonged administration of ethanol the adaptive mechanism for synaptic alteration of phospholipids becomes impaired (perhaps because synaptic phospholipid turnover is grossly slowed) so that the neurones are relatively 'fixed' in the state of cellular tolerance.

(d) Removal of ethanol from an animal in this 'fixed' tolerant state will produce a functional change which will continue until the neurones can resume their normal condition. This causes the ethanol withdrawal syndrome.

Just as in the case of an acute physical effect of ethanol on neuronal membranes this sequence of events could produce the wide variety of neurochemical changes which are associated with ethanol tolerance and dependence (see Littleton, 1978). What I have termed the 'basic science

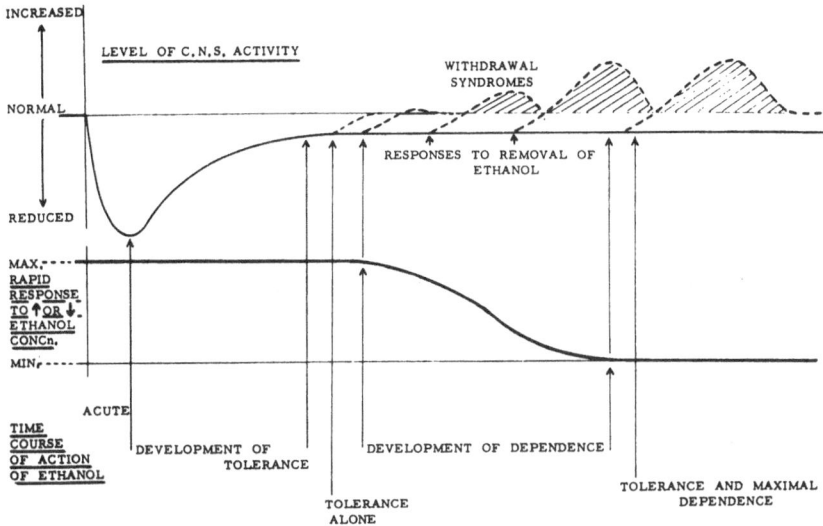

Figure 4 The relationship between tolerance and dependence is seen as a continuum in which the gradual loss of the ability to respond rapidly to an altered drug situation eventually confers the state of physical dependence. Removal of ethanol now exposes the state of cellular tolerance and subsequent readaptations of the cell are insufficiently rapid to prevent the occurrence of a functional change in neuronal activity. This causes the physical withdrawal syndrome

approach' offers a hope of understanding the often apparently conflicting biochemical findings reported during an uncoordinated approach to the problem. The hypotheses put forward here may be incorrect, but at least they represent a logical approach to the problem. Research into the basic pharmacology of alcohol should precede attempts to understand alcoholism at the clinical level, rather than following clinical hypotheses in a haphazard manner.

CONCLUSIONS

The parallels between alcoholism and schizophrenia are many. Research on alcoholism is now beginning to benefit from the application of basic research methods to animal models of alcohol tolerance and dependence, and the worth of this approach should soon be tested in clinical medicine. In my opinion the most exciting line of investigation is that centred around the fundamental properties of cell membranes, and the ability of cells to alter these properties in response to pharmacological, hormonal and dietary stimuli.

The situation in schizophrenia research seems to me to be much less coherent. The inevitable lack of an adequate animal model for the condition makes a logical research programme much less easy to design, but the extremely fragmented approach suggested by the current literature is difficult for an outsider to understand. There are a large number of suggestive leads for the basic defect in schizophrenia: the success of antipsychotic drugs; the reported differences in dopamine receptor binding; the genetic predispositon; the usual age of onset; the relation to food allergies; and so on. I believe it to be important to take all of these leads into consideration before deciding on a likely area for research. My own interests in alcohol research now lie in the area of membrane lipid biochemistry, and I am not ashamed to advance this as a field which has been relatively neglected in schizophrenia research. The ability of organisms to alter neuronal membrane lipids fits the bill as a fundamental process which may be influenced by genetics, diet, age and hormones, and which could produce changes in a variety of transmitter-related enzymes and receptors. It is likely that changes similar to those produced by alcohol are too crude to underlie such a subtle disease as schizophrenia, but more precise defects in the ability to synthesize membrane lipid components in response to normal and abnormal stimuli may be worth consideration.

Whatever happens in schizophrenia research, and the distressing nature of the disease makes one hope that something will happen soon; the action of the Schizophrenia Association of Great Britain in bringing together workers from different disciplines to discuss their research can only be applauded. The promising lines of investigation now being pursued in the field will be helped and encouraged by the informed comment and criticism of scientists and doctors in the same and related fields.

Acknowledgements

Much of the work described was performed with the aid of grants from the Medical Council on Alcoholism, the Mental Health Research Fund and the Medical Research Council. I am grateful to the Schizophrenia Association of Great Britain for the opportunity to air my somewhat controversial views.

References

Alpert, M. and Silvers, K. N. (1970). Perceptual characteristics distinguishing auditory hallucinations in schizophrenia and acute alcoholic psychoses. *Am. J. Psychiatry*, **127**, 298
Barboriak, J. J., Anderson, A. J., Rimm, A. A. and Tristani, F. E. (1979). Alcohol and coronary arteries. *Alcoholism Clin. Exp. Res.*, **3**, 29
Blum, K., Hamilton, M. G. and Wallace, J. E. (1977). Alcohol and opiates: a review of common neurochemical and behavioural mechanisms. In Blum, K. (ed.) *Alcohol and Opiates*, p. 203. (New York: Academic Press)

Bretscher, M. S. and Raff, M. C. (1975). Mammalian plasma membranes. *Nature*, **258**, 43

Chin, J. H. and Goldstein, D. B. (1977a). Effects of low concentrations of ethanol on the fluidity of spin-labelled erythrocyte and brain membranes. *Mol. Pharmacol.*, **13**, 435

Chin, J. H. and Goldstein, D. B. (1977b). Drug tolerance in biomembranes: a spin label study of the effects of ethanol. *Science*, **196**, 684

Chin, J. H., Parsons, L. M. and Goldstein, D. B. (1978). Increased cholesterol content of erythrocyte and brain membranes in ethanol-tolerant mice. *Biochim. Biophys. Acta*, **513**, 358

Cronan, Jr., J. E. and Gelmann, E. P. (1975). Physical properties of membrane lipids: biological relevance and regulation. *Bacteriol. Rev.*, **39**, 232

Edwards, G. and Gross, M. M. (1976). Alcohol dependence: provisional description of a clinical syndrome. *Br. Med. J.*, **1**, 1058

Farias, R. N., Bloj, B., Morero, R. D., Sineriz, F. and Trucco, R. E. (1975). Regulation of allosteric membrane-bound enzymes through changes in membrane lipid composition. *Biochim. Biophys. Acta*, **415**, 231

Friedman, H. J. and Lester, D. (1977). A critical view of progress towards an animal model of alcoholism. In Blum, K. (ed.) *Alcohol and Opiates*, p. 1. (New York: Academic Press)

Grieve, S. J., Littleton, J. M., Jones, P. A. and John, G. R. (1979). Functional tolerance to ethanol in mice; relationship to lipid metabolism. *J. Pharm. Pharmacol.* (In press)

Haut, M. J. and Cowan, D. H. (1974). The effect of ethanol on haemostatic properties of human blood platelets. *Am. J. Med.*, **56**, 22

Hill, M. W. and Bangham, A. D. (1975). General depressant drug dependency: a biophysical hypothesis. *Adv. Exp. Med. Biol.*, **59**, 1

Hirst, M., Hamilton, M. G. and Marshall, A. M. (1977). Pharmacology of isoquinoline alkaloids and ethanol interactions. In Blum, K. (ed.) *'Alcohol and Opiates'*, pp. 167–188. (London: Academic Press)

Hoffman, P. L. and Tabakoff, B. (1977). Alterations in dopamine receptor sensitivity by chronic ethanol treatment. *Nature (London)*, **268**, 551

Johnson, D. A., Lee, N. M., Cooke, R. and Loh, H. H. (1979). Ethanol induced fluidization of brain lipid bilayers: role of cholesterol in expression of tolerance. *Mol. Pharmacol.* **15**, 739

Littleton, J. M. (1978). Alcohol and Neurotransmitters. *Clin. Endocrinol. Metab.*, **7**, 369

Littleton, J. M. (1979a). The assessment of rapid tolerance to ethanol. In Rigter, H. and Crabbe, J. (eds.) *Experimental Handbook of Alcohol Tolerance and Dependence*, (Amsterdam: Elsevier) (In press)

Littleton, J. M. (1979b). Neuropharmacological aspects of alcohol tolerance and dependence. *Adv. Biol. Psychiatry.*, **3**, 75

Littleton, J. M. and John, G. R. (1977). Synaptosomal membrane lipids of mice during continuous exposure to ethanol. *J. Pharm. Pharmacol.*, **29**, 579

Littleton, J. M., John, G. R. and Grieve, S. J. (1979). Alterations in phospholipid composition in ethanol tolerance and dependence. *Alcoholism Clin. Exp. Res.*, **3**, 50

Littleton, J. M., John, G. R. and Jones, P. A. (1980). Feeding diets containing lipids of different composition to mice during development alters sensitivity and subsequent development of tolerance to ethanol. *Life Sci.* (In press)

Mendelson, J. H. (1971). Biochemical mechanisms of alcohol addiction. In *Biology of alcoholism*, Vol I. Biochemistry, pp. 513–544. (London: Plenum Press)

Michaelson, D. M., Horwitz, A. F. and Klein, M. P. (1974). Headgroup modulation of membrane fluidity in sonicated phospholipid dispersions. *Biochemistry*, **13**, 2605

Seeman, P. (1972). The membrane actions of anaesthetics and tranquillizers. *Pharm. Rev.*, **24**, 583

Shields, J. (1977). Genetics and alcoholism. In Edwards, G. and Grant, M. (eds.) *Alcoholism: New Knowledge and New Responses*, pp. 117–135. (London: Croom Helm)

Tabakoff, B. (1977). Neurochemical aspects of ethanol dependence. In Blum, K. (ed.) *Alcohol and Opiates*, pp. 21–40. (London: Academic Press)

Ulett, G. A. Itil, E. and Perry, S. G. (1974). Cytotoxic food testing in alcoholics. *Q. J. Stud. Alcohol*, **35**, 930

Victor, M. (1970). The alcohol withdrawal syndrome: theory and practice. *Postgrad. Med.*, **4**, 68

17
Opiate dependence and tolerance: a pharmacological analysis

D. L. FRANCIS

The capacity of opiates to induce, upon continued administration, a state of physiological dependence is possibly the most characteristic feature of this class of compounds. The existence of such a state of dependence is usually only discernible when administration of the drug is terminated, at which time a spectrum of gross physiological disturbances occurs, which constitutes the 'abstinence' or 'withdrawal' syndrome. Such disturbances occur following the cessation of chronic administration of other drugs, such as alcohol or barbiturates, or lesser effects may occur following the termination of chronic administration of drugs such as nicotine or caffeine. The nature of the abstinence syndrome seen when opiates are withdrawn from an opiate-dependent individual is, however, readily distinguishable from that seen in individuals dependent upon drugs of other classes. Avoidance of the intense discomfort experienced by a heroin addict when levels of heroin in his body are insufficient to prevent onset of the withdrawal syndrome is believed to be a powerful motivating factor for continued abuse of heroin.

The nature of the processes involved in the establishment of physiological dependence on opiates has been actively pursued for more than a century (Terry and Pellens, 1928). The last twenty years has, however, seen a steady escalation in the number of such studies, particularly in studies of analgesia, tolerance and dependence.

The discovery by Pert and Snyder (1973) of binding sites in the central nervous system (CNS) with a high specificity for opiates, and the identification by Hughes (1975) of endogenous substances (peptides) with actions similar to morphine, encouraged investigators from many areas of research to interest themselves in the action of these endogenous opioid peptides. A recent scan of the literature revealed that during 1975 and 1976 there were only five publications on endogenous opioid peptides, whereas since then over 750 have been listed. During each of these same two time periods there were 2000–3000 publications on opiate drugs. This amount of effort, although adding vastly to our understanding of the properties and actions of these substances, has still not led to a clear understanding of processes mediating opioid analgesia, tolerance or dependence. It has not yet been established that processes associated with the most familiar acute action of opioids – analgesia – are directly related to those processes associated with subacute actions – tolerance and dependence – or even that these two subacute actions are representative of a common process.

THEORIES OF OPIATE TOLERANCE AND PHYSICAL DEPENDENCE

Several theories of opiate tolerance/dependence have been postulated and can be roughly classified according to one of two basic concepts. The first of these, proposed by Tatum, Seevers and Collins (1929) was the 'dual action' hypothesis. According to Tatum *et al.*, tolerance and dependence arise as a direct result of an interaction between stimulant and depressive effects of opiates on the CNS. Tolerance develops to the depressive effects but not to the stimulant effects. Chronic treatment leads to greater periods of excitability as the stimulant effects progressively outlast the depressive effects and larger doses are therefore required to produce the desired depressive effect such as analgesia. Within this framework dependence was seen as a state of physiological balance between stimulation and depression and the withdrawal syndrome as a state of hyperexcitability due to the unopposed direct stimulant effects of residual opiate. This hypothesis was largely rejected (Seevers and Deneau, 1968) when it was found that narcotic antagonists, which did not inhibit the direct excitatory actions of opiates, did inhibit the development of dependence when administered chronically with the dependence-inducing opiate.

Recently, however, new interest in the 'dual action' theory has been shown by Jacquet (Jacquet *et al.*, 1977; Jacquet, 1978) whose experiments suggest the existence of two classes of narcotic receptors, one set associated with stimulant effects and not antagonizable by naloxone (narcotic antagonist), and another, associated with depressive effects of opiates that is antagonized by naloxone.

A new light has also been thrown on this theory by Villarreal and Castro (1979) who proposed a reformulation of the 'dual action' hypothesis in which they liken the development of dependence to the process of 'neuronal kindling' (see review by Wada and Ross, 1976). Villarreal and Castro suggest that the latent hyperexcitability of dependence arises from activation, by the opiate, of a pathway that establishes or sensitizes a kindling mechanism within opioid sensitive neurones. When this mechanism is kindled it can then be triggered by various excitatory stimuli, such as administration of naloxone or chair restraint, to give the gross physiological disturbances seen as the withdrawal syndrome.

Other hypotheses of tolerance/dependence are largely based on the proposal of Himmelsbach (1943) that dependence arises as a homeostatic reaction to the depressive effects of opiate administration. Himmelsbach suggested that morphine affects the hypothalamus – important in the control of the internal environment – by initiating a reaction to its presence that increases in efficiency with chronic administration. A condition then arises in which the presence of morphine is required to maintain homeostatic equilibrium.

Other theories, revolving about some kind of homeostatic adaptation to the depressive effects of opiates include: (1) disuse supersensitivity (Jaffe and Sharpless, 1968); (2) enzyme expansion (Goldstein and Goldstein, 1961, 1968; Shuster, 1961); (3) changes in the number or efficiency of receptors (Collier, 1965, 1966, 1969, 1972); (4) a surfeit of transmitters and pharmacological denervation (Paton, 1969; Crossland, 1970); (5) pharmacological redundancy (Martin, 1968); and (6) immunological processes (Cochin and Kornetsky, 1968). More recently Kosterlitz and Hughes (1975, 1978) suggested that tolerance and dependence may arise from a reduction in the synthesis of endogenous opioid peptides as, with continued administration, the exogenous opiate takes over the functions normally controlled by the endogenous opioid peptide.

Collier (1979a,b) in a recent critical review of evidence relating to opiate tolerance and dependence made the point that the neurone possessing specific opiate receptors is the primary and sufficient site for opiate tolerance and dependence to occur. When making this proposal Collier listed several lines of experimental support which included: (a) in the dependent rat, drugs affecting neurotransmitter function have differential effects on signs of withdrawal when given shortly before naloxone challenge, whereas the effects of opiates and specific opiate antagonists are uniform; (b) tolerance and dependence can be demonstrated in single neurones *in situ* of rat cerebral cortex and myenteric plexus of guinea pig ileum; (c) these phenomena can be induced in segments of guinea pig ileum exposed to opiate *in vitro* in conditions of transmitter blockade, both to the ganglion and the neuromuscular junction; and (d) tolerance and dependence develops in cultured, opiate sensitive neuroblastoma × glioma hybrid cells.

MECHANISMS OF OPIATE TOLERANCE AND
PHYSICAL DEPENDENCE

Science, like other areas of human interest, has periods when particular ideas are, for one reason or another, in vogue. Studies of mechanisms of opiate action have concentrated, for the best part of the last 25 years, on interactions with classical neurotransmitters. A literature review soon reveals an abundance of evidence for effects of opioids on levels, turnover, or action of acetylcholine (ACh), 5-hydroxytryptamine (5-HT), noradrenaline (NA) and dopamine (DA). There is also a wealth of information on the often pronounced effects that drugs, capable of modifying the function of these neurotransmitters, have on acute and subacute actions of opiates. These studies, possibly due to their sheer abundance, appear to have done little to lead to a clear understanding of the basic mechanism of opiate action, but as with scientific investigations in general, have left us with many unanswered questions. Some excellent reviews of biochemical and behavioural interactions between opioids and neurotransmitters have been written (Clouet and Iwatsubo, 1975b; Kuschinsky, 1977; Sewell and Spencer, 1977; Takemori, 1974, 1975, 1976).

The wealth of sometimes contradictory evidence led Collier, Francis and Schneider (1972) to propose that the magnitude and direction of action that a drug may have on morphine withdrawal is related to the withdrawal sign observed and to the time in the course of dependence/withdrawal when the drug is given. This was explored experimentally in rats in which dependence was induced by a single injection of morphine in a sustained release preparation. A narcotic agonist (heroin), given before morphine, increased the incidence of some signs of withdrawal without reducing the incidence of any, whereas, given before naloxone challenge, heroin reduced the incidence of most withdrawal signs without increasing the incidence of any. Others have confirmed these observations (Blasig and Herz, 1974; Iorio et al., 1975; Cochin and Mushlin, 1976), whereas it has been shown that narcotic antagonists given before or during the development of dependence, produce a uniform reduction in the incidence of signs of withdrawal (Frederickson and Smits, 1973; Bhargava, 1978).

Such uniformity of effect could not be demonstrated by Collier et al. with drugs affecting neurohumoral systems. Atropine (ACh antagonist), given before morphine, intensified withdrawal jumping and headshakes but lessened irritability, whereas when given before naloxone, atropine decreased jumping, diarrhoea and chewing but increased irritability and paw tremor. An inhibitor of 5-HT synthesis, parachlorophenylalanine (pCPA), given before morphine, increased the incidence of jumping and reduced head shakes, whereas given before naloxone, pCPA reduced jumping and diarrhoea. Indomethacin (an inhibitor of prostaglandin biosynthesis), given before morphine, reduced the incidence of irritability and diarrhoea, whereas given before naloxone challenge, indomethacin increased irritability but decreased the incidence of chewing.

Although somewhat large doses of modifying drugs were used in this study it did demonstrate that, with the exception of opiates, drugs affecting neurohumoral systems may appear to enhance or inhibit the development of dependence or the expression of withdrawal dependent upon the withdrawal sign observed. The 'multipartite' nature of dependence and withdrawal proposed in this study has since been confirmed by others (Jhamandas *et al.*, 1973; Jhamandas and Dickinson, 1973; Herz *et al.*, 1974; Frederickson, 1975).

This multiplicity of interactions between opiates and neurotransmitters points out some of the difficulties in interpretation of such studies in a way leading to an understanding of dependence. These arise partly because one is trying to interpret results obtained *in vivo* with whole populations of neurones, some of which will be devoid of opiate receptors, and partly because a unifying principle is required to help interpret the sometimes contradictory observations.

A POSSIBLE UNIFYING MECHANISM:
THE CYCLIC NUCLEOTIDE 'SECOND MESSENGER' SYSTEM

The involvement of cholinergic, serotonergic, catecholaminergic and other neurohumoral systems, and interactions between these systems, in the development of dependence and in the expression of withdrawal suggests that there must be some underlying, unifying process through which these interactions are mediated. Such a unifying process must be capable of mediating or modulating the action of a wide variety of neurotransmitters or neurohormones. As the action of neurohumoral substances is generally believed to be initiated through their interaction with receptors, which show a high degree of specificity for their ligands, it is unlikely that a unifying process could act at this level. It is to the mechanism(s) that enable the interaction of the substance with its receptor to be transduced into the appropriate physiological response that we must look for a unifying process.

In recent years a great deal of research has centred on the role of cyclic nucleotides in cellular function. Work pioneered by Sutherland and colleagues (Sutherland *et al.*, 1968) has shown that many hormonal actions in various systems are mediated by cyclic 3′,5′-adenosine monophosphate (cyclic AMP). This function of cyclic AMP fits that necessary for the hypothesized unifying process, and as such makes it an attractive candidate for a mediator of opioid action. The role of cyclic AMP in the CNS has been the subject of an enormous number of investigations during the last decade (see reviews by Daly, 1975, 1977; Makman, 1977; Nathanson, 1977; Skolnick and Daly, 1977). Figure 1 shows the metabolism of cyclic AMP and the ways by which cyclic AMP may regulate cellular activity, and the factors influencing this process.

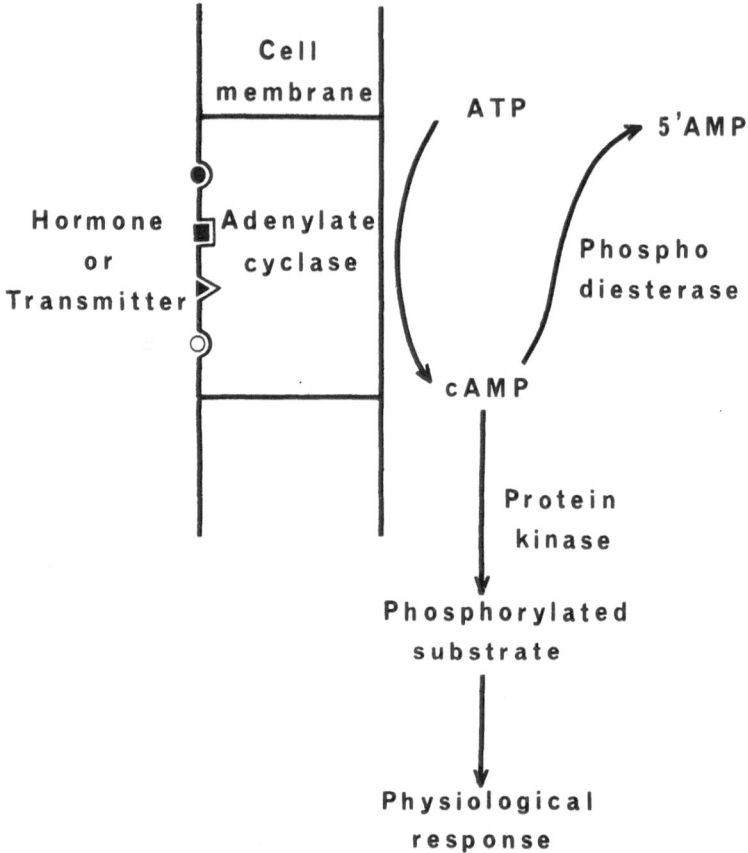

Figure 1   Schematic diagram of cyclic AMP system. ATP, adenosine triphosphate; 5'-AMP, 5'-adenosine monophosphate; cAMP, cyclic 3',5'-adenosine monophosphate

The level of cyclic AMP is determined by the activity of two complex enzymes (see Figure 1) responsible respectively for its formation from adenosine triphosphate (adenylate cyclase) and for its hydrolysis to 5'-AMP (phosphodiesterase, PDE). Adenylate cyclase is a membrane-bound enzyme with at least three components: a receptor unit located on the outer wall of the cell membrane; a catalytic unit on the inner surface of the membrane; and a coupling unit which directly or indirectly connects the two. Activity of adenylate cyclase is regulated by the interaction of various hormones with the receptor unit and is dependent on, or regulated by magnesium, calcium, guanosine nucleotides and adenosine, and at least one regulatory protein. Once formed, cyclic AMP mediates cellular activity by binding to a specific protein kinase that, when activated, specifically phosphorylates enzymes and other functional proteins, altering their properties so as to initiate the appropriate physiological response. The physiological response is in turn terminated by the action of specific phosphoprotein phosphatases which hydrolyse the phosphorylated proteins. Cyclic AMP activity is stopped by the action of specific phosphodiesterases which exist in several forms in membrane and cytosol; they show specificity for substrate (cyclic AMP or cyclic 3', 5'-guanosine monophosphate – cyclic GMP) and substrate concentration and react differentially to endogenous and exogenous inhibitors and activators.

Cyclic AMP expansion as a mechanism of opiate tolerance and physical dependence

Several laboratories have studied the part played by cyclic nucleotides in opiate action. From studies carried out (see below), an hypothesis of opiate action, associated with an interaction between opiates and cyclic AMP formation, has developed. The essential feature of this concept is that opiate tolerance and physiological dependence represent the increased capacity or effectiveness of a neuronal cyclic AMP-generating mechanism, which develops in response to the acute inhibition, by opioids, of adenylate cyclase activity (Collier and Francis, 1978).

Collier and Roy (1974a,b) proposed that:

> 'The ability of opiates to inhibit the stimulation by E prostaglandins of cyclic AMP formation in rat brain homogenate, presumably by inhibiting stimulation of a neuronal adenyl cyclase, represents a biochemical mechanism that could account for the analgesic and allied effects of these drugs . . . If this is how opiates act, then tolerance and dependence . . . may represent a compensating hypertrophy of a part of the inhibited PGE-cyclic AMP mechanism'.

From observations of the effects of PDE inhibitors (caffeine, 3-isobutyl-1-methylxanthine (IBMX) and theophylline), a PDE stimulant (imidazole) and centrally administered cyclic AMP, on the naloxone precipitated withdrawal syndrome in morphine-dependent rats. Collier and Francis (1975) extended this proposal by stating that:

> 'Opiate dependence is a state of potential increase in activity of a neuronal cyclic AMP mechanism, held in check by the presence of opiate, which inhibits an adenyl cyclase of morphine-sensitive neurones'.

This hypothesis has since been restated and extended by those working with neuroblastoma × glioma hybrid cells in culture (Sharma *et al.*, 1975a, 1975b, 1977; Traber *et al.*, 1975b). For example Sharma and colleagues (Sharma *et al.*, 1975a) stated that:

'Narcotics affect adenylate cyclase in two opposing ways, both mediated by the opiate receptor. The first process is the readily reversible inhibition of the enzyme by narcotics; the second is a compensatory increase in enzyme activity which is delayed in onset and relatively stable. Late positive regulation of this enzyme counteracts the inhibitory influence of morphine and is responsible for narcotic dependence and tolerance'.

Experimental evidence, giving support to this hypothesis, comes from several sources.

Behavioural studies

(a) *Analgesia and induction of tolerance and dependence* – Leong Way and colleagues were possibly first to demonstrate an interaction between cyclic AMP and morphine (Loh *et al.*, 1971; Ho *et al.*, 1971). They reported that cyclic AMP antagonised three acute effects of morphine in mice, (antinociception, increased locomotory activity and Straub tail) and accelerated the development of opiate tolerance/dependence.

These initial studies were extended (Ho *et al.*, 1972, 1973a, 1973b, 1975) to show that cyclic AMP or its dibutyryl analogue given intravenously (i.v.) or intracerebroventricularly (i.c.v.) to mice or rats antagonized the antinociceptive effects of morphine. This effect was also observed after the PDE inhibitor, theophylline. The action of cyclic AMP appeared to be dependent on the integrity of the noradrenergic system, as pargyline or DOPS (dihydroxyphenylserine) (NA precursor) reversed the effects of cyclic AMP whereas L-dopa was without effect. The 5-HT precursor L-tryptophan augmented the ability of cyclic AMP to antagonise morphine analgesia in morphine tolerant mice. Cyclic AMP given by either a single injection before the implantation of pellets of morphine, or before and during the pellet implantation period, accelerated the development of tolerance/dependence in mice and rats. These latter effects could be blocked by cycloheximide or by the β-adrenergic blocking agents, dichloroisoproterenol, pronethalol or propranalol. These β-blockers were only effective when given i.c.v. shortly before cyclic AMP. Theophylline accelerated the development of morphine tolerance/dependence in mice whereas other cyclic nucleotides such as 2'3'-cyclic AMP or cyclic GMP were without effect.

(b) *Expression of withdrawal* – If the acute action of opiates that leads to the development of dependence is the inhibition of the activity of an adenylate cyclase, and if there is a compensatory increase in cyclic AMP production to counteract this inhibition, then one would expect an increase in cyclic AMP levels to occur during withdrawal, once the opioid has left the system; that is, the withdrawal syndrome would be associated with an increase in levels of cyclic AMP. If this is so, then compounds capable of elevating cyclic AMP levels in the CNS would potentiate the withdrawal syndrome. Evidence in support of this hypothesis was reported by Collier and Francis (1975) who demonstrated that the withdrawal syndrome precipitated by naloxone in rats that had been treated 24 h previously with morphine in a sustained release preparation, was potentiated by the administration, shortly before naloxone, of compounds known to elevate the levels of cyclic AMP. These compounds, which effectively potentiated the naloxone-precipitated withdrawal syndrome were caffeine, theophylline and 3-isobutyl-1-methylxanthine (IBMX), which have each

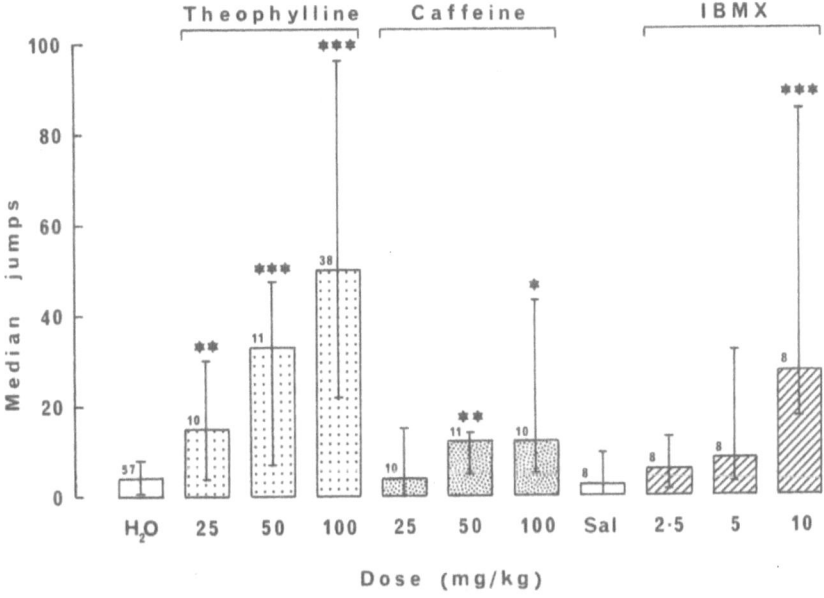

Figure 2 Effect of methylxanthines on naloxone-precipitated jumping in morphine dependent rats. Rats given morphine (150 mg/kg s.c.) in a sustained-release preparation were treated 22 h later with theophylline, caffeine or water, given orally, or 23 h later with IBMX or saline, given s.c. All rats were challenged with naloxone (1.0 mg/kg s.c.), 24 h after treatment with morphine. Immediately after challenge rats were placed in plastic cylinders and observed for a 15 min period during which the number of vertical jumps made were recorded. For significance of difference from appropriate controls; *, $p < 0.05$; **, $p < 0.01$; ***, $p < 0.001$. Each histogram shows the median number of jumps made with vertical bars giving the interquartile range. Numbers above each column show number of rats tested

been shown to inhibit the hydrolysis of cyclic AMP by its phospho-diesterase in homogenates of rat whole brain (Beer *et al.*, 1972; review by Daly, 1977) or in the case of theophylline, to increase the levels of brain cyclic AMP when given *in vivo* (Chiu *et al.*, 1977).

Theophylline and IBMX increased the intensity of the total withdrawal syndrome and caffeine, theophylline and IBMX produced a marked potentiation of the frequency of jumping (Figure 2). That the overall with-drawal score was not increased to a greater extent was probably because jumping was increased so dramatically, and being a dominant sign (Francis and Schneider, 1971; Blasig *et al.*, 1973) this excluded the occur-rence of other mutually exclusive, less dominant signs. In another experi-ment, in which jumping was physically restricted, IBMX significantly increased the incidence of several other signs of withdrawal. Collier and Francis also reported that imidazole, a stimulant of cyclic AMP phospho-diesterase, which might be expected to reduce cyclic AMP levels in the CNS, completely reversed the effects of theophylline on jumping, and, given alone before naloxone challenge, reduced the incidence of jump-ing. Of particular importance to the hypothesis that cyclic AMP plays a unifying role in mediating dependence was the observation that in no case was the incidence of any signs reduced by administration of these methylxanthines. Other experiments showed that cyclic AMP, or its dibutyryl analogue, given i.c.v. shortly before naloxone challenge, increased the incidence of several signs of withdrawal without decreas-ing the incidence of any signs, whereas cyclic GMP given i.c.v. increased the incidence of some signs but decreased the incidence of others.

This series of experiments gives strong support to the hypothesis that the expression of withdrawal is associated with an increase in levels of cyclic AMP in opioid sensitive neurones. In support of this, others have shown that, during naloxone precipitated withdrawal, the cyclic AMP content of whole brain of rats increased (Mehta and Johnson, 1974). Recently Bonnet *et al.*, (1978) reported that cyclic AMP levels in the tha-lamus, and to a lesser extent the periaqueductal grey (PAG), was signifi-cantly increased after naloxone challenge to morphine dependent rats.

(c) *Heroin seeking behaviour* – In another series of experiments carried out in our laboratories, the effects of compounds known to alter cyclic AMP levels were determined on steady state heroin self-administration in heroin dependent rats. Rats, prepared for intravenous heroin self-administration (Weeks, 1962, 1972; Francis, D. L., Schneider, C. and Collier, H. O. J., unpublished), were given free access to heroin in a situ-ation where the operation of a lever switch resulted in the delivery of 0.125 mg/kg of heroin in 0.1 ml of saline delivered over a 10 second period. The ratio of the number of times the rat was required to press the bar to get a dose of heroin was steadily increased from one to ten over a

3–4 week period until the rats were exhibiting a very stable pattern of heroin intake within and between 24 hour periods. The rats were on a 12 hour day/night cycle and test drugs were given i.v. immediately prior to the onset of darkness. Theophylline, as its more soluble preparation, aminophylline (theophylline ethylenediamine), was given in order to raise cyclic AMP levels, and imidazole was given in order to lower levels of cyclic AMP.

Table 1 Effect of aminophylline or imidazole on heroin-seeking behaviour in heroin-dependent rats

Treatment	Mean number of heroin infusions taken per hour ± SE mean				
	(Time period in hours since treatment)				
(dose, mg/kg)	(0–3)	(3–6)	(6–9)	(9–12)	(12–24)
Saline	1.6 ± 0.6	2.3 ± 0.6	2.7 ± 0.7	2.6 ± 0.9	1.4 ± 0.2
Aminophylline (20)	2.5 ± 0.5	4.7 ± 1.2	3.2 ± 1.2	2.9 ± 1.0*	1.3 ± 0.2
Saline	2.2 ± 0.7	3.1 ± 1.0	3.6 ± 1.4	2.5 ± 0.5	1.3 ± 0.3
Aminophylline (40)	3.5 ± 0.9***	3.2 ± 1.2	3.9 ± 2.1	4.0 ± 1.0	1.4 ± 0.3
Saline	1.7 ± 0.3	3.0 ± 0.7	3.2 ± 0.7	3.1 ± 0.4	1.2 ± 0.2
Aminophylline (80)	2.6 ± 0.4*	3.0 ± 0.4	3.5 ± 1.0	3.3 ± 0.8	1.8 ± 0.3**
Saline	2.6 ± 0.5	3.3 ± 0.6	2.8 ± 0.5	3.4 ± 0.7	1.8 ± 0.4
Imidazole (40)	1.7 ± 0.2*	2.7 ± 0.5**	3.6 ± 0.8	2.7 ± 0.4	1.5 ± 0.4*
Saline	2.2 ± 0.3	3.4 ± 0.5	3.0 ± 0.3	2.8 ± 0.5	1.5 ± 0.4
Imidazole (80)	1.1 ± 0.5*	1.9 ± 0.4*	2.3 ± 0.6	2.9 ± 0.4	1.4 ± 0.3
Saline	1.7 ± 0.3	3.3 ± 0.6	2.4 ± 0.5	2.9 ± 0.7	1.4 ± 0.5
Imidazole (160)	1.4 ± 0.4	1.2 ± 0.4***	1.3 ± 0.4	1.5 ± 0.6*	1.3 ± 0.4

For significance of difference from saline-treated controls; *, $p < 0.05$; **, $p < 0.025$; ***, $p < 0.01$

Aminophylline increased the number of heroin reinforcements taken within the 24 hour period following its administration, whereas imidazole decreased the number of reinforcements taken (Table 1). Lower doses of each compound had somewhat less pronounced effects over the time course studied.

If one makes the assumption that the onset of withdrawal has an influence on heroin seeking behaviour by rats which have become physically dependent on the drug, then the observations that aminophylline consistently increased and imidazole consistently reduced the frequency of heroin self-administration are consistent with the hypothesis that withdrawal is associated with an increase in cyclic AMP in opiate sensitive neurones.

It would be interesting to repeat these experiments using more potent inhibitors and stimulators of cyclic AMP PDE which could be given by continuous slow infusion. It would also be necessary to determine whether any observed effects on heroin self-administration relate to this behaviour in particular or are seen when reinforcers other than heroin (e.g. food, water, cocaine) are used to maintain operant behaviour.

These experiments, unfortunately, do not increase to any significant degree our understanding of mechanisms mediating the reinforcing properties of opiates. They have at most indicated that heroin seeking behaviour can be modified by drugs known to act on the cyclic AMP metabolising system. In addition they do suggest that a high intake of caffeine is inadvisable in cases of narcotic addiction, during maintenance therapy or during controlled withdrawal.

(d) *The 'quasi-morphine withdrawal' syndrome* – There can be little doubt that the morphine withdrawal syndrome is mediated by a central biochemical process, or series of processes, triggered by the removal of morphine from cells or cellular systems that have become dependent upon the presence of the opiate for normal functioning. Tolerance to morphine and physical dependence on it presumably arise through adaptations within existing neurohumoral systems within which the recently identified endogenous opioid peptides may normally function. If this is so it should be possible to mimic the withdrawal syndrome in opiate naive animals by modifications to the appropriate neurohumoral system in a direction opposite to that in which opiates exert their acute effects.

Collier (1974) used the term 'quasi-abstinence' to describe such a phenomenon, defining quasi-abstinence effects as:

'an effect resembling one elicited by withdrawal of a drug on which an animal has been made dependent, but produced by another treatment in a naive animal never exposed to the drug nor to a like-acting congener that induces such dependence'.

Since many drugs elicit, in opiate naive animals, single signs like those seen in withdrawal, quasi-withdrawal phenomena become impressive when a drug produces many or all of the signs of withdrawal and no other behavioural signs. The resulting pattern of behaviour is termed a quasi-withdrawal syndrome. The literature reveals many studies that have demonstrated effects that resemble behaviourally some aspects of the morphine withdrawal syndrome. Apomorphine induces rats to jump (Weissman, 1971), an effect which, it is suggested, is related to DA receptor stimulation. That DA is involved in the jumping response was supported by the observation that jumping, elicited in mice by a combination of amphetamine and L-dopa (Lal *et al.*, 1975), was blocked by pimozide or haloperidol but not by phentolamine. Jumping in mice elicited by α-naphthyloxyacetic acid (α-NOAA), was blocked by chlorpromazine, reserpine or chlordiazepoxide (Weissman, 1973), but no relationship was found between α-NOAA elicited jumping and that elicited by naloxone in morphine dependent mice. Weissman (1973) tested several central stimulants and reported that none elicited a significant amount of jumping, although caffeine (100 mg/kg) induced a low incidence (30%) of jumping.

'Wet dog shakes' are another response frequently observed during naloxone precipitated withdrawal in morphine dependent rats. Rats treated with 1-(2-hydroxyphenyl)-4-(3-nitrophenyl)-1,2,3,6-tetra-hydro-pyrimidine-2-one (AG-3-5) show an excessive amount of vigorous 'wet dog shakes' (Burford and Chappel, 1972; Wei, 1976), together with ptosis, hypothermia, intense grooming and some escape attempts. Body shakes induced by AG-3-5 were not reduced by codeine, methadone, reserpine, atropine or pentobarbitone but were decreased by high doses of morphine (Burford and Chappel, 1972). Wei (1976) reported that AG-3-5 elicited 'wet dog shakes' were blocked by haloperidol, perphenazine, clonidine, morphine and methadone. In our laboratory (Cuthbert, N. J. and Francis, D. L., unpublished) jumping and shaking elicited by AG-3-5 was blocked by morphine and by naloxone.

A recent study (Glick and Crane, 1978) showed that histamine, injected into the dorsal hippocampus of drug naive rats elicted teeth chattering, facial tremors, head shakes, 'wet dog shakes', writhing, salivation, yawning, chewing, grooming and irritability. Unfortunately these workers did not determine the effects of narcotic agonists or antagonists on the phenomenon, although histamine injected into the dorsal raphe nucleus or PAG produced a state of analgesia. Boer et al. (1977) showed that n-dipropylacetate (DPA), which elevates GABA levels, produced a spectrum of behavioural signs resembling the morphine withdrawal syndrome that could be blocked by morphine, but the effects of DPA were not potentiated by naloxone.

None of the studies discussed above demonstrated effects that could be described as a complete 'quasi-withdrawal syndrome'. When applying the concept of 'quasi-withdrawal' to opioid dependence it is essential that the test drug inducing the quasi-morphine withdrawal syndrome (QMWS) should produce an effect meeting at least the following criteria: (a) the syndrome induced by the test drug should consist of a spectrum of behavioural and other signs resembling, as near as possible, that elicited by naloxone in morphine dependent rats; (b) the effects induced by the test drug should, like the real morphine withdrawal syndrome, be potentiated by naloxone and like-acting drugs; (c) the effects induced by the test drug should, like the real morphine withdrawal syndrome, be suppressed by opiates and morphine-like drugs with agonist activity and this effect of agonists should show specificity of action (reversal by naloxone); (d) narcotic antagonist or agonist activity in potentiating or suppressing the effects induced by the test drug, should, if the effect is associated with morphine sensitive neurones and opiate receptors, show stereospecificity of action; (e) drugs from other classes known to affect the morphine withdrawal syndrome should have similar effects on the syndrome induced by the test drug, and likewise drugs that do not affect the morphine withdrawal syndrome should not affect the syndrome induced by the test drug; and (f) the test drug should not only induce the quasi-withdrawal syndrome, but should also potentiate the true morphine withdrawal syndrome.

These essential criteria gave the framework upon which a study of the induction of the QMWS by agents modifying the cyclic nucleotide system was structured. If the expression of the opiate withdrawal syndrome is associated with an increase in the level of cyclic AMP then, according to the concept of quasi-withdrawal, the elevation of cyclic AMP levels in appropriate neurones would be expected to induce a quasi-withdrawal syndrome in opiate naive rats. Based on this assumption we tested several PDE inhibitors for their potential as inducers of the QMWS. In a long series of experiments, reported in detail elsewhere (Collier et al., 1974; Francis et al., 1975; Collier and Francis, 1976; Cuthbert et al., 1976; Francis et al., 1976; Collier et al., 1977; Collier et al., 1978; Francis et al., 1978; Butt et al., 1979) we demonstrated that a spectrum of behavioural and other signs can be induced in drug naive rats by treatment with methylxanthines (caffeine, theophylline or IBMX) and certain other PDE inhibitors (ICI 63197 and Ro 201724). The similarity of this spectrum of responses to the very characteristic withdrawal syndrome precipitated by naloxone in morphine dependent rats, indicates that methylxanthines and like-acting drugs are capable of inducing a QMWS. Characterisation studies of this methylxanthine (IBMX)-induced QMWS indicate that its resemblance to the naloxone-precipitated withdrawal syndrome is very close indeed.

Primarily, the pattern of behavioural and other signs induced in opiate naive rats by IBMX and naloxone was indistinguishable from that precipitated by naloxone in morphine dependent rats (Table 2). This spectrum of signs included jumping, a characteristic and dominant sign of opiate withdrawal in the rat. Other signs observed included rearing on hind legs, restlessness, head shakes, body shakes, squeak on touch, diarrhoea and ptosis. The intensity of the IBMX-induced QMWS was, like the morphine withdrawal syndrome, directly related to the dose of naloxone given. Rats treated 24 h previously with a single dose of morphine in a sustained-release preparation were however, more sensitive to the effects of naloxone challenge than were rats treated 1 h before challenge, with IBMX. Naloxone was not the only narcotic antagonist shown to potentiate the QMWS; naltrexone and the active (−)-isomers of two pairs of synthetic narcotic antagonists were also effective, indicating that narcotic antagonist potentiation of the QMWS was a stereospecific effect. This was confirmed by studies showing that whereas (−)-naloxone inten-

Table 2   Signs induced by treatment with IBMX in opiate-naive rats or elicited by naloxone in morphine-dependent rats

Sign	% Incidence of signs after treatment		
	S + N	IBMX + N	SRM + N
Jumping	0	50*	67***
Teeth Chattering	0	58*	92***
Squeak on touch	0	50**	75***
Squeak on handling	15	100***	100***
Diarrhoea	0	92***	92***
Chewing	0	83***	92***
Ptosis	0	100***	92***
Body shakes	0	50*	50**
Head shakes	15	33	8
Paw tremor	0	50**	33*
Rearing	62	100*	100*
Restlessness	38	83	58
Salivation	0	33*	33*
Licking penis	50	67	42
Median withdrawal score (IQR)	5 (4–6)	9 (8–11)	10 (8–12)
No. rats tested	12	12	12

S, saline; N, naloxone, 1 mg/kg s.c.; IBMX, 3-isobutyl-l-methylxanthine, 10 mg/kg s.c. given 1 h before saline or naloxone challenge; SRM, 150 mg/kg morphine given s.c. in a sustained-release preparation 24 h before naloxone challenge. Signs were recorded during 15 min after challenge. For significance of difference from controls (S + N); *, $p < 0.05$; **, $p < 0.01$; ***, $p < 0.001$. IQR, interquartile range.

sified the IBMX-induced QMWS, the recently synthesized (+)-isomer of naloxone was ineffective.

These findings would suggest that IBMX, and other compounds active in this test, interact with a natural cyclic AMP mechanism that is inhibited by endogenous opioids. Giving IBMX raises the level of cyclic AMP, and this is restrained by endogenous opioid as a negative feedback which is in turn overcome by the administration of a narcotic antagonist.

The opiate withdrawal syndrome is readily suppressed by treatment with opiates, an effect exploited as a means of determining addiction liability of new compounds of the narcotic type. This characteristic is another shared with the QMWS. Narcotic agonists specifically and stereospecifically suppress the spectrum of responses induced by IBMX. This suppression of the QMWS by narcotic agonists was readily reversed by naloxone. Moreover, the order of potency of a large range of narcotic agonists in suppressing the QMWS correlated well with their potency as analgesics in man and rodents and with their ability to inhibit electrically evoked contractions of the guinea pig ileum and to act as ligands for the opiate receptor.

The closeness of the similarity between the QMWS and the morphine withdrawal syndrome was further enhanced by the effects of several non-opiate drugs on IBMX treated rats. Haloperidol, which reduces several signs of withdrawal in morphine dependent rats (Lal and Numan, 1976), suppressed the effects of IBMX, but this effect was not significantly reversed by naloxone. Pentobarbitone reduced the intensity of the QMWS but again this effect was not reversed by naloxone. Diazepam and chlorpromazine, which did not reduce the intensity of the IBMX-induced QMWS increased the incidence of jumping in IBMX treated rats; this action of these two compounds could be related to their ability to inhibit cyclic AMP phosphodiesterase (Beer et al., 1972; Chiu et al., 1977). Additionally, lanthanum, which inhibits naloxone induced jumping in morphine-dependent mice and has analgesic activity that is cross tolerant with morphine (Harris et al., 1975a, 1975b, 1976) effectively suppressed the IBMX-induced QMWS. Of possible relevance to this effect of lanthanum is that, whereas it antagonises many actions of calcium, lanthanum also inhibits rat brain adenylate cyclase activity independent of an interaction with calcium (Nathanson et al., 1976). Such an effect of lanthanum could, according to the hypothesis that opiate actions are mediated via inhibition of adenylate cyclase, explain the similarity of some effects of morphine and lanthanum.

Another drug tested was cycloheximide which effectively inhibits the induction of opiate dependence. Cycloheximide significantly intensified the QMWS indicating a point of difference between the induction of QMWS on the one hand and the induction of morphine dependence on the other. This suggests that protein synthesis is not required for the QMWS and suggests that the effects of IBMX would be greater but for the synthesis of a protein or peptide that inhibits it. This could be the synthesis of new PDE to replace that inhibited by IBMX or of an opioid peptide that would antagonise the effects of IBMX.

The observations that methylxanthines induce a QMWS in opiate naive animals and potentiate the naloxone precipitated withdrawal syndrome in morphine dependent animals are supported by two recent studies. Jacob et al. (1976) observed that theophylline produced several signs of withdrawal in drug naive rats, and, more recently Aceto et al. (1978) reported that caffeine or IBMX precipitated signs of withdrawal when given to morphine dependent Rhesus monkeys.

(e) *Biochemical events mediating these interactions* – The establishment of a quasi-morphine withdrawal syndrome with methylxanthines and other PDE inhibitors, combined with the effects of methylxanthines on the

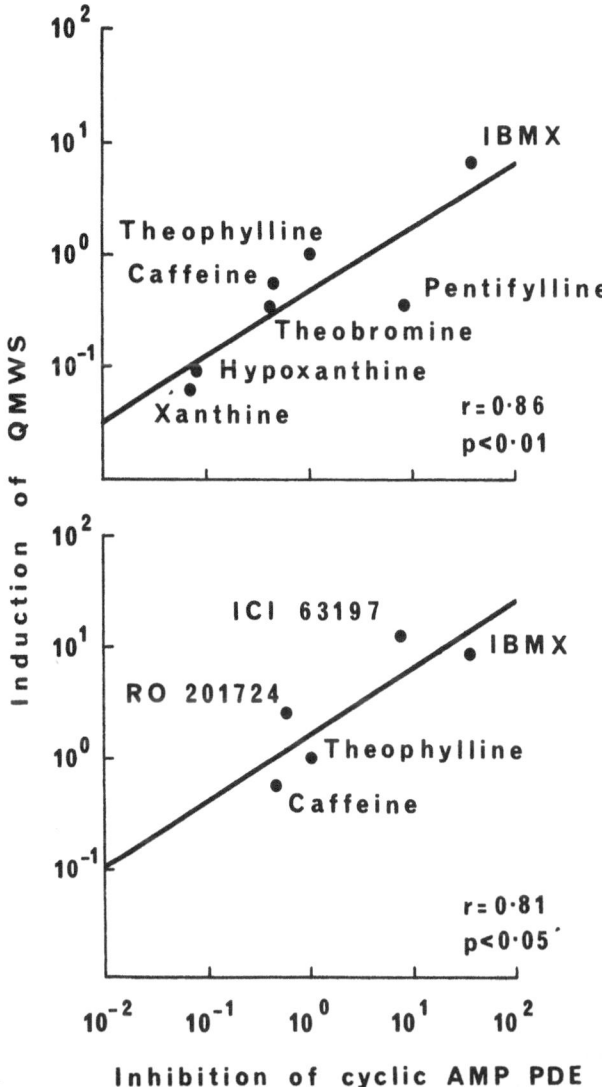

Figure 3 Relationships between the effectiveness of compounds at inducing a QMWS and at inhibiting cyclic AMP phosphodiesterase. The relationship between the effectiveness of several compounds at inducing a QMWS in drug naive rats and at inhibiting low K_m cyclic AMP phosphodiesterase in homogenates of rat whole brain was determined using a least-squares linear regression analysis. Potencies were calculated relative to that of theophylline which was given a value of unity. (*Top*) relationship for a series of seven xanthine derivatives. (*Bottom*) relationship for five compounds most effective at inducing a QMWS

withdrawal syndrome in rats treated with opiates, indicates a very close association between the mechanism of action of these compounds and those processes mediating the expression of withdrawal in opiate dependent animals. Therefore, by determining the mechanism of this action of the methylxanthines we may come to a closer understanding of the opiate withdrawal syndrome and thereby of the mechanism of opioid dependence.

Methylxanthines have a wide range of actions including: (a) inhibition of cyclic AMP PDE; (b) inhibition of cyclic GMP PDE; (c) inhibition of 5'-nucleotidase (Tsuzuki and Newburgh, 1975); (d) antagonism of the effects of adenosine (Phillis and Kostopoulos, 1975; Mah and Daly, 1976); (e) interaction with neurotransmitters (Fredholme et al., 1976); (f) stimulation of the release of ACTH (Vernikos-Danellis and Harris, 1968); (g) interactions with the cellular activity of calcium (Ritchie, 1975); and (h) antagonism of prostaglandins (Horrobin et al., 1977).

The most widely studied of these actions of methylxanthines has been their capacity to inhibit phosphodiesterase. Numerous studies have shown that cyclic nucleotide PDE activity, in crude or purified homogenates of rat brain, is inhibited by the compounds theophylline, caffeine, IBMX, ICI 63197 and RO 201724 that induce a QMWS (Beer et al., 1972; Chasin et al., 1972; Weinryb et al., 1972; Stefanovich et al., 1974; Francis et al., 1975; Fredholme et al., 1976). Recent experiments have shown that rat brain PDE is inhibited in vivo by administration of ICI 63197 or theophylline, (Chiu et al., 1977). Theophylline produced a significant increase in cyclic AMP content of rat brain, when rats were killed 1 h after treatment (Stefanovich, 1978).

Experiments from our laboratories have confirmed the findings of other workers and established an order of potency for these compounds as inhibitors of cyclic AMP or cyclic GMP hydrolysis (Butt et al., 1979). In a group of seven xanthines tested, their relative potencies in eliciting the QMWS correlated highly ($r = 0.86$, $p < 0.01$) with their relative potencies as inhibitors of low K_m cyclic AMP phosphodiesterase in rat whole brain homogenate in vitro (Figure 3). The rank order of potency of five compounds – three xanthines: (caffeine, theophylline and IBMX) and two non-xanthines (RO 201724 and ICI 63197) – so far found to produce an unmistakable QMWS was not significantly different from their order of potency as inhibitors of low K_m cyclic AMP phosphodiesterase ($r = 0.81$, $p > 0.05$). Of these five compounds, IBMX and theophylline also inhibited cyclic GMP PDE (at higher concentrations than required to inhibit cyclic AMP PDE), but caffeine, RO 201724 and ICI 63197 were virtually ineffective. The results of these experiments indicated that caffeine, IBMX, theophylline, ICI 63197 and RO 201724 contribute to the QMWS by inhibiting a low K_m cyclic AMP, and not through an action on cyclic GMP PDE. It should be stressed that as RO 201724 and ICI 63197 induce a recognisable QMWS, when given to opiate naive rats in the presence of naloxone, then any explanations (other than inhibition of cyclic AMP PDE) such as those listed above, given to account for the ability of the methylxanthines to induce the QMWS, should also be shown to be an action of these two compounds.

Extrapolation of results from experiments using whole brain homogenates to situations *in vivo* is complicated by the distribution and specificity of cyclic nucleotide phosphodiesterase. It is well established that there are several forms of PDE in rat brain. They exhibit substrate specificity for cyclic AMP or for cyclic GMP (Thompson and Appleman, 1971a, 1971b). They are inhibited or activated selectively by various endogenous proteins or exogenous substances and their activity is closely related, via feedback mechanisms, to the levels of cyclic AMP or cyclic GMP (Cheung, 1971; Harris et al., 1973; Gnegy et al., 1976a). They also vary in proportion in different brain areas and show changes in distribution and activity dependent upon the age of the animal (Weiss and Strada, 1972; Strada et al., 1974). It seems probable that the ability of IBMX and like-acting drugs to produce a QMWS may depend on their selective inhibition of a particular phosphodiesterase associated with the cyclic AMP, the production of which is inhibited by opiates.

Brain preparations in vitro

Shortly after the reports of Leong Way and colleagues, Collier and Roy reported that opioids inhibited cyclic AMP formation in preparations of rat brain *in vitro*. They reported that morphine inhibited, in a dose and time dependent manner, the stimulation by E prostaglandins (PG) of cyclic AMP formation in homogenates of whole rat brain (Collier and Roy, 1974a, 1974b; Roy and Collier, 1975; Collier et al., 1976). They demonstrated that this was a stereospecific effect of narcotic agonists; the potency of several narcotic agonists in this situation compared favourably with their potency in analgesic and other tests, and the effects could be blocked by naloxone. Additionally the endogenous opioid peptides – β-endorphin and N-methyl-methionine enkephalin amide – effectively inhibited PGE_1-stimulated cyclic AMP formation, although they, unlike the opiates, also but more weakly, inhibited basal cyclic AMP formation (Collier, H.O.J., Roy, A.C. and Smyth, D.G., unpublished). Although several laboratories have been unable to repeat or support these observations (Tell et al., 1975; Van Inwegan et al., 1975; Katz and Catravas, 1977; Von Voigtlander and Losey, 1977; Schmidt and Leong Way, 1976) support has been provided by Laduron (1975) and more recently Kuschinsky and Havemann (Havemann and Kuschinsky, 1978a, 1978b; Kuschinsky and Havemann, 1978) have reported that opiates and endogenous opioids specifically and stereospecifically inhibited PGE_2

stimulated cyclic AMP formation in rat striatal slices (but not homogenates). Support for the observations of Collier and Roy has also come from those working with neuroblastoma × glioma hybrid cells in culture.

The question of whether the adenylate cyclase sensitive to prostaglandins is intimately associated with the action of opiates or is merely representative of a class of adenylate cyclases with which opiates interact is not yet answered. A great deal of attention has been paid to the DA-sensitive adenylate cyclase, located in DA rich brain areas and thought by many to represent the DA receptor. Although morphine does not affect DA-sensitive adenylate cyclase activity either after *in vivo* administration or in rat brain homogenates (Minneman, 1977; Tell *et al.*, 1975) it effectively inhibits the activity of this enzyme in whole cell preparations using slices of primate amygdala (Wilkening *et al.*, 1976) or rat striatum (Minneman, 1977). Morphine did not affect adenosine, isoprenaline or PGE_1-stimulated adenylate cyclase in rat striatal slices (Minneman, 1977).

Guinea-pig ileum

Experiments using isolated segments of guinea-pig ileum have provided some evidence for opioid–cyclic AMP interactions. Opioids specifically and stereospecifically inhibit electrically induced contractions of the ileum by inhibiting the release of ACh at the neuronal–muscular junction between the myenteric plexus and longitudinal muscle. That cyclic AMP might mediate this opiate action is suggested by observations that caffeine, and IBMX reversed the inhibitory action of morphine in this preparation, as did E prostaglandins (Hammond *et al.*, 1976).

Others, however, have shown that whereas theophylline antagonises the inhibitory effects of morphine and other narcotic agonists on the guinea-pig ileum, it also reversed the effects of high doses of cyclic AMP, its dibutyryl analogue and adenosine which all had actions similar to those of the opiates (Sawynok and Jhamandas, 1976; Jhamandas and Sawynok, 1976). These workers initially believed that the antagonism by theophylline, of opiate inhibition of the evoked contraction of the guinea pig ileum, was due to its effectiveness in antagonising adenosine (Sawynok and Jhamandas, 1976), but later studies showed that this was not so (Jhamandas and Sawynok, 1976). Recently these workers, from experiments on the effects of methylxanthines and opioids on the release of ACh in rat cerebral cortex, have postulated that the action of methylxanthines in reversing the inhibitory effects of opioids is due to their action on the mobilization of calcium (Jhamandas *et al.*, 1978).

Others reported that cyclic AMP and dibutyryl cyclic AMP inhibited electrically induced contractions and ACh release from guinea-pig ileum (Takagi and Takayanagi, 1972). Of several PDE inhibitors tested, RO 201724 and dipyridamole potentiated the inhibitory action of morphine or adenosine on the guinea-pig ileum longitudinal muscle–myenteric plexus preparation, SQ 20006 was without effect, and theophylline antagonised the effects of adenosine but did not affect the inhibitory action of morphine (Gintzler and Musacchio, 1975). Ehrenpreis (Ehrenpreis *et al.*, 1976), who reported that cyclic AMP produced a marked inhibition of the electrically induced contraction of the longitudinal muscle preparation, and that this effect was partially reversed by PGE$_2$, believes that the acute action of opioids on the guinea-pig ileum is unlikely to be mediated via the cyclic nucleotide system.

These contradictions will only be resolved when the answers to two questions are provided: (a) does cyclic AMP, or inhibition of cyclic AMP PDE, increase the release of ACh in the longitudinal muscle–myenteric plexus preparation – and (b) does morphine induce a decrease of cyclic AMP formation in this preparation? In these studies the significant effects on the neuronal elements of the preparation must be separated from effects on the larger muscular elements. This has been done, to some extent, by electrophysiological studies of single opioid sensitive neurons in this preparation. Recently, North (1979; Karras and North, 1979) reported that opioids inhibited the electrical activity of these cells but the effect could not be reversed by cyclic AMP, its dibutyryl analogue or by the PDE inhibitor, IBMX. The question of the interaction on neurotransmitter release at the single neuron level still remains unanswered.

Hybrid cells in culture

The wealth of contradictory evidence relating to the effects of opioids on brain biochemistry is hardly surprising when one considers the complexity of the tissue involved. Very few studies have related the biochemical effects of opioids on tissue from within a very well defined area of the brain to the behavioural effects of applying the opioid directly to that area. Cultured cells, derived from hybrids of mouse neuroblastoma and rat glioma cells lines (NGL08–15), which have many properties characteristic of neurons and which possess opioid receptors (Klee and Nirenberg, 1974), have provided several findings relevant to the understanding of opioid action (see reviews by Klee, 1976, 1977; Hamprecht, 1977). These cultures have advantages over brain preparations in being homogenous collection of cells. In these cells, narcotic agonists specifically and stereospecifically inhibit adenylate cyclase activity and reduce basal and PGE- or adenosine-stimulated cyclic AMP formation (Traber *et al.*, 1974, 1975a, 1975b; Klee *et al.*, 1975; Sharma *et al.*, 1975b; Klee, 1976; Sharma, 1976; Hamprecht, 1977). This effect of opiates is not found in all cultured cells responsive to prostaglandins but only in those cells of neuronal origin (Traber et al., 1974). Furthermore, the sensitivity of these cells to opiate inhibition of cyclic AMP formation is dependent upon a functional interaction between opiate receptors and adenylate cyclase (Sharma et al., 1975b). Recent experiments have shown that the endogenous opioid peptides interact in the same way as narcotic agonists with the cyclic AMP forming system in these cells (Brandt et al., 1976a, 1976b; Klee and Nirenberg, 1976; Goldstein et al., 1977). The potency of several narcotic agonists at inhibiting cyclic AMP formation in these cells correlated with their agonist activity in other situations and with their affinity for the opiate receptor.

As neuroblastoma × glioma hybrid cells show responsiveness to opioid action they present a useful model for the study of opioid tolerance and dependence. Experiments carried out in two laboratories have revealed that in these cultures tolerance develops to the inhibitory action of morphine on adenylate cyclase activity. The formation of cyclic AMP in cells incubated in the presence of morphine returned to normal and was not affected by additional morphine (Klee et al., 1975; Sharma et al., 1975a; Traber et al., 1975b; Sharma, 1976). That these cells were also dependent upon morphine for normal functioning was shown by the finding that when morphine was removed from the incubation medium the adenylate cyclase activity increased dramatically, an effect considerably enhanced by the addition of naloxone and/or PGE_1 (Klee et al., 1975; Sharma et al., 1975a; Traber et al., 1975b). Cells incubated in the presence of morphine were also more responsive to PGE stimulation of cyclic AMP formation and this process could be partly blocked by the protein synthesis inhibitor cycloheximide (Sharma et al., 1975a, 1977; Traber et al., 1975b). Similar changes in cyclic AMP formation, adenylate cyclase activity and the sensitivity of PGE_1 stimulated cyclic AMP formation occurred following continued treatment of neuroblastoma × glioma hybrid cells with the endogenous opioid peptides (Brandt et al., 1976a; Klee et al., 1976; Lampert et al., 1976).

Site of hypertrophy within cyclic AMP system

Evidence for opiate inhibition of cyclic AMP formation and for an increase in cyclic AMP being associated with the withdrawal phenomena indicates that chronic opiate administration leads to a hypertrophy within the cyclic AMP system of opioid sensitive neurons. Cyclic AMP activity could be enhanced in several ways, including: (a) the amount or activity of adenylate cyclase might increase; (b) protein kinase, which acts as a receptor for cyclic AMP might increase in amount or activity; or (c) the amount or activity of cyclic AMP phosphodiesterase could be diminished.

Adenylate cyclase

The functional generation of cyclic AMP is believed to be dependent on the interaction of two components of the enzyme adenylate cyclase, a receptor unit situated on the outer cell surface, and a catalytic unit situated on the inner surface of the cell membrane. The relationship of receptor to catalytic units is not yet fully understood and several hypotheses have been proposed (Perkins, 1973; Cuatrecasas, 1975; Greaves, 1977; Levitzki, 1978; Rimon *et al.*, 1978). One hypothesis suggests that the receptor unit may be part of a regulating subunit of the enzyme that is bound, directly or indirectly or through an intermediate component (coupling unit) to the catalytic unit which is normally in a state of low activity. This concept sees the adenylate cyclase complex as a relatively fixed unit extending across the cell membrane. The binding of a neurotransmitter or hormone to the receptor unit induces a configurational change resulting in activation of the enzyme. Another hypothesis suggests that the receptor and catalytic units are completely independent entities situated on the outer and inner surfaces of the cell membrane respectively. In the inactivated state they are free to move about within the membrane. In this case the consequence of a neurotransmitter or hormone binding to the receptor unit is a configurational change that allows the receptor unit to bind to the catalytic unit (maybe via a coupling unit) and thus activate the enzyme. In addition, enzyme activity is dependent upon the presence of ionic cofactors, phospholipids and guanosine nucleotides and is controlled by at least one endogenous protein.

Given this complexity of structure there are several ways by which adenylate cyclase could adapt to opioid inhibition of activity. These include: (a) an increase in amount of receptors for substances stimulating enzyme activity or a decrease in amount of receptors for substances inhibiting activity; (b) the absolute amount of adenylate cyclase molecules (receptor and/or catalytic units) could increase; (c) there could be an improved efficiency of the coupling mechanism; (d) there could be an increase in the amount or activity of an endogenous activator of the enzyme; or (e) the amount or activity of other cofactors (ions, phospholipids, or guanosine nucleotides) could increase. That changes in adenylate cyclase activity are associated with the acute and subacute actions of opiates is supported by the demonstration (Hosein and Lau, 1977) that adenylate cyclase activity in rat brain synaptosomes, which decreased after acute morphine, an effect to which tolerance developed, was elevated following withdrawal of the opioid. Others have shown that in the morphine dependent rat the basal level of adenylate cyclase activity increases for up to 72 h after the last injection of morphine (Lal *et al.*, 1976). Kuriyama *et al.* (1978) showed that chronic morphine administration led to an increase in adenylate cyclase activity of mouse cerebral cortex. These studies suggest that an adaptation to opioid depression of cyclic AMP formation *in vivo* does occur and probably does so at the level of adenylate cyclase.

If we assume that an interaction between opioid (endogenous or exogenous) and its receptor is associated with adenylate cyclase in such a way as to have an inhibitory influence on the activity of the enzyme, then a reduction in the number or density of opioid receptors or a reduction in the affinity of these sites for the opioid, would lead to a hypertrophy of the cyclic AMP generating system. Studies to date however have shown that the number and affinity of receptors for opioids remain unchanged during chronic opioid administration (Klee and Streaty, 1974; Hollt *et al.*, 1975; Pert *et al.*, 1976).

Few studies have yet established a clear relationship between opioid dependence and sensitivity of adenylate cyclase to stimulation. In one experiment it was reported that PGE stimulated cyclic AMP formation was significantly greater in brain homogenates from rats made dependent on heroin and then withdrawn for a few hours (at which time the rats were jumping) than was cyclic AMP formation in brain homogenates from non-dependent control rats (Collier *et al.*, 1975). Recently Llorens *et al.* (1978) reported that opiate receptors were closely associated with β-adrenergic receptors situated presynaptically on noradrenergic neurones. Chronic morphine induced an increased responsiveness of slices of rat cortex to NA-stimulated cyclic AMP formation and this was due, in part, to an increase in the number of postsynaptic β-receptors. Kuriyama *et al.* (1978) showed that cerebral cortical slices, from morphine dependent mice undergoing levallorphan (narcotic antagonist) precipitated withdrawal, showed an increased responsiveness of the cyclic AMP generating system to stimulation by NA.

Experiments with neuroblastoma × glioma hybrid cells have provided valuable information on adaptations within the adenylate cyclase enzyme. Sharma *et al.* (1977) demonstrated that in neuroblastoma × glioma hybrid cells the adaptation to opioid inhibition of cyclic AMP formation is brought about by a change in adenylate cyclase from a low activity form to a form with high activity. They found no evidence for a change in absolute amount of enzyme, nor for a change in sensitivity at the receptor level to inhibition by opioids or to stimulation by PGE₁ or 2-chloro-adenosine. They found some evidence indicating that the opioid dependent increase in adenylate cyclase activity could be reversed by agents that are thought to uncouple adenylate cyclase from receptors. Cycloheximide blocked most, but not all of the opioid dependent increase in adenylate cyclase, indicating that protein synthesis is necessary for the adaptation to occur. They suggested that the activity of adenylate cyclase (cyclic AMP formation) determines the rate of conversion of the enzyme from one form to the other and that opiates, by inhibiting adenylate cyclase, alter the relative proportions in favour of the high activity form. Traber et al. (1975b) also found that cycloheximide blocked the development of increased responsiveness to PGE_1 in morphine treated cells.

Tolerance to and physical dependence on opioids can be measured in ileum removed from opioid dependent guinea-pigs (Goldstein and Schulz, 1973; Schulz and Goldstein, 1973; Frederickson et al., 1976; Schulz and Herz, 1976) or in ileum from a drug naive guinea-pig that has been incubated for several hours in a physiological medium containing an opioid (Hammond et al., 1976; Villarreal et al., 1977). This preparation has presented us with an extremely useful model for studying the induction of opioid tolerance/dependence. The nature of tolerance/dependence seen in the tissue resembles in many ways that seen in vivo and furthermore, evidence indicates that the effect occurs in opioid sensitive neurones of the myenteric plexus. That this is so was confirmed byNorth and Karras (1978) who reported the development of tolerance/dependence in single neurones of the myenteric plexus.

In ileum incubated for up to 22 h in the presence of morphine the development of tolerance was attenuated by the addition of PGE_2 or dibutyryl cyclic AMP to the incubation medium (Hammond et al., 1976). This supported the concept that tolerance arises in response to opioid inhibition of neuronal cyclic AMP formation that is probably effected by an E prostaglandin sensitive adenylate cyclase. That ileum removed from morphine dependent guinea-pigs showed, after naloxone challenge, an increased responsiveness to the stimulatory effects of PGE_1 (Schulz and Herz, 1976) supports the concept that an adenylate cyclase sensitive to E prostaglandins is involved in the development of tolerance and dependence. That the morphine tolerant neuroblastoma cells showed an increased responsiveness to PGE_1 and to 2-chloroadenosine, and that the ileum from morphine dependent guinea-pigs showed an increased responsiveness to PGE_1 and to 5-HT suggests a lack of specificity of increased responsiveness and makes it unlikely that an increase in the number of receptors for the excitatory transmitter can account for the hypertrophy of the cyclic AMP generating system.

The argument for an involvement of coupling mechanisms in producing an hypertrophy of the cyclic AMP generating system relies on experiments with NaF and is based largely on the assumption that NaF preferentially stimulates the catalytic unit of adenylate cyclase and therefore acts independently of any coupling mechanism. That opioids inhibit the formation of PGE stimulated cyclic AMP formation but do not affect the stimulation by NaF (Collier and Roy, 1974a, 1974b; Sharma et al., 1975b, 1977; Havemann and Kuschinsky, 1978a, 1978b) and that adenylate cyclase of morphine dependent neuroblastoma × glioma hybrid cells shows increased responsiveness to PGE_1 and 2-chloroadenosine, but not to NaF, suggests that the adenylate cyclase unit as a whole, including the coupling mechanism, is involved in acute and chronic actions of opioids. Changes in the coupling mechanism could account for the non-specificity of the increased responsiveness of adenylate cyclase to excitatory neuro-humoral substances. The nature of the coupling mechanism is not yet fully understood, but is believed to involve phospholipids and guanosine nucleotides. For example, guanosine triphosphate (GTP) decreases the affinity of a number of receptors for their agonists. This includes PG receptors (Lefkowitz et al., 1977), opiate receptors (Childers and Snyder, 1978) and DA receptors (Zahniser and Molinoff, 1978). The latter workers suggested that this action of GTP is associated with the coupling of the DA-receptor to adenylate cyclase. Others have shown that phospholipids such as phosphatidylserine enhance the binding of opiates to their receptors (Abood and Hoss, 1975).

Another factor controlling adenylate cyclase activity that may be of great importance to mechanisms of tolerance and dependence is the calcium dependent regulator (CDR) of adenylate cyclase and of phosphodiesterase (Chasin and Harris, 1976; Wang, 1977; Brostrom et al., 1978; Cheung et al., 1978). Although there is as yet no evidence for a role of CDR in opioid tolerance/dependence, it has been shown that chronic DA blockade results in an increase in the CDR controlling the activity of adenylate cyclase and PDE (Gnegy et al., 1976b, 1977a, 1977b).

The concept that opioid tolerance and physical dependence may develop as a response to opioid inhibition of cyclic AMP formation has received support from experiments in other areas. Several recent studies in vitro have demonstrated the development of relatively specific supersensitivity or subsensitivity of the cyclic AMP generating system in brain slices or homogenates to catecholamine stimulation following chronic treatment with agents reducing (reserpine, haloperidol, 6-OHDA) or elevating, d. amphetamine, L-dopa, isoproterenol, bromocriptine) CA activity (Baudry et al., 1976; Sporn et al., 1976; Costa et al., 1977; Gnegy et al., 1977a, 1977b; Mishra et al., 1978; Nahorski, 1977; Palmer et al., 1976; Quik and Iversen, 1978; Skolnick et al., 1978). In these studies it was suggested that this altered cyclic AMP formation developed as a result of (a) an increase or decrease in number of receptors for the neurotransmitter (Baudry et al., 1976; Sporn et al., 1976; Mishra et al., 1978; Quik and Iversen, 1978), (b) an increase in the affinity of the receptor for the agonist (Palmer et al., 1976), (c) an increased efficiency of the adenylate cyclase or its coupling unit (Nahorski, 1977; Skolnick et al., 1978) or (d) an increase in the protein activator of adenylate cyclase (Gnegy et al., 1977a, 1977b). Subsequent studies (Gnegy et al., 1977b) confirmed that chronic dopaminergic blockade produces an increase in the endogenous calcium-dependent protein activator of adenylate cyclase and PDE in synaptic membranes of rat striatum.

Protein kinase

One way in which the cyclic AMP system could compensate for inhibition of adenylate cyclase activity would be by increased levels or synthesis of the specific protein kinase through which cyclic AMP mediates its messenger function. Few experiments have investigated protein kinase activity in cycles of opioid dependence, but one study (Clark *et al.*, 1972) showed that protein kinase activity was depressed in chronically morphinized rats and elevated during spontaneous withdrawal. Recently (Kuriyama *et al.*, 1978) reported that chronic morphine administration resulted in an increase in protein kinase activity in mouse cortical synaptosomes. More investigations are obviously called for in this area.

Phosphodiesterase

Numerous studies (Chou *et al.*, 1971; Naito and Kuriyama, 1973; Van Inwegan *et al.*, 1975; Badger and Cicero, 1977) have shown that neither acute nor subacute opioid administration has any effects on cyclic AMP PDE. That this is an area that needs further investigation is indicated by the complexity of PDE and by the recent observations of endogenous substances that inhibit or activate cyclic AMP PDE (Chasin and Harris, 1976; Cheung *et al.*, 1978; Kakiuchi *et al.*, 1978); for instance, chronic dopaminergic blockade has been shown to increase the amount of the calcium dependent protein activator of PDE in rat brain (Gnegy *et al.*, 1977a).

SUMMARY AND CONCLUSIONS

A unifying mechanism for opioid dependence is proposed. It is suggested that cyclic AMP plays an important mediatory role in the development of this phenomenon. Dependence arises as a state of increased activity or effectiveness of a neuronal cyclic AMP or its generating system in homeostatic response to the inhibition, by opiate, of the activity of adenylate cyclase. In the presence of opiate the increased activity of the cyclic AMP mechanism is held in check, but once the opiate has left the system, or a narcotic antagonist is administered, the withdrawal syndrome, associated with an increase in activity of this cyclic AMP system occurs. Experimental evidence supporting this concept comes from several sources:–

(1) Opiates inhibit cyclic AMP formation in homogenates of rat whole brain, in slices of rat striatum, and in neuroblastoma × glioma hybrid cells in culture.

(2) Methylxanthines – caffeine, theophylline and IBMX – which are capable of elevating cyclic AMP levels by inhibiting its hydrolysis by phosphodiesterase, potentiate the withdrawal syndrome in morphine dependent rats and monkeys.

(3) These methylxanthines and two other PDE inhibitors – RO 201724 and ICI 63197 – induce, in opiate naive rats, in the presence of naloxone, a quasi-morphine withdrawal syndrome, and do so with an order of potency that correlates highly with their order of potency as inhibitors of low K_m cyclic AMP phosphodiesterase in rat whole brain homogenate.

(4) In rat brain, in preparations of rat brain *in vitro* and in neuroblastoma × glioma hybrid cells in culture, the removal of opiate after prolonged administration results, in certain circumstances in increases in cyclic AMP levels and in the activity of adenylate cyclase, or an increase in the responsiveness of adenylate cyclase to stimulation by protaglandins or noradrenaline.

Experimental evidence suggests that the adaptation occurs within the adenylate cyclase enzyme but the precise nature of the adaptation has yet to be determined.

References

Abood, L. G. and Hoss, W. (1975). Stereospecific morphine adsorption to phosphatidyl serine and other membranous components of brain. *Eur. J. Pharmacol.*, **32**, 66

Aceto, M. D., Carchman, R. A., Harris, L. W. and Flora, R. E. (1978). Caffeine elicited withdrawal signs in morphine-dependent Rhesus monkeys. *Eur. J. Pharmacol.*, **50**, 203

Badger, T. M. and Cicero, T. J. (1977). Norepinephrine-sensitive adenylate cyclase in rat hypothalamus: Effects of adrenergic blockers and narcotics. *Res. Commun. Chem. Pathol. Pharmacol.*, **18**, 175

Baudry, M., Martres, M -P. and Schwartz, J. -C. (1976). Modulation in the sensitivity of noradrenergic receptors in the CNS studied by the responsiveness of the cyclic AMP system. *Brain Res.*, **116**, 111

Beer, B., Chasin, M., Clody, D. E., Vogel, J. R. and Horovitz, Z. P. (1972). Cyclic adenosine monophosphate phosphodiesterase in brain: Effect on anxiety. *Science*, **176**, 428

Bhargava, H. (1978). The effects of naltrexone on the development of physical dependence on morphine. *Eur. J. Pharmacol.*, **50**, 193

Blasig, J. and Herz, A. (1974). Suppression of precipitated morphine withdrawal by opiates in rats. *J. Pharmacologie*, **5**, 8

Blasig, J., Herz, A., Reinhold, K. and Zieglgansberger, S. (1973). Development of physical dependence on morphine in respect to time and dosage and quantification of the precipitated withdrawal syndrome in rats. *Psychopharmacologia* , **33**, 19

de Boer, T., Metselaar, H. J. and Bruinvels, J. (1977). Suppression of GABA-induced abstinence behaviour in naive rats by morphine and bicuculline. *Life Sci.*, **20**, 933

Bonnet, K. A., Gusik, S. A. and Sunshine, A. G. (1978). Multiple opiate receptors reflected in region-specific alterations in brain cyclic nucleotides. In van Ree, J. M. and Terenius, L. (eds.) *Characteristics and Function of Opioids*, pp. 453–464. (Amsterdam: Elsevier/North-Holland Biomedical Press)

Brandt, M., Fischer, K., Moroder, L., Wunsch, E. and Hamprecht, B. (1976a). Enkephalin evokes biochemical correlates of opiate tolerance and dependence in neuroblastoma × glioma hybrid cells. *Febs Lett.*, **68**, 38

Brandt, M., Gullis, R. J., Fischer, K., Buchen, C., Hamprecht, B., Moroder, L. and Wunsch, E. (1976b). Enkephalin regulates the levels of cyclic nucleotides in neuroblastoma × glioma hybrid cells. *Nature*, **262**, 311

Brostrom, M. A., Brostrom, C. O., Breckenridge, B. McL., and Wolff, D. J. (1978). Calcium-dependent regulation of brain adenylate cyclase. *Adv. Cyclic Nucleotide Res.*, **9**, 85

Burford, R. G. and Chappel, C. I. (1972). 'Wet dog shake' induction in rats by a novel compound. In *Fifth Int. Congr. Pharmac.*, p33. (San Francisco: IUPHAR)

Butt, N. M., Collier, H. O. J., Cuthbert, N. J., Francis, D. L. and Saeed, S. A. (1979). Mechanism of quasi-morphine withdrawal behaviour induced by methylxanthines. *Eur. J. Pharmacol.*, **53**, 375

Chasin, M. and Harris, D. N. (1976). Inhibitors and activators of cyclic nucleotide phosphodiesterase. *Adv. Cyclic Nucleotide Res.*, **7**, 225

Chasin, M., Harris, D. N., Phillips, M. B. and Hess, S. M. (1972). 1-ethyl-4-(isopropylidenehydrazino)-1H-pyrazolo-(3,4,-b)-pyridine-5-carboxylic acid, ethyl ester, hydrochloride (SQ 20009) – a potent new inhibitor of cyclic 3′,5′-nucleotide phosphodiesterases. *Biochem. Pharmacol.*, **21**, 2443

Cheung, W. Y. (1971). Cyclic 3′,5′-nucleotide phosphodiesterase: evidence for and properties of a protein activator. *J. Biol. Chem.*, **246**, 2859

Cheung, W. Y., Lynch, T. J. and Wallace, R. W. (1978). An endogenous Ca^{2+}-dependent activator protein of brain adenylate cyclase and cyclic nucleotide phosphodiesterase. *Adv. Cyclic Nucleotide Res.*, **9**, 233

Childers, S. R. and Snyder, S. H. (1978). Guanine nucleotides differentiate agonist and antagonist interactions with opiate receptors. *Life Sci.*, **23**, 759

Chiu, A., Eccleston, D. and Palomo, T. (1977). A model to test the relative potencies of phosphodiesterase inhibitors in brain (*in vivo*). *Br. J. Pha:m.*, **61**, 119

Chou, W. S., Ho, A. K. S. and Loh, H. H. (1971). Effect of acute and chronic morphine and norepinephrine on brain adenyl cyclase activity. *Proc. West. Pharmacol. Soc.*, **14**, 42

Clark, A. G., Jovic, R., Ornellas, M. R. and Weller, M. (1972). Brain microsomal protein kinase in the chronically morphinized rat. *Biochem. Pharmacol.*, **21**, 1989

Clouet, D. H. and Iwatsubo, K. (1975)a. Dopamine-sensitive adenylate cyclase of the caudate nucleus of rats treated with morphine. *Life Sci.*, **17**, 35

Clouet, D. H. and Iwatsubo, K. (1975b). Mechanisms of tolerance to and dependence on narcotic analgesic drugs. *Annu. Rev. Pharmacol.*, **15**, 49

Cochin, J. and Kornetsky, C. (1968). Factors in blood of morphine-tolerant animals that attenuate or enhance effects of morphine in non-tolerant animals. In Wikler, A. (ed.) *The Addictive States*, pp. 268–279. (Baltimore: Williams and Wilkins)

Cochin, J. and Mushlin, B. E. (1976). Effect of agonist–antagonist interaction on the development of tolerance and dependence. *Ann. N. Y. Acad. Sci.*, **281**, 244

Collier, H. O. J. (1965). A general theory of the genesis of drug dependence by induction of receptors. *Nature*, **205**, 181

Collier, H. O. J. (1966). Tolerance, physical dependence and receptors. *Adv. Drug Res.*, **3**, 171

Collier, H. O. J. (1969). Humoral transmitters, supersensitivity, receptors and dependence. In Steinberg, H. (ed.) *Scientific Basis of Drug Dependence*, pp. 49–66. (London: Churchill)

Collier, H. O. J. (1972). A pharmacological analysis of drug dependence. In van Praag, H. M., de Erven, F. and Bohn, N. V. (eds.) *Biochemical and Pharmacological Aspects of Dependence and Reports on Marihuana Research*. (Amsterdam: Haarlem)

Collier, H. O. J. (1974). The concept of the quasi-abstinence effect and its use in the investigation of dependence mechanisms. *Pharmacology*, **11**, 58

Collier, H. O. J. (1979a). Dependence within the opiate-sensitive neurone. In Harris, L. S. (ed.) *41st Meeting of the Committee on Problems of Drug Dependence.* (Washington D.C.: National Institute for Drug Abuse)

Collier, H. O. J. (1979b). Dependence within the opiate sensitive neurone. *Nature (London),* **283,** 625

Collier, H. O. J., Butt, N. M., Francis, D. L., Roy, A. C. and Schneider, C. (1978). Mechanism of opiate dependence elucidated by analysis of the interaction between opiates and methylxanthines, In Deniker, P., Radouco-Thomas, C. and Villeneuve, A. (eds.) *Neuropsychopharmacology,* pp. 1331–1338. (Oxford: Pergamon)

Collier, H. O. J. and Francis, D. L. (1975). Morphine abstinence is associated with increased brain cyclic AMP. *Nature (London),* **255,** 159

Collier H. O. J. and Francis, D. L. (1976). Stereospecific suppression by opiates of the quasi-morphine abstinence syndrome induced by 3-isobutyl-1-methylxanthine (IBMX). *Br. J. Pharmacol.,* **56,** 382P

Collier, H. O. J. and Francis, D. L. (1978). A pharmacological analysis of opiate tolerance/dependence. In Fishman, J. (ed.) *The Bases of Addiction,* pp. 281–298. (Berlin: Dahlem Konferenzen)

Collier, H. O. J., Francis, D. L., Henderson, G. and Schneider, C. (1974). Quasi morphine-abstinence syndrome. *Nature,* **249,** 471

Collier, H. O. J., Francis, D. L., McDonald-Gibson, W. J., Roy, A. C. and Saeed, S. A. (1975). Prostaglandins, cyclic AMP and the mechanism of opiate dependence. *Life Sci.,* **17,** 85

Collier, H. O. J., Francis, D. L. and Roy, A. C. (1976a). Opiates, cyclic nucleotides and xanthines. In Costa, E., Giacobini, E. and Paoletti, R. (eds.) *Adv. Biochem. Pharmacol.,* **15,** pp. 337–345. (New York: Raven Press)

Collier, H. O. J., Francis, D. L. and Schneider, C. (1972). Modification of morphine withdrawal by drugs interacting with humoral mechanisms: some contradictions and their interpretation. *Nature (London),* **237,** 220

Collier, H. O. J. and Roy, A. C. (1974a). Morphine-like drugs inhibit the stimulation by E prostaglandins of cyclic AMP formation by rat brain homogenate. *Nature (London),* **248,** 24

Collier, H. O. J. and Roy, A. C. (1974b). Hypothesis: Inhibition of E prostaglandin-sensitive adenyl cyclase as the mechanism of morphine analgesia. *Prostaglandins,* **7,** 361

Costa, E., Gnegy, M. E. and Uzunov, P. (1977). Regulation of dopamine receptor sensitivity by an endogenous protein activator of an adenylate cylase. *Naunyn-Schmiedeberg's Arch. Pharmacol.,* **297,** 547

Crossland, J. (1970). Acetylcholine and morphine abstinence syndrome. In Heilbronn, E. and Winter, A. (eds) *Drugs and Cholinergic Mechanisms in the CNS,* pp. 634–635. (Stockholm: Forsvarets-Forsk)

Cuatrecasas, P. (1975). Hormone receptors; their function in cell membranes and some problems related to methodology. *Adv. Cyclic Nucleotide Res.,* **5,** 79

Cuthbert, N. J., Dinneen, L. C., Francis, D. L. and Schneider, C. (1976). A rapid *in vivo* test for dependence potential of analgesic drugs. *Br. J. Pharmacol.,* **56,** 386P

Daly, J. W. (1975). Cyclic adenosine 3',5'-monophosphate role in the physiology and pharmacology of the central nervous system. *Biochem. Pharmacol.,* **24,** 159

Daly, J. (1977). *Cyclic Nucleotides in the Nervous System.* (New York: Plenum Press)

Ehrenpreis, S., Greenberg, J. and Comaty, J. (1976). Evidence for a role of prostaglandin in the synaptic effects of opiates and other analgesics on guinea-pig ileum. In Ford, D. H. and Clouet, D. H. (eds.) *Tissue Responses to Addictive Drugs,* pp. 273–295. (New York: Spectrum Publications)

Francis, D. L., Cuthbert, N. J., Dinneen, L. C., Schneider, C. and Collier, H. O. J. (1976). Methylxanthine-accelerated opiate dependence in the rat. In Kosterlitz, H. W. (ed.) *Opiates and Endogenous Opioid Peptides,* pp. 177–184. (Amsterdam: Elsevier/North-Holland Biomedical Press)

Francis, D. L., Cuthbert, N. J., Saeed, S. A., Butt, N. M. and Collier, H. O. J. (1968). Meaning of quasi-withdrawal phenomena for the cellular mechanism of abstinence. In van Ree, J. M. and Terenius, L. (eds.) *Characteristics and Function of Opioids*, pp. 37–49. (Amsterdam: Elsevier/North-Holland Biomedical Press)

Francis, D. L., Roy, A. C. and Collier, H. O. J. (1975). Morphine abstinence and quasi-abstinence effects after phosphodiesterase inhibitors and naloxone. *Life Sci.*, **16**, 1901

Francis, D. L. and Schneider, C. (1971). Jumping after naloxone precipitated withdrawal of chronic morphine in the rat. *Br. J. Pharm.*, **41**, 424

Frederickson, R. C. A. (1975). Morphine withdrawal response and central cholinergic activity. *Nature*, **257**, 131

Frederickson, R. C. A., Hewes, C. R. and Aiken, J. W. (1976). Correlation between the *in vivo* and an *in vitro* expression of opiate withdrawal precipitated by naloxone: Their antagonism by 1-(−)-Δ^9-tetrahydrocannabinol. *J. Pharmacol. Exp. Ther.*, **199**, 375

Frederickson, R. C. A. and Smits, S. E (1973). Time course of dependence and tolerance development in rats treated with 'slow release' morphine suspensions. *Res. Commun. Chem. Pathol. Pharmacol.*, **5**, 867

Fredholme, B. B., Fuxe, K. and Agnati, L. (1976). Effect of some phosphodiesterase inhibitors on central dopamine mechanisms. *Eur. J. Pharmacol.*, **38**, 31

Gintzler, A. R. and Musacchio, J. M. (1975). Interactions of morphine, adenosine, adenosine triphosphate and phosphodiesterase inhibitors in the field stimulated guinea-pig ileum. *J. Pharmacol. Exp. Therr.*, **194**, 575

Glick, S. D. and Crane, L. A. (1978). Opiate-like and abstinence-like effects of intracerebral histamine administration in rats. *Nature (London)*, **273**, 547

Gnegy, M. E., Costa, E. and Uzunov, P. (1976a). Regulation of trans-synaptically elicited increase of 3':5'-cyclic AMP by endogenous phosphodiesterase activator. *Proc. Natl. Acad. Sci. USA*, **73**, 352

Gnegy, M. E., Lucchelli, A. and Costa, E. (1977a). Correlation between drug-induced supersensitivity of dopamine dependent striatal mechanisms and the increase in striatal content of the Ca^{2+} regulated protein activator of cAMP phosphodiesterase. *Naunyn-Schmiedeberg's Arch. Pharmacol.*, **301**, 121

Gnegy, M. E., Uzunov, P. and Costa, E. (1976b). Regulation of dopamine stimulation of striatal adenylate cyclase by an endogenous Ca^{++}-binding protein. *Proc. Natl. Acad. Sci. USA*, **73**, 3887

Gnegy, M., Uzunov, P. and Costa, E. (1977b). Participation of an endogenous Ca^{++}-binding protein activator in the development of drug-induced supersensitivity of striatal dopamine receptors. *J. Pharmacol. Exp. Ther.*, **202**, 558

Goldstein, A., Cox, B. M., Klee, W. A. and Nirenberg, M. (1977). Endorphin from pituitary inhibits cyclic AMP formation in homogenates of neuroblastoma × glioma hybrid cells. *Nature (London)*, **265**, 362

Goldstein, A. and Goldstein, D. B. (1968). Enzyme expansion theory of drug tolerance and physical dependence. In A. Wikler (ed.) *The Addictive States*, pp. 265–267. (Baltimore: Williams & Wilkins)

Goldstein, A. and Schulz, R. (1973). Morphine-tolerant longitudinal muscle strip from guinea-pig ileum. *Br. J. Pharm.*, **48**, 655

Goldstein, D. B. and Goldstein, A. (1961). Possible role of enzyme inhibition and repression in drug tolerance and addiction. *Biochem. Pharmacol.*, **8**, 48

Greaves, M. F. (1977). Membrane receptor – adenylate cyclase relationships. *Nature (London)*, **265**, 681

Hammond, M. D., Schneider, C. and Collier, H. O. J. (1976). Induction of opiate tolerance in isolated guinea-pig ileum and its modification by drugs. In Kosterlitz, H. W. (ed.) *Opiates and Endogenous Opioid Peptides*, pp. 169–176. (Amsterdam: Elsevier/North-Holland Biomedical Press)

Hamprecht, B. (1977). Structural, electrophysiological, biochemical and pharmacological properties of neuroblastoma–glioma cell hybrids in cell culture. *Int. Rev. Cytology*, **49**, 99

Harris, D. N., Chasin, M., Phillips, M. B., Goldenberg, H., Samaniego, S. and Hess, S. M. (1973). Effect of cyclic nucleotides on activity of cyclic 3′, 5′-adenosine monophosphate phosphodiesterase. *Biochem. Pharmacol.*, **22**, 221

Harris, R. A., Iwamoto, E. T., Loh, H. H. and Leong Way, E. (1975a). Site dependent analgesia after microinjection of morphine or lanthanum in rat brain. *Proc. West. Pharmacol. Soc.*, **18**, 275

Harris, R. A., Iwamoto, E. T., Loh, H. H. and Leong Way, E. (1975b). Analgetic effects of lanthanum: cross-tolerance with morphine. *Brain Res.*, **100**, 221

Harris, R. A., Loh, H. H. and Leong Way, E. (1976). Antinociceptive effects of lanthanum and cerium in non-tolerant and morphine tolerant-dependent animals. *J. Pharmacol. Exp. Ther.*, **196**, 288

Havemann, U. and Kuschinsky, K. (1978a). Interactions of opiates and prostaglandins E with regard to cyclic AMP in striatal tissue of rats in vitro. *Naunyn-Schmiedeberg's Arch. Pharmacol.*, **302**, 103

Havemann, U. and Kuschinsky, K. (1978b). Effect of morphine on prostaglandin E_2 (PGE_2-sensitive adenylate cyclase in corpus striatum of rats and its cellular localization by using kainic acid. *Brain Res.*, **150**, 441

Herz, A., Blasig, J. and Papeschi, R. (1974). Role of catecholaminergic mechanisms in the expression of the morphine abstinence syndrome in rats. *Psychopharmacologia*, **39**, 121

Himmelsbach, C. K. (1943). With reference to physical dependence. *Fed. Proc.*, **2**, 201

Ho, I. K., Loh, H. H., Bhargava, H. N. and Leong Way, E. (1975). Effect of cyclic nucleotides and phosphodiesterase inhibition on morphine tolerance and physical dependence. *Life Sci.*, **16**, 1895

Ho, I. K., Loh, H. H. and Leong Way, E. (1972). Effect of cyclic AMP on morphine, analgesia tolerance and physical dependence. *Nature (London)*, **238**, 397

Ho, I. K., Loh, H. H. and Leong Way, E. (1973a). Cyclic adenosine monophosphate antagonism of morphine analgesia. *J. Pharmacol. Exp. Ther.*, **185**, 336

Ho, I. K., Loh, H. H. and Leong Way, E. (1973b). Effects of cyclic 3′,5′-adenosine monophosphate on morphine tolerance and physical dependence. *J. Pharmacol. Exp. Ther.*, **185**, 347

Hollt, V., Dum, J., Blasig, J., Schubert, P. and Herz, A. (1975). Comparison of *in vivo* and *in vitro* parameters of opiate receptor binding in naive and tolerant/dependent rodents. *Life Sci.*, **16**, 1823

Horrobin, D. F., Manku, M. S., Franks, D. J. and Hamet, P. (1977). Methylxanthine phosphodiesterase inhibitors behave as prostaglandin antagonists in a perfused rat mesenteric artery preparation. *Prostaglandins*, **13**, 33

Hosein, E. A. and Lau, A. (1977). Adenylate cyclase activity during tolerance and dependence to morphine. *Trans. Am. Soc. Neurochem.*, **8**, 83

Hughes, J. (1975). Isolation of an endogenous compound from the brain with pharmacological properties similar to morphine. *Brain Res.*, **88**, 295

van Inwegan, R. G., Strada, S. J. and Robison, G. A. (1975). Effects of prostaglandins and morphine on brain adenylyl cyclase. *Life Sci.*, **16**, 1875

Iorio, L. C., Deacan, M. A. and Ryan, E. A. (1975). Blockade by narcotic drugs of naloxone-precipitated jumping in morphine-dependent mice. *J. Pharmacol. Exp. Ther.*, **192**, 58

Jacob, J. J., Tremblay, E. C. and Michand, G. M. (1976). Antagonism of precipitated abstinence by narcotics, narcotic antagonists and mixed agonist-antagonists. In Kosterlitz, H. W. (ed.) *Opiates and Endogenous Opioid Peptides*, pp. 377–384. (Amsterdam: Elsevier/North-Holland Biomedical Press)

Jacquet, Y. (1978). 'Opioid' behavioural effects following ACTH or ß-endorphin injections in periaqueductal gray of drug-naive rats: A dual mechanism of drug dependence. In van Ree, J. M. and Terenius, L. (eds.) *Characteristics and Function of Opioids*, pp. 429–430.

(Amsterdam: Elsevier/North-Holland Biomedical Press)

Jacquet, Y. F., Klee, W. A., Rice, K. C., Iijima, I. and Minamikawa, J. (1977). Stereospecific and non-stereospecific effects of (+) and (−) morphine: Evidence for a new class of receptors. *Science*, **198**, 842

Jaffe, J. H. and Sharpless, S. K. (1968). Pharmacological denervation sensitivity in central nervous system: A theory of physical dependence. In Wikler, A. (ed.) *The Addictive States*, pp. 226–246. (Baltimore: Williams & Wilkins)

Jhamandas, K. and Dickinson, G. (1973). Modification of precipitated morphine and methadone abstinence in mice by acetylcholine antagonists. *Nature (London)*, **245**, 219

Jhamandas, K. and Sawynok, J. (1976). Methylxanthine antagonism of opiate and purine effects on the release of acetylcholine. In Kosterlitz, H. W. (ed.) *Opiates and Endogenous Opioid Peptides*, pp. 161–168. (Amsterdam: Elsevier/North-Holland Biomedical Press)

Jhamandas, K., Sawynok, J. and Sutak, M. (1978). Antagonism of morphine action on brain acetylcholine release by methylxanthines and calcium. *Eur. J. Pharmacol.*, **49**, 309

Jhamandas, K., Sutak, M. and Bell, S. (1973). Modification of precipitated morphine withdrawal syndrome by drugs affecting cholinergic mechanisms. *Eur. J. Pharmacol.*, **24**, 296

Kakiuchi, S., Yamazaki, R., Teshima, Y., Uenishi, K., Yasuda, S., Kashiba, A., Sobue, K., Ohshima, M. and Nakajima, T. (1978). Membrane-based protein modulator and phosphodiesterase. *Adv. Cyclic Nucleotide Res.*, **9**, 253

Karras, P. J. and North, R. A. (1979). Inhibition of neuronal firing by opiates: Evidence against the involvement of cyclic nucleotides. *Br. J. Pharmacol.*, **65**, 647

Katz, J. B. and Catravas, G. N. (1977). Absence of morphine antagonism of prostaglandin E_1-stimulated [^{3}H]3′,5′-cyclic adenosine monophosphate accumulation in a rat brain mince system. *Brain Res.*, **120**, 263

Klee, W. A. (1976). Interactions of opiate receptors with adenylate cyclase. In Beers, R. F. and Bassett, E. G. (eds.) *Cell Membrane Receptors for Viruses, Antigens and Antibodies, Polypeptide Hormones and Small Molecules*, pp. 451–466. (New York: Raven)

Klee, W. A. (1977). Opiates and cyclic AMP. In Blum, K. (ed.) *Alcohol and Opiates. Neurochemical and Behavioural Mechanisms*. pp. 299–308. (New York: Academic Press)

Klee, W. A., Lampert, A. and Nirenberg, M. (1976). Dual regulation of adenylate cyclase by endogenous opioid peptides. In Kosterlitz, H. W. (ed.). *Opiates and Endogenous Opioid Peptides*, pp. 153–159. (Amsterdam: Elsevier/North-Holland Biomedical Press)

Klee, W. A. and Nirenberg, M. (1974). A neuroblastoma × glioma hybrid cell line with morphine receptors. *Proc. Natl. Acad. Sci. USA*, **71**, 3474

Klee, W. A. and Nirenberg, M. (1976). Mode of action of endogenous opiate peptides. *Nature (London)*, **263**, 609

Klee, W. A., Sharma, S. K. and Nirenberg, M. (1975). Opiate receptors as regulators of adenylate cyclase. *Life Sci.*, **16**, 1869

Klee, W. A. and Streaty, R. A. (1974). Narcotic receptor sites in morphine-dependent rats. *Nature (London)*, **248**, 61

Kosterlitz, H. W. and Hughes, J. (1975). Some thoughts on the significance of enkephalin, the endogenous ligand. *Life Sci.*, **17**, 91

Kosterlitz, H. W. and Hughes, J. (1978). Endogenous opioid peptides. In J. Fishman (ed.) *The Bases of Addiction*, pp. 411–430. (Berlin: Dahlem Konferenzen)

Kuriyama, K., Nakagawa, K., Naito, K. and Muramatsu, M. (1978). Morphine-induced changes in cyclic AMP metabolism and protein kinase activity in the brain. *Jpn. J. Pharmacol.*, **28**, 73

Kuschinsky, K. (1977). Opiate dependence. *Prog. Pharmacol.*, **1**, 1

Kuschinsky, K. and Havemann, U. (1978). Antagonism by opiates against prostaglandin E_2-stimulated adenylate cyclase in the corpus striatum. *Naunyn-Schmiedeberg's Arch. Pharmacol.*, **302**, (Suppl.), R62

Laduron, P. (1975). Adenyl cyclase: A possible target for morphine-like compounds and neuroleptics. In *Sixth Int. Congr. Pharmacol.*, Abstract No. 1477. (Helsinki: IUPHAR)

Lal, H., Colpaert, F. C. and Laduron, P. (1975). Narcotic withdrawal-like jumping produced by amphetamine and l-dopa. *Eur. J. Pharmacol.*, **30**, 113

Lal, H. and Numan, R. (1976). Blockade of morphine-withdrawal body shakes by haloperidol. *Life Sci.*, **18**, 163

Lal, H., Puri, S. K. and Volicer, L. (1976). A comparison between narcotics and neuroleptics: Effects on striatal dopamine turnover, cyclic AMP, and adenylate cyclase. In D. H. Ford and D. H. Clouet (eds.) *Tissue Responses to Addictive Drugs*, pp. 187–207. (New York: Spectrum Publications)

Lampert, A., Nirenberg, M. and Klee, W. A. (1976). Tolerance and dependence evoked by an endogenous opioid peptide. *Proc. Natl. Acad. Sci. USA.*, **73**, 3165

Lefkowitz, R. J., Mullikin, D., Wood, C. L., Gore, T. B. and Mukherjee, C. (1977). Regulation of prostaglandin receptors by prostaglandin and guanine nucleotides in frog erythrocytes. *J. Biol. Chem.*, **252**, 5295

Levitzki, A. (1978). The mode of coupling of adenylate cyclase to hormone receptors and its modulation by GTP. *Biochem. Pharmacol.*, **27**, 2083

Llorens, C., Martres, M. P., Baudry, M. and Schwartz, J. C. (1978). Hypersensitivity to noradrenaline in cortex after chronic morphine: relevance to tolerance and dependence. *Nature (London)*, **274**, 603

Loh, H. H., Ho, I. K., Lu, S. E. and Leong Way, E. (1971). Effect of c-AMP on morphine analgesia. *Pharmacologist*, **13**, 313

Mah, H. D. and Daly, J. W. (1976). Adenosine-dependent formation of cyclic AMP in brain slices. *Pharmacol. Res. Commun.*, **8**, 65

Makman, M. H. (1977). Actions of cyclic AMP and its relationship to transmitter function in nervous tissue. In Litwach, G. (ed.) *Biochemical Actions of Hormones*. Vol. IV, pp. 407–496. (London: Academic Press)

Martin, W. R. (1968). A homeostatic and redundancy theory of tolerance to and dependence on narcotic analgesics. In Wikler, A. (ed.) *The Addictive States*, pp. 206–225. (Baltimore: Williams & Wilkins)

Mehta, C. S. and Johnson, W. (1974). Elevation of brain cyclic adenosine 3′ :5′ monophosphate during naloxone precipitated withdrawal in morphine dependent rats. *Fed. Proc.*, **33**, 493

Minneman, K. P. (1977). Morphine selectively blocks dopamine-stimulated cyclic AMP formation in rat neostriatal slices. *Br. J. Pharmacol.*, **59**, 480

Mishra, R. K., Wong, Y-W., Varmuza, S. and Tuff, L. (1978). Chemical lesion and drug induced supersensitivity and subsensitivity of caudate dopamine receptors. *Life Sci.*, **23**, 443

Nahorski, S. R. (1977). Altered responsiveness of cerebral beta adrenoceptors assessed by adenosine cyclic 3′,5′-monophosphate formation and ^{3}H-propranolol binding. *Mol. Pharmacol.*, **13**, 679

Naito, K. and Kuriyama, K. (1973). Effect of morphine administration on adenyl cyclase and 3′,5′-cyclic nucleotide phosphodiesterase activities in the brain. *Jpn. J. Pharmacol.*, **23**, 274

Nathanson, J. A. (1977). Cyclic nucleotides and nervous system function. *Physiol. Rev.*, **57**, 157

Nathanson, J. A., Freedman, R. and Hoffer, B. J. (1976). Lanthanum inhibits brain adenylate cyclase and blocks noradrenergic depression of Purkinje cell discharge independent of calcium. *Nature (London)*, **261**, 330

North, R. A. (1979). Studies of opioid action on single neurons. In Beers, R. F. and Bassett, E. G. (eds.) *Mechanism of Pain and Analgesic Compounds*, pp. 373–381. (New York: Raven Press)

North, R. A. and Karras, P. J. (1978). Opiate tolerance and dependence induced *in vitro* in single myenteric neurones. *Nature (London)*, **272**, 73

Palmer, G. C., Wagner, H. R. and Putman, R. W. (1976). Neuronal localization of the enhanced adenylate cyclase responsiveness to catecholamines in the rat cerebral cortex following reserpine injections. *Neuropharmacology*, **15**, 695

Paton, W. D. M. (1969). A pharmacological approach to drug dependence and drug tolerance. In Steinberg, H. (ed.) *Scientific Basis of Drug Dependence*, pp. 31–47. (London: Churchill)

Perkins, J. P. (1973). Adenyl cyclase. *Adv. Cyclic Nucleotide Res.*, **3**, 1

Pert, C. B. and Snyder, S. H. (1973). Opiate receptor: demonstration in nervous tissue. *Science*, **179**, 1011

Pert, C. B., Snyder, S. H. and Kuhar, M J. (1976). Opiate receptor binding in intact animals. In Ford, D. H. and Clouet, D. H. (eds.) *Tissue Responses to Addictive Drugs*, pp. 89–101. (New York: Spectrum Publications)

Phillis, J. W. and Kostopoulos, G. K. (1975). Adenosine as a putative transmitter in the cerebral cortex: Studies with potentiators and antagonists. *Life Sci.*, **17**, 1085

Quik, M. and Iversen, L. L. (1978). Subsensitivity of the rat striatal dopaminergic system after treatment with bromocriptine: effects on [³H]spiperone binding and dopamine-stimulated cyclic AMP formation. *Naunyn-Schmiedeberg's Arch. Pharmacol.*, **304**, 141

Raman, G. and Ahmed, M. (1977). Amelioration of withdrawal symptoms in morphine addicted albino rats. *Indian J. Exp. Biol.*, **15**, 238

Rimon, G., Hanshi, E., Braun, S. and Levitzki, A. (1978). Mode of coupling between hormone receptors and adenylate cyclase elucidated by modulation of membrane fluidity. *Nature (London)*, **276,**, 394

Ritchie, J. M. (1975). The xanthines. In Goodman, L. S. and Gilman, A (eds.) *The Pharmacological Basis of Therapeutics*, (5th edition), pp. 367–378. (New York: MacMillan)

Robinson, G. A., Butcher, R. W. and Sutherland, E. W. (1967). Adenyl cyclase as an adrenergic receptor. *Ann. N. Y. Acad. Sci.*, **139**, 703

Roy, A. C. and Collier, H. O. J. (1975). Prostaglandins, cyclic AMP and the biochemical mechanism of opiate agonist action. *Life Sci.*, **16**, 1857

Sawynok, J. and Jhamandas, K. G. (1976). Inhibition of acetylcholine release from cholinergic nerves by adenosine, adenine nucleotides and morphine: antagonism by theophylline. *J. Pharmacol. Exp. Ther.*, **197**, 379

Schmidt, W. K. and Leong Way, E. (1976). Does morpine inhibit prostaglandin-stimulated adenylate cyclase in the rat brain? *Proc. West. Pharmacol. Soc.*, **19**, 55

Schulz, R. and Goldstein, A. (1973). Morphine tolerance and supersensitivity to 5-hydroxytyptamine in the myenteric plexus of the guinea-pig. *Nature (London)*, **244**, 168

Schulz, R. and Herz, A. (1976). Aspects of opiate dependence in the myenteric plexus of the guinea-pig. *Life Sci.*, **19**, 1117

Seevers, M. H. and Deneau, G. A. (1968). A critique of the 'dual action' hypothesis of morphine physical dependence. In Wikler, A. (ed.) *The Addictive States*, pp. 199–205. (Baltimore: Williams & Wilkins)

Sewell, R. D. E. and Spencer, P. S. J. (1977). The role of biogenic amines in the actions of centrally acting analgesics. *Prog. Med. Chem.*, **14**, 249

Sharma, S. K. (1976). Modulation of adenylate cyclase activity by narcotics in neuroblastoma × glioma hybrid cells. In Kosterlitz, H. W. (ed.) *Opiates and Endogenous Opioid Peptides*, pp. 257–260. (Amsterdam: Elsevier/North-Holland Biomedical Press)

Sharma, S. K., Klee, W. A. and Nirenberg, M. (1975a). Dual regulation of adenylate cyclase accounts for narcotic dependence and tolerance. *Proc. Natl. Acad. Sci. USA.*, **72**, 3092

Sharma, S. K., Klee, W. A. and Nirenberg, M. (1977). Opiate-dependent modulation of adenylate cyclase. *Proc. Nat. Acad. Sci. USA.*, **74**, 3365

Sharma, S. K., Nirenberg, M. and Klee, W. A. (1975b). Morphine receptors as regulators of adenylate cyclase activity. *Proc. Natl. Acad. Sci. USA.*, **72**, 590

Shuster, L. (1961). Repression and de-repression of enzyme synthesis as a possible explanation of some aspects of drug action. *Nature (London)*, **189**, 314

Skolnick, P. and Daly, J. W. (1977). Regulation of cAMP formation in brain tissue by putative neurotransmitters. In Cramer, H. and Schultz, J. (eds.) *Cyclic 3',5'-Nucleotides: Mechanisms of Action*, pp. 289–315. (London: John Wiley & Sons)

Skolnick, P., Stalvey, L. P., Daly, J. W., Hoyler, E. and Davis, J. N. (1978). Binding of α- and ß-adrenergic ligands to cerebral cortical membranes: Effect of 6-hydroxydopamine treatment and relationship to the responsiveness of cyclic AMP-generating systems in two rat strains. *Eur. J. Pharmacol.*, **47**, 201

Sporn, J. R., Harden, T. K., Wolfe, B. B. and Molinoff, P. B. (1976). ß-Adrenergic receptor involvement in 6-hydroxydopamine induced supersensitivity in rat cerebral cortex. *Science*, **194**, 624

Stefanovich, V. (1978). Concerning the influence of theophylline on cAMP concentration in rat brain. In G. Folco and R. Paoletti (eds.). *Molecular Biology and Pharmacology of Cyclic Nucleotides*. pp. 225–226. (Amsterdam: Elsevier/North-Holland Biomedical Press)

Stefanovich, V., Von Polnitz, M. and Reiser, M. (1974). Inhibition of various cyclic AMP phosphodiesterases by pentifylline and theophylline. *Arzneim-Forsch. (Drug Res.)*, **24**, 1747

Strada, S. J., Uzunov, P. and Weiss, B. (1974). Ontogenetic development of a phosphodiesterase activator and the multiple forms of cyclic AMP phosphodiesterase of rat brain. *J. Neurochem.*, **23**, 1097

Sutherland, E. W., Robison, G. A. and Butcher, R. W. (1968). Some aspects of the biological role of adenosine 3',5'-monophosphate (cyclic AMP). *Circulation*, **37**, 279

Takagi, K. and Takayanagi, I. (1972). Effect of N^6, 2'-0-dibutyryl 3',5'-cyclic adenosine monophosphate, 3',5',-cyclic adenosine monophosphate and adenosine triphosphate on acetylcholine output from cholinergic nerves in guinea-pig ileum. *Jpn. J. Pharmacol.*, **22**, 33

Takemori, A. E. (1974). Biochemistry of drug dependence. *Ann. Rev. Biochem.*, **43**, 15

Takemori, A. E. (1975). Neurochemical bases for narcotic tolerance and dependence. *Biochem. Pharmacol.*, **24**, 2121

Takemori, A. E. (1976). Pharmacologic factors which alter the action of narcotic analgesics and antagonists. *Ann. N. Y. Acad. Sci.*, **281**, 262

Tatum, A. L., Seevers, M. H. and Collins, K. G. (1929). Morphine addiction and its physiological interpretation based on experimental evidence. *J. Pharmacol. Exp. Ther.*, **36**, 447

Tell, G. P., Pasternak, G. W. and Cuatrecasas, P. (1975). Brain and caudate nucleus adenylate cyclase: Effects of dopamine, GTP, E prostaglandins and morphine. *Febs. Lett.*, **51**, 242

Terry, C. E. and Pellens, M. (1928). *The Opium Problem*. (New York: Bureau of Social Hygiene)

Thompson, W. J. and Appleman, M. M. (1971a). Characterization of cyclic nucleotide phosphodiesterases of rat tissues. *J. Biol. Chem.*, **246**, 3145

Thompson, W. J. and Appleman, M. M. (1971b). Multiple cyclic nucleotide phosphodiesterase activities from rat brain. *Biochem.*, **10**, 311

Traber, J., Fischer, K., Latzin, S. and Hamprecht, B. (1974). Morphine antagonises the action of prostaglandins in neuroblastoma cells but not of prostaglandin and noradrenaline in glioma and glioma × fibroblast hybrid cells. *Febs. Lett.*, **49**, 260

Traber, J., Fischer, K., Latzin, S. and Hamprecht, B. (1975a). Morphine antagonises action of prostaglandin in neuroblastoma and neuroblastoma × glioma hybrid cells. *Nature (London)*, **253**, 120

Traber, J., Gullis, R. and Hamprecht, B. (1975b). Influence of opiates on the levels of adenosine 3':5'-cyclic monophosphate in neuroblastoma × glioma hybrid cells. *Life Sci.*, **16**, 1863

Tsuzuki, J. and Newburgh, R. W. (1975). Inhibition of 5'-nucleotidase in rat brain by methylxanthines. *J. Neurochem.*, **25**, 895

Vernikos-Danellis, J. and Harris, C. G. (1968). The effect of *in vitro* and *in vivo* caffeine, theophylline and hydrocortisone on the phosphodisterase activity of the pituitary, median eminence, heart, and cerebral cortex of the rat. *Proc. Soc. Exp. Biol. Med.*, **128**, 1016

Villarreal, J. E. and Castro, A. (1979). A reformulation of the dual-action model of opioid-dependence. In Beers, R. F. and Bassett, E. G. (eds.) *Mechanisms of Pain and Analgesic Compounds*, pp. 407–428. (New York: Raven Press)

Villarreal, J. E., Martinez, J. M. and Castro, A. (1977). Validation of a new procedure to study narcotic dependence in the isolated guinea-pig ileum. In *36th Meeting of Committee on Problems of Drug Dependence*, pp. 305–314. (Washington D.C.: CPDD Inc.)

von Voigtlander, P. F. and Losey, E. G. (1977). Prostaglandin E_2, cyclic adenosine monophosphate and morphine analgesia. *Brain Res.*, **128**, 275

Wada, J. A. and Ross, R. T. (1976). *Kindling*. (New York: Raven Press)

Wang, J. H. (1977). Calcium-regulated protein modulator in cyclic nucleotide systems. In Cramer, H. and Schultz, J. (eds.) *Cyclic 3',5'-nucleotides: Mechanisms of Action*, pp. 37–56. (London: John Wiley & Sons)

Weeks, J. R. (1962). Experimental morphine addiction: method for automatic intravenous injections in unrestrained rats. *Science*, **138**, 143

Weeks, J. R. (1972). Long-term intravenous infusion. In Myers, R. D. (ed.) *Methods in Psychobiology*, Vol.2, pp. 155–168. (New York: Academic Press)

Wei, E. T. (1976). Chemical stimulants of shaking behaviour. *J. Pharm. Pharmacol.*, **28**, 722

Weinryb, I., Chasin, M., Free, C. A., Harris, D. N., Goldenberg, H., Michel, I. M., Paik, V. S., Phillips, M., Samaniego, S. and Hess, S. M. (1972). Effects of therapeutic agents on cyclic AMP metabolism *in vitro*. *J. Pharm. Sci.*, **61**, 1556

Weiss, B. and Strada, S. J. (1972). Neuroendocrine control of the cyclic AMP system of brain and pineal gland. *Adv. Cyclic Nuclotide Res.*, **1**, 357

Weissman, A. (1971). Cliff jumping in rats after intravenous treatment with apomorphine. *Psychopharmacologia*, **21**, 60

Weissman, A. (1973). Jumping in mice elicited by α-naphthyloxyacetic acid (α-NOAA). *J. Pharmacol. Exp. Ther.*, **184**, 11

Wilkening, D., Mishra, R. K. and Makman, M. H. (1976). Effects of morphine on dopamine-stimulated adenylate cyclase and on cyclic GMP formation in primate brain amygdaloid nucleus. *Life Sci.*, **19**, 1129

Zahniser, N. R. and Molinoff, P. B. (1978). Effect of guanine nucleotides on striatal dopamine receptors. *Nature (London)*, **275**, 453

Section 4:
PUERPERAL PSYCHOSES

18
Puerperal schizophrenia?

I. F. BROCKINGTON, E. SCHOFIELD and K. GREGORY

Although many psychiatrists believe that schizophrenia and manic depression are aetiologically distinct conditions, it is also held that both can be precipitated by parturition. That the same provoking event should affect them equally seems rather improbable. The association with the manic depressive diathesis is well founded on the work of Bratfos and Haug (1966) and Reich and Winokur (1970) who showed high puerperal breakdown rates in these patients, but there is no such evidence in schizophrenia. Is it possible that the apparent occurrence of puerperal schizophrenia is spurious, another consequence of the muddle over the diagnosis of schizophrenia? In theory this should be a simple epidemiological question to answer; all we need do is to define 'puerperal psychosis' and 'schizophrenia' and study a series of postpartum psychoses to see whether the form of the illness is schizophrenic.

The definition of puerperal psychosis is epidemiological. The only reason for using this term is the sharp rise in the incidence of mental hospital admissions in the immediate puerperium, demonstrated for example by Paffenbarger in his studies in Cincinatti and Hamilton County, Ohio (Paffenbarger, 1964). He found that 164 patients were admitted during the first puerperal month compared with monthly rates of 8 during pregnancy and 16 during the 2nd to 6th months postpartum. Our figures from the Mothers and Babies Unit at Manchester are similar: of 241 patients admitted in 7 years, 43 became ill before delivery, 148 within one month and 44 in the remaining 11 months of the first post-partum year (six patients giving no information about time of onset). Looking more closely at the timing of onset (Figure 1), 81 began during the first week and 46 during the second, so that over half the admissions (127/241 = 53%) fell ill within two weeks. In view of this steep gradient it seems wise to define puerperal psychotics in terms of an onset of illness within two weeks of delivery.

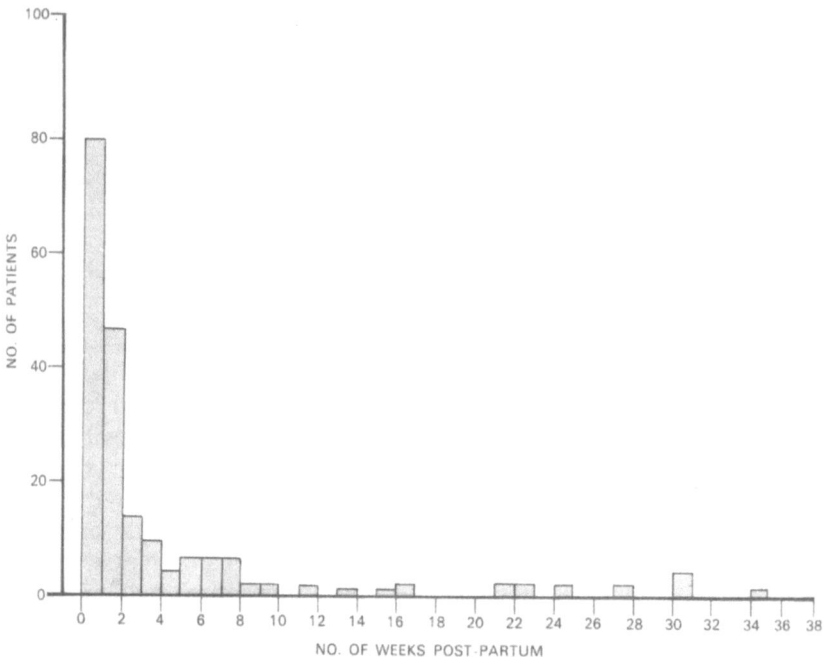

Figure 1 Onset of symptoms in 241 patients admitted to the Mothers and Babies Unit in Manchester

It must, however, be borne in mind that the onset of illness cannot be established with the same precision as the date of admission to hospital. Patients' accounts are distorted by their illness and husbands may not notice the early signs, so that the history is obscure in a proportion of cases. We have measured the inter-rater concordance in determining the time of onset and it is well short of unity; for illnesses beginning within two weeks it was 0.61 (Cohen's kappa), for those beginning during pregnancy itself it was 0.66 and for those beginning more than 2 weeks after delivery it was 0.75. It is essential therefore to use all available information and two raters when deciding time of onset, but even then there is bound to be contamination by patients who did not in fact start within two weeks of childbirth.

Another problem in defining puerperal psychosis is that there is an excess of cases beginning between the 3rd and the 8th week postpartum (Figure 1). Almost all these patients are depressed and it is possible that they are also puerperal psychoses in whom the emergence of symptoms has been more gradual. We may, therefore, be selecting a group biased against depression when we choose onset within two weeks as the defining criterion.

Thirdly, any series defined purely in temporal terms will be contaminated by sporadic cases starting by chance within that interval. In the case of schizophrenia this contamination will be small. The incidence is only about 10/100 000 per year, and the proportion of the population giving birth is about 1% each year. Among the 1.5 million inhabitants served by our Mother and Baby Unit, there would be about 105 000 giving birth in 7 years and within this number one would expect only 0.4 new cases of schizophrenia starting in any two week interval; if we add those patients with previous attacks who relapse we can still expect only one or two patients presenting with schizophrenia beginning fortuitously in the puerperium.

A final problem is contamination by mental illness aetiologically linked to childbirth by mechanisms different from puerperal psychosis, just as heart failure appearing in the puerperium may be due to postpartum hypertension, bacterial endocarditis or thromboembolic pulmonary hypertension. The puerperium is certainly a major life event and a stressful one in some women, especially when the baby is not wanted; depressive episodes arising from this may start within two weeks and, if you believe that schizophrenia is related to life events, this stressful event could precipitate schizophrenia.

These four sources of error are minor in themselves but cumulatively they must produce a degree of contamination which will blur the findings.

With schizophrenia the matter is very much more difficult. There is no agreement at present on the meaning of the term. Originally it was derived by Kraepelin from long term studies of the natural history of mental illness, and he described the clinical manifestations of patients considered to be suffering from dementia praecox at all stages of the disease. By a sleight of hand the disease came to be defined in terms of those clinical features, even though there is no evidence that a group of patients with such a 'syndrome' can be marked off from the mass of psychotics (Kendell and Gourlay, 1970). This first major difficulty – whether schizophrenia should be defined in terms of its clinical picture or its course – is unresolved at the present time. The second difficulty is that the best definitions in use have a rather low mutual concordance. The mean concordance between Catego, Schneider, Langfeldt, Carpenter, Spitzer and Astrachan's definitions in a recent study of psychotic patients was 0.59 (Cohen's Kappa). If an outcome definition was employed it is unlikely that the agreement would be any better. Brockington *et al.* (1978) achieved concordances of 0.67 and 0.55 in making outcome diagnoses in the US/UK and schizoaffective series. Furthermore these low levels of agreement have been achieved using an agreed data base, usually a standardized mental state examination. But much error is involved in establishing such a data base. Mental state examinations are known to be deficient in the rating of objective phenomena which may be important, for example, in distinguishing between schizophrenia and mania. The level of error involved in establishing the phenomena on which schizophrenia is diagnosed has been assessed by Helzer *et al.* (1978), who interviewed patients on two occasions and applied standard defining criteria; they found a concordance of only 0.58 for schizophrenia. So we have 0.59 and 0.58 as estimates of the disagreement in two separate stages of making a diagnosis. Taking both these sources of error into account, Helzer measured the agreement between a research diagnosis and the hospital diagnosis and found it to be 0.37.

From all this it is obvious that it is not going to be easy to determine whether or not puerperal psychotics are schizophrenic. Rigorous clinical methods will be required and it will be necessary to employ a number of different concepts and definitions of schizophrenia. Since July 1976, we have been collecting new cases of postpartum psychosis admitted to the Mothers and Babies Unit at Manchester and studying their phenomenology by standardized mental state interviews administered to patients and next of kin, nurse rating, videotape interviews and self rating, and then reviewing all the available information about the clinical state to establish consensus ratings (3 raters) and applying a number of operational definitions of schizophrenia (2 raters). In this publication we can give only the preliminary results in 58 puerperal psychotics and 38 nonpuerperal controls.

Table 1 shows the diagnoses made when some well accepted definitions of schizophrenia are applied. They show no differences between puerperal psychotics and the comparison series. Fourteen out of 58 (24%) had Schneider's first rank symptoms, and thirteen (22%) had one of the symptom complexes which Langfeldt identified as indicative of poor

Table 1   Diagnoses in puerperal psychosis, using various definitions of schizophrenia

	Puerperal psychosis (N = 58)	Controls (N = 38)
Schneider's first rank symptoms	14	13
Langfeldt's poor prognosis schizomania	13	15
Carpenter's flexible system:		
5 symptoms	25	17
6 symptoms	12	10
Leff's WHO definition of mania	25	9

prognosis, including: passivity phenomena; primary delusions; chronic hallucinosis; catatonic features; and hebephrenia. Twenty-five (43%) had five out of twelve of the symptoms included in Carpenter's list, which are derived from a discriminant function analysis of data from the International Pilot Study of Schizophrenia; and twelve (21%) had six Carpenter symptoms, elsewhere found to be a relatively strict definition of schizophrenia. Our work, therefore, appears at first sight to confirm the prevailing view that many puerperal patients are typical schizophrenics. Indeed the number diagnosed as schizophrenic (21–43%) is more than the number of schizophrenics in a Camberwell first admission study of psychotics (18–24%) using these same criteria (Brockington and Leff, 1979), and the 18–36% found in the Netherne series (Brockington *et al.*, 1978).

Table 2 Diagnoses in puerperal psychosis, using Spitzer's Research Diagnostic Criteria

	Puerperal psychosis (N = 58)	Controls (N = 38)
Mania (11), hypomanic (1)	12	6
Schizoaffective, manic type	10	1
Major depressive disorder (23) or episodic minor depressive disorder (3)	26	9
Schizoaffective, depressed type	4	12
Schizophrenia (4) or probable schizophrenia (1)	5	9
Undiagnosed	2	1
Totals	59*	38

* One patient manic and depressed

When we employ Spitzer's Research Diagnostic Criteria, however, we get a different result. We now find (Table 2): 12 puerperals diagnosed manic; 10 schizoaffective (manic type); 26 with depressive disorders; 4 schizoaffective (depressed type); and only 5 schizophrenic. Thus a high proportion (38%) were either manic or schizomanic, and only 9% had schizophrenic symptoms without affective disorder. When compared with a control series of 38 non-puerperal psychotic women of the same age, they show an excess of manic or schizomanic women and a deficit of schizodepressive and schizophrenics, these differences being significant at the 5% level of significance. The excess of manics is confirmed when the criteria of Leff *et al.* (1976) are applied.

How is it possible to reconcile these divergent results? It cannot be done by discounting some definitions because of their lack of validity, e.g. their failure to predict outcome. This is only true of Schneider's first rank symptoms, which were shown to have poor predictive validity in a recent study (Brockington *et al.*, 1978). Langfeldt's and Carpenter's did not appear less effective than Spitzer's in predicting outcome. Further studies (Brockington, in preparation) have shown that they are relatively good in predicting treatment response while Spitzer's criteria are peculiar in selecting a group of patients with very poor outcome who do not respond to neuroleptic drugs.

One solution to the mystery may be in the schizoaffective quality of these puerperal patients. Table 1 shows that 14/58 (24%) met Spitzer's definitions of schizoaffective disorder, which is much higher than the number considered schizoaffective in other general psychotic series (e.g. 7% in the Camberwell first admission series using the same definitions). Spitzer's criteria are alone among the definitions in the careful attention given to the presence of affective symptoms; using Spitzer's criteria it was evident that 90% of the puerperal patients had very marked affective symptoms, and the majority of patients considered schizophrenic by the other definitions were classed as schizoaffective by Spitzer's. The nosology of the puerperal disorders is therefore closely linked with the riddle of the schizoaffective psychoses. Brockington, Wainwright and Kendell have recently completed a study of some 108 schizoaffectives and, in outline, the results showed that most 'schizomanic' patients followed a benign course, but that in 'schizodepressive' patients it was hard to predict outcome and only a long term follow-up could resolve the conundrum of diagnosis.

Inevitably we are forced to the conclusion that outcome studies are necessary to answer the question of whether or not schizophrenia is truly associated with the puerperium. Our evidence, therefore, will not be complete without a follow-up study, which is now in progress.

References

Bratfos, O. and Haug, J. O. (1966). Puerperal mental disorders in manic depressive females. *Acta Psychiatr. Scand.*, **42**, 285

Brockington, I. F., Kendell, R. E. and Leff, J. P. (1978). Definitions of schizophrenia: concordance and prediction of outcome. *Psychol. Med.*, **8**, 387

Brockington, I. F. and Leff, J. P. (1979). Schizo-affective psychosis: definition and incidence. *Psychol. Med.*, **9**, 91

Helzer, J. E., Clayton, P. J., Pambakian, R. and Woodruff, R. A. (1978). Concurrent diagnostic validity of a structured psychiatric interview. *Arch. Gen. Psychiatry*, **35**, 849

Kendell, R. E. and Gourlay, J. (1970). The clinical distinction between affective psychoses and schizophrenia. *Br. J. Psychiatry*, **117**, 261

Kraepelin, E. (1919) 'Dementia Praecox' trans. Barclay, Edinburgh, Livingstone.

Leff, J. P., Fischer, M. and Bertelsen, A. (1976). A cross national epidemiological study of mania. *Br. J. Psychiatry*, **129**, 428

Paffenbarger, R. S. (1964). Epidemiological aspects of parapartum mental illness. *Br. J. Preventive Soc. Med.*, **18**, 189

Reich, T. and Winokur, G. (1970). Postpartum psychoses in patients with manic depressive disease. *J. Nerv. Ment. Dis.*, **151**, 60

Section 5:
ENZYMOLOGY

19
The digestion and absorption of dietary protein

J. F. WOODLEY, E. E. STERCHI, J. F. BRIDGES, T. FORSYTH,
L. FAULKNER, J. LUCY and A. MAKIN

The ability of the human gastrointestinal tract to digest protein was first demonstrated by Spallanzani in 1783. He showed that if he swallowed some meat enclosed in a muslin bag, and then withdrew the bag from his stomach sometime later, then the meat had 'dissolved'. This was essentially the first demonstration of the action of the proteolytic enzyme pepsin.

Since then many advances have been made in the understanding of the digestive process, but there remain many unanswered questions. The purpose of this paper is to discuss some of the important information that is known about protein digestion and then to focus on some of the anomalies and seeming contradictions which are becoming increasingly evident, and to discuss their possible significance.

ENZYMOLOGY OF PROTEIN DIGESTION

It is now well established that the degradation of dietary protein takes place by a series of attacks by proteolytic enzymes from firstly the stomach, and then the pancreas. These enzymes are of two categories: the endopeptidases, which hydrolyse peptide bonds in the interior of the protein, and the exopeptidases which hydrolyse the terminal amino acids from protein chains. The combined action in terms of specificity and products of hydrolysis is summarised in Table 1.

The end products of the combined action of the enzymes is a mixture of

Table 1 Breakdown of proteins by proteases from stomach and pancreas

Enzyme	Location	Specificity	Products
Endopeptidases			
Pepsin	Stomach	Aromatic, small aliphatic, and glutamic acid residues	Peptides with C-terminal aromatics, aliphatics and glutamate
Trypsin	Pancreatic juice	Arginine, lysine	Peptides with C-terminal arginine and lysine
Chymotrypsin	Pancreatic juice	Aromatic amino acids	Peptides with C-terminal tyrosine, phenylalanine and tryptophan
Elastase	Pancreatic juice	Broad specificity. Mainly neutral aliphatic amino acids	Peptides with C-terminal aliphatic amino acids
Exopeptidases			
Carboxypeptidase A	Pancreatic juice	Cleaves off C-terminal tyrosine, phenylalanine and tryptophan	Free tyr, phe, trp and peptides
Carboxypeptidase B	Pancreatic juice	Cleaves off C-terminal arginine and lysine	Free arg and lys and peptides

free amino acids, and small peptides of varying chain lengths. Free amino acids will be actively transported into the enterocytes, by the four specific amino acid transport systems located in the brush border.

The fate of small peptides is less clear. There is evidence (Silk, 1977) that in man, di- and tripeptides can be absorbed intact by the cells of small intestinal epithelium. Alternatively peptides may be further hydrolysed at the lumenal surface of the enterocytes, if there are active peptidases located at that site.

We have been studying peptidases of purified brush border membranes from human small intestine (Sterchi and Woodley, 1977). Purified brush borders have been prepared from sections of human small intestine, obtained at surgery, frozen immediately, and stored deep frozen until required. The preparation of brush borders obtained shows an enrichment or purification factor of 24-fold with respect to the brush border marker enzyme α-glucosidase. The preparation was free from contamination with lysosomal or cytosol enzymes. The brush border preparation showed hydrolytic activity against a range of peptide substrates. Table 2 shows the activity of the brush border membranes against a range of natural peptide substrates and some naphthylamide derivatives used to measure peptide activity. It can be seen the brush border contains substantial peptidase activity especially against the tetrapeptide and the tri-

Table 2 Specific activities of peptidase hydrolase activities in purified brush border membranes

Substrate	Specific activity
phe-gly-gly-phe	8.15
leu-leu-leu	6.28
leu-2-naphthylamide	4.1
phe-gly-gly	2.83
leu-leu	1.9
leu-gly-gly	1.88
gly-pro-2-naphthylamide	1.73
leu-gly	1.41
tyr-gly-gly	1.37
tyr-tyr-tyr	1.21
phe-gly	0.83
γ-gly-2-naphthylamide	0.76
tyr-gly	0.69
tyr-tyr	0.52
α-glu-2-naphthylamide	0.38

Specific activity is μ moles of substrate hydrolysed min $^{-1}$ mg protein $^{-1}$. (Each is mean of 3–6 fractionations.)

peptide substrates. Welsh *et al.* (1972) showed that human brush border membranes possess endopeptidase activity against the B chain of insulin. This and the results presented here, is convincing evidence for the concept of protein and peptide digestion taking place at or on the brush border membrane.

Thus the combined action of all these enzymes from stomach, pancreas, and brush border membrane should ensure that any dietary protein is hydrolysed to its constituent amino acids or at least to very small peptides which may be absorbed and hydrolysed intracellularly.

ABSORPTION OF UNDIGESTED PROTEIN

Despite the evidence cited above that the mammalian gastrointestinal tract contains considerable capacity for the hydrolysis of dietary proteins, it is now clear from numerous studies (e.g. Hemmings and Williams, 1978) that large protein fragments can pass across the small intestine intact in adult animals. Recent studies from our laboratory have confirmed these observations. Using an *in vitro* gut sac system (Bridges and Woodley, 1979), the uptake of the macromolecule polyvinylpyrrolidone has been observed both into the epithelial cells of the sac, and across the gut wall to the serosal side.

This work has now been extended to the study of the uptake of the enzyme horseradish peroxidase (HRP). Figure 1 shows the rate of transfer of HRP into the serosal space of adult rat gut sacs. As the presence of the protein is detected by its enzymatic activity, it is assumed that this represents the transfer of intact protein. Clearly, there may be large fragments of the molecule being transported, but not detected in the system used.

FACTORS AFFECTING UPTAKE OF PROTEINS BY SMALL INTESTINE

If, as evidence now suggests, intact proteins can be taken up across the small intestine, then it may be of considerable importance in relation to inflammatory disease of the intestine, and other disease with an immunological aetiology. It is of importance to establish whether the nature of the protein may affect its uptake. A protein which is taken up readily either because of its resistance to proteolytic degradation or because of some inherent structural feature which favours uptake, could be potentially damaging to the individual.

Following the suggestions by Dohan that the wheat protein gliadin may be harmful to schizophrenic patients, studies have shown that glia-

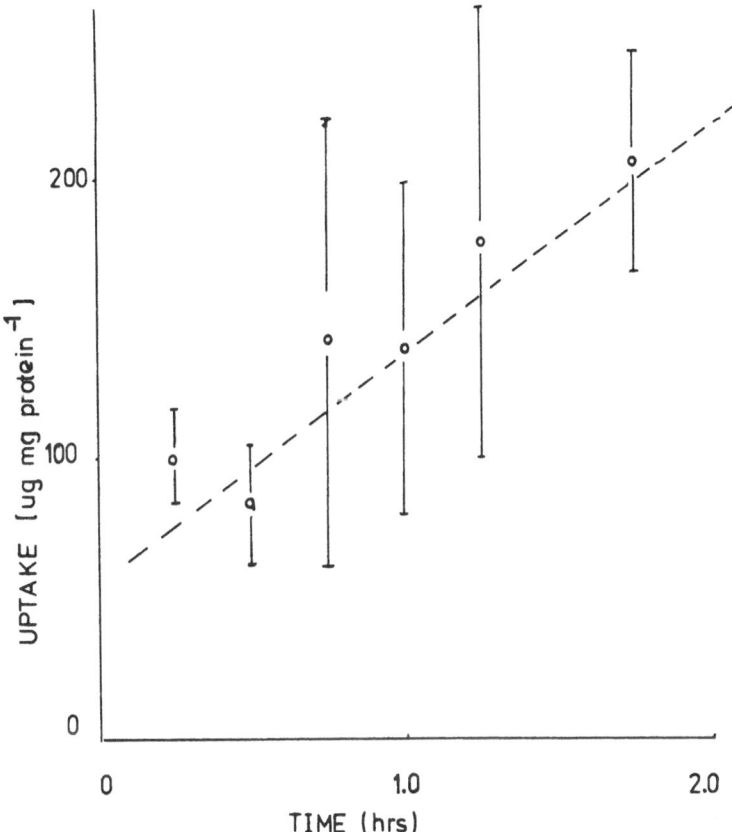

Figure 1 The transport of horseradish peroxidase into the serosal space of everted gut sacs from adult rats. The sacs are incubated in TC 199 medium containing 10% calf serum with a substrate concentration of 400 µg ml^{-1}. Transport is expressed as µg protein translocated mg^{-1} tissue protein. Graph is computer plotted best fit line

din can be absorbed intact (or at least large fragments of it) by adult rats (Hemmings *et al.*, 1977; Hemmings and Williams, 1978). ^{125}I-labelled gliadin was fed to adult rats, and acid precipitable labelled fragments detected in various tissues. Preliminary experiments in this laboratory have shown that the method of labelling used to attach the radioactive iodide to the gliadin alters the distribution of the labelled fragments found in the tissues after feeding the preparations to adult rats. Gliadin was labelled by the chloramine T method of McFarlane (1958) and by the electrolytic method of Rosa *et al.* (1964). The former method is an oxidative method which may cause a number of changes to the protein molecule including oxidation of methionine and cystine residues and partial denaturation.

Table 3 Tissue distribution of radioactivity after the feeding of ^{125}I-labelled gliadin to rats

Tissue	Electrolytically labelled		Chloramine T labelled	
	% of dose	% TCA soluble	% of dose	% TCA soluble
Blood	~0.6	55.0	~0.7	55.0
Brain	0.11	29.8	0.0	–
Faeces	4.5	55.8	82.0	88.0
Intestine	0.9	67.0	0.2	n.d.
Intestinal wash	2.3	76.8	6.15	36.1
Kidneys	0.19	80.7	0.02	n.d.
Liver	1.22	79.5	0.3	n.d.
Stomach	0.5	77.8	0.06	61.0
Stomach wash	4.71	83.7	1.07	74.0
Thyroid	6.6	5.3	2.5	7.6
Urine	41.5	91.5	6.64	92.4

The electrolytic method is far more gentle and results in a higher degree of labelling of the protein molecule. Equal doses of labelled gliadin (2 mg) were administered to adult rats perorally by fine tube directly into the stomach of the animal. The animals were kept for 24 hours with free access to food and water. The animals were then sacrificed and tissues removed and homogenized. Tissues were counted for radioactivity and samples precipitated with trichloroacetic acid and protein bound activity measured. Table 3 shows that the distribution of the radioactivity in the rats is different depending on the labelling procedure used.

In each case radioactivity appears in a bound form in a number of tissues, but it can be seen clearly that the chloramine T labelled gliadin is much less readily absorbed. With this material 82% of the dose is recovered in the faeces, whereas with the electrolytically labelled gliadin the figure is 4.5%. The recoveries in the urine substantiate this observation. The implication of this result is that the physical chemical state of the indigested protein may have a profound influence on its absorption. Clearly the different treatments of the protein gliadin alter its absorption and subsequent distribution in tissues. From such *in vivo* studies it is not possible to say whether the effect is on the digestion of the protein or the mechanism of uptake by the epithelial cells. Further studies on the effect of protein composition on the uptake mechanism are in progress in our laboratory using the *in vitro* sac system.

EFFECT OF GLIADIN ON BEHAVIOUR IN RATS

Following reports (Dohan, 1969; Singh and Kay, 1976) suggesting that the wheat protein gliadin may be deleterious to schizophrenics, much interest has focussed on the effects this protein may or may not have on neurological function. We decided, in a preliminary study, to see whether any behavioural changes could be seen in rats fed high doses of the protein. It was decided to look at behaviour during development of young rats, as it is well established that neonates can absorb large amounts of intact proteins for up to 21 days following birth. Thus it could be assumed that a proportion of any protein fed to animals during this period would be absorbed intact or in large fragments.

Two pregnant rats were handled by experimenters and placed on a gliadin free diet a few days before they were due to give birth. After birth the pups were numbered and divided into three groups. From day 5 the pups were fed daily by mouth tube with either a dose of gliadin (4 mg/ml + sucrose trace); bovine serum albumin (4 mg/ml + sucrose trace) or dilute sucrose, and returned to the mothers. The dose of protein was started at 0.025 ml per animal and gradually increased to 0.2 ml by day 28. All groups received the same dose of material. The experimenters did not know the identity of the three solutions until the experiment was terminated.

The animals were studied daily for a number of behavioural parameters. These included motor development, such as posturing, pivoting, eye opening etc., complex motor skills (rope climbing), and a simple learning avoidance test. The latter test involved placing the animals in a box, and, following sudden exposure to a very bright light, measuring the latency of avoidance (by jumping through a hole into a dark box). After 28 days the animals were sacrificed, the brains removed and weighed and analysed for protein content and acetyl cholinesterase activity.

While most of the simple parameters of motor development showed no significant difference between groups, some differences were observed in the more complex skills, when comparing the gliadin fed animals with the animals fed the non-suspect protein bovine serum albumin. For example in one litter clinging time was significantly different ($p < 0.10$) and total time spent on the rope ($p < 0.05$). For the avoidance learning test there was a significant difference in both litters, between the gliadin and the albumin fed animals. Table 4 shows the mean latency time for the groups of animals.

Biochemical studies showed that while brain to body weight ratios and brain protein levels were similar for all animals, the gliadin fed groups always showed twice the acetyl cholinesterase activity of all the other groups.

Table 4 Avoidance learning test. Mean latency times of avoidance of sudden exposure to bright light (in seconds) of the groups of pups

Age (days)	Litter 1		Litter 2	
	Gliadin-fed	BSA-fed	Gliadin-fed	BSA-fed
23	161	196	160	201
24	133	217	78	205
25	97	191	160	240
26	95	156	145	142
27	47	92	40	152
28	99	87	88	65
	$p < 0.05$		$p < 0.10$	

These preliminary studies indicate that gliadin in the diet of young rats may alter their brain development when fed from an early age. It should be stressed that these results are preliminary, but that the experimental design described may be a useful one for further studies on the effect of diet on development and behaviour.

CONCLUSION

While the small intestine of mammals contains a vast array of enzymes involved in protein digestion, evidence is now accumulating to indicate that small amounts of intact proteins may cross the mucosa to reach the serosal side. The transport of these proteins may be very dependent on the structure and chemical properties of the proteins, at least in the case of the wheat protein gliadin. Gliadin may also affect the neural development of young rats, when included in their diet from a very early age.

Acknowledgement

We wish to thank Hazel Cable for technical support.

References

Bridges, J. F. and Woodley, J. F. (1979). The uptake of ^{125}I-labelled polyvinylpyrrolidone by adult rat gut *in vitro*. In Hemmings, W. A. (ed.) *Protein Transmission through Living Membranes*, pp. 249–257. (Amsterdam: Elsevier/North Holland Biomedical Press)

Dohan, F. C. (1969). Is coeliac disease a clue to the pathogenesis of schizophrenia? *Ment. Hyg.*, **53**, 525

Hemmings, C., Hemmings, W. A., Patey, A. L. and Wood, D. (1977). The ingestion of dietary protein as large molecules mass degradation products in adult rats. *Proc. R. Soc. London,* **198**, 439

Hemmings, W. A. and Williams, E. W. (1978). Transport of large breakdown products of dietary protein through the gut wall. *Gut*, **19**, 715

McFarlane, A. S. (1958). Efficient trace-labelling of proteins with iodine. *Nature (London)*, **182**, 53

Rosa, U., Scassellati, G. A., Pennisi, F., Riccioni, N., Giagnoni, P. and Giordani, R. (1964). Labelling of human fibrinogen with ^{131}I by electrolytic iodination. *Biochim. Biophys. Acta*, **86**, 519

Silk, D. B. A. (1977). Amino acid and peptide absorption in man. In *Peptide Transport and Hydrolysis, CIBA Symposium No. 50*, pp. 15–29

Singh, M. M. and Kay, S. R. (1976). Wheat gluten as a pathogenic factor in schizophrenia. *Science*, **191**, 401

Sterchi, E. E. and Woodley, J. F. (1977). Peptidases of the human intestinal brush border membrane. In McNicholl, B., McCarthy, C. F. and Fottrell, P. F. (eds.) *Perspectives in Coeliac Disease*, pp. 437–449. (Lancaster: MTP Press)

Welsh, J. D., Preiser, H., Woodley, J. F. and Crane, R. K. (1972). An enriched microvillous membrane preparation from frozen specimens of human small intestine. *Gastroenterology*, **62**, 572

Section 6:
PHYSIOLOGY

20

Correlation between behavioural responses and cardiovascular changes and the central nervous mechanisms responsible for them

S. M. HILTON

Any study of behaviour and its central nervous control is inevitably concerned with the whole, intact organism. Physiologists are becoming increasingly aware of the challenge that studies of this kind represent. It is not just a matter of developing new and more appropriate experimental techniques; it is also, and even more important, a question of finding the right ideas to work with. In the particular case of my present topic, it may be asked whether emotion is indeed a proper subject for physiological study. However, we have realised since the work of Cannon (1929) in the early part of this century that, in the case of fear and rage reactions, the responses of the internal organs as well as the skeletal muscles may properly be regarded as adaptive, for they enable the organism to deal with particular types of emergency, engendered by a potential threat to which the animal (or man) may best respond by flight or fight. In the light of this hypothesis, the challenge to the physiologist is to unravel the changes occurring within the organism and to test whether they really would contribute to its maximum efficiency if severe muscular exertion were to be called for. Pursuance of this goal goes hand in hand with another one, which is to define those regions of the central nervous system which integrate the whole pattern of response and to study the nervous pathways by which they are activated or inhibited on the one hand, and by which they exert their effects on the other.

Cannon's student, Bard (1928), was the first to define the special role of the hypothalamus in both driving and integrating fear and rage responses. Some time later, mostly in the 1940s, Hess (1949) carried out a monumental series of experiments, largely concerned with observing the effects of electrical stimulation of restricted regions of the hypothalamus and midbrain in the cat, which enabled him to map separate regions concerned with alimentary and sexual behaviour as well as fear and rage behaviour, which he called the defence reaction (Hess and Brugger 1943). This reaction begins as alerting, with threshold stimulation, and culminates, if stimulation is sufficiently intense, in flight or attack, the behaviour being indistinguishable from the animal's natural response to environmental stimuli. This was a major step forward in the way of clarifying the neurological basis of instinctive behaviour; for it enabled these activities to be seen as little different in principle from, say, temperature regulation, which is also a patterned response with internal visceral and overt motor components and an organizing region in the hypothalamus. The defence reaction is more like temperature regulation than alimentary or sexual responses in that these are only intermittently expressed whereas the defence response is really a particularly strong involvement of the brainstem activating or arousal system which is continuously expressed in the waking state.

Together with a number of colleagues I have been working on the defence reaction for some twenty years, particularly on its cardiovascular components and central nervous organization, and these are what I want to deal with in more detail. Firstly, we know the precise location of regions in the hypothalamus, mid-brain and medulla (Abrahams et al., 1960; Coote et al., 1973) which, by their concerted action, integrate the pattern of cardiovascular response. The response itself is characterized by dilatation of resistance vessels in skeletal muscle with vasoconstriction in the gastro-intestinal tract, kidney and skin, which effects an appropriate redistribution of circulating blood; venous reservoirs are mobilized which, with increased heart-rate and contractility, ensure a significant rise in cardiac output. All these effects lead to an increase in mean arterial pressure and pulse pressure (for references, see Hilton, 1965). In this way, the cardiovascular adjustments are made which may have to meet the urgent demands of struggle or escape. In several animal species and in man, special vasodilator nerve fibres play an important part in bringing about the muscle vasodilatation. As these nerve fibres are not involved in any other cardiovascular response, their activation has proved to be a most useful index of the whole response in all our mapping studies in experimental animals; they enabled us to show the exact location of the integrating regions and the efferent pathway leading from them. When stimulating within these integrating regions in conscious animals, we could show that the cardiovascular response occurs in the early alerting stage of the behavioural reaction when the animal shows no more than pupillary dilatation, pricking of the ears and an increase in respiration (Abrahams *et al.*, 1964). The same changes occur after any sudden novel stimulus in the animal's environment and the whole response may therefore be classed as a preparatory reflex.

Although most of the experimental work so far has been carried out on cats, enough has been done on other mammalian species, including monkeys (Schramm *et al.*, 1971), for us to be sure that in all of them analogous regions of the brain perform a similar function. In man, too, mild electrical stimulation in the medial hypothalamus has produced feelings variously recorded as restlessness, anxiety, depression, fright and horror, while stronger stimulation in the posterior hypothalamus can produce rage (Heath and Mickle, 1960; Sem Jacobsen and Torkildsen, 1969). It is a fact with interesting neurophysiological implications that electrical stimulation in these areas of the brain can produce changes apparently identical with those occurring on natural stimulation. The only apparent difference is the suddenness of onset and the abrupt termination of the response as the stimulus is switched on and off; maybe even this is reproduced in neuropathological conditions.

Under natural conditions, the response is evoked by inputs of several modalities – auditory, visual and noxious, in particular – and by any signal associated with a threatening situation. It is readily elicited in man by a problem in mental arithmetic (Brod *et al.*, 1959). Before considering such naturally occurring responses in further detail, the idea that there is a simple reflex integrated in the brainstem has to be qualified, as the central nervous system acts as a whole. There is no convincing evidence that alerting or defence response can be initiated from the neocortex, (Hilton *et al.*, 1979) although they can be modulated from particular areas of the frontal cortex (Timms, 1977). There is, however, no doubt of the significance of the limbic system, which comprises the structures surrounding the hilus of the cerebral hemisphere and which are almost identical in all mammals. The region most directly connected with the hypothalamus and midbrain resides in the amygdala, a group of nuclei subjacent to the hippocampus, within the temporal lobe. Stimulation of a localized region of the amygdala synaptically activates the defence areas of the hypothalamus and midbrain by a direct pathway (Hilton and Zbrozyna, 1963). In addition, the stria terminalis contains a group of nerve fibres which course from the anterior hypothalamus to the amygdala to activate it. This anatomical arrangement is suggestive of a circuit with positive feedback, and indeed, the effect of stimulation of the stria terminalis or the amygdala differs from that of brainstem stimulation in that the response builds up gradually and persists for minutes after stimulation has ceased. There have been a few studies of amygdala stimulation in man which have pointed in the same direction, even to the extent of causing increases in blood pressure and heart rate (Heath *et al.*, 1955; Chapman, 1960; Bovard, 1962).

Patients suffering chronic anxiety states show the cardiovascular features of the defence response, including a large increase in muscle blood flow (Kelly and Walter, 1968). Moreover, a return of muscle blood flow to normal may be the best early indication of successful therapy. Suddenly provoked defence reactions, including their cardiovascular components show the usual type of waning, or habituation, with repetition of any particular stimulus, in man and experimental animals; however, they are also readily conditioned (for references, see Martin *et al.*, 1976), and these conditioned responses seem to be especially stable. The habituation and conditioning of the responses are particularly interesting because of the different time courses that may be taken by the various cardiovascular and behavioural components. With repetition of a stimulus, moreover, there are individuals in whom, while some components are habituated, other components show the converse and are sensitized. Thus either behavioural or cardiovascular responsiveness might increase with stimulus repetition in different individuals; even single components of the cardiovascular response might show such sensitization. In brief, while it is correct to emphasize that the central nervous control of the cardiovascular system is indissolubly bound up with the control of behavioural responses and that this is nowhere clearer than in the case of the defence reaction (Hilton, 1979), the possible fragmentation of the reaction is an important subject for study, especially under circumstances in which apparently inappropriate responses appear.

Mention must be made, in this connection, of other components of the whole defence reaction. In particular, there is the well known release of catecholamines from the adrenal medulla in sufficient amounts to mobilise liver glycogen and give rise to glycosuria; as discussed by Cannon (1929) they will also improve the performance of fatigued muscle, and can reduce coagulation time (and increase fibrinolytic activity). Adrenocorticotrophic hormone (ACTH) has also been known for some time to be regularly released in response to stimuli leading to arousal or distress, in monkeys and men (Mason, 1959; for review, see Leshner, 1977). Evidence from neurophysiological experiments supports the conclusion that it is released as part of the defence reaction (see Hilton, 1965). Plasma levels of 17-hydroxycorticoids approaching those observed in acute reactions in aircrew, and more persistently in patients during the first week after major thoracic surgery (approximately a doubling of the normal level), have been reported in subjects with anxiety states (e.g. Hamburg *et al.*, 1958). ACTH itself may appear in the blood of medical students after oral examinations, at levels as high as those found in Cushing's disease (Hodges *et al.*, 1962). A particular point regarding these hormonal changes is that they are incompatible with short term homoeostasis.

Their powerful effects can greatly disturb the internal milieu, particularly if no muscular exertion occurs, and they are by no means conducive to a feeling of well being. As a feature of the cardiovascular component of the defence reaction, there is a further disturbance of homoeostasis by virtue of a powerful inhibition of the baroreceptor reflex, which enables a concomitant increase of mean arterial pressure, pulse pressure and heart rate. It has been natural to discuss this particular anti-homoeostatic effect as a contributory factor in the evolution of essential hypertension.

The defence reaction – or, at least its alerting stage – is a common feature of the waking life of animals and man. Indeed, it is a constant feature of the waking state. Because of the ubiquity of its various components, the ease of conditioning, and the abrogation of homoeostatic mechanisms which it imposes, it could give rise to a variety of disturbances if unduly intense or prolonged. As we know the precise location of the areas of the brain which, when activated, by whatever means, actually arouse the subjective emotional responses as well as eliciting a group of well defined objective manifestations, both autonomic and hormonal, the way seems open for the development of a new understanding of both normal and disturbed central nervous function. This could lead to new ways of categorising disturbed function, and to increasingly specific pharmacological approaches towards its alleviation.

References

Abrahams, V. C., Hilton, S. M. and Zbrożyna, A. W. (1960). Active muscle vasodilatation produced by stimulation of the brainstem: its significance in the defence reaction. *J. Physiol.*, **154**, 491

Abrahams, V. C., Hilton, S. M. and Zbrożyna, A. W. (1964). The role of active muscle vasodilatation in the alerting stage of the defence reaction. *J. Physiol.*, **171**, 189

Bard, P. (1928). A diencephalic mechanism for the expression of rage with reference to the sympathetic nervous system. *Am. J. Physiol.*, **84**, 490

Bovard, E. W. (1962). The balance between negative and positive brain system activity. *Perspect. Biol. Med.*, **6**, 116

Brod, J., Fencl, V., Hejl, Z. and Jirka, J. (1959). Circulatory changes underlying blood pressure elevation during acute emotional stress (mental arithmetic) in normotensive and hypertensive subjects. *Clin. Sci.*, **18**, 269

Cannon, W. B. (1929). *Bodily changes in Pain, Hunger, Fear and Rage.* 2nd Edn. (New York: Appleton)

Chapman, W. P. (1960). In Ramey, E. R. and O'Doherty, D. S. (eds) *Electrical Studies on the Unanaesthetized Brain*, p. 334. (New York: Paul B. Hoeber)

Coote, J. H., Hilton, S. M. and Zbrożyna, A. W. (1973). The ponto-medullary area integrating the defence reaction in the cat and its influences on muscle blood flow. *J. Physiol.*, **229**, 257

Hamburg, D. A., Sabshin, M. A., Board, F. A., Grinker, R. R., Korchin, S. J., Basowitz, H., Heath, H. and Persky, H. (1958). Classification and rating of emotional experiences. *Arch. Neurol. Psychiatry*, **79**, 415

Heath, R. G. and Mickle, W. A. (1960). In Ramey, E. R. and O'Doherty, D. S. (eds.) *Electrical Studies on the Unanaesthetized Brain*, p. 214 (New York: Paul B. Hoeber)

Heath, R. G., Monroe, R. R. and Mickle, W. A. (1955). Stimulation of the amygdaloid nucleus in a schizophrenic patient. *Am. J. Psychiatry*, **111**, 862

Hess, W. R. (1949). *Das Zwischenhirn*. (Basel: Schwabe)

Hess, W. R. and Brügger, M. (1943). Das Subkorticale Zentrum der affectiven Abwehrreaktion. *Helv. Physiol. Acta*, **1**, 33

Hilton, S. M. (1965). Hypothalamic control of the cardiovascular responses in fear and rage. *Sci. Basis Med. Annu. Rev.*, 217

Hilton, S. M. (1979). The defence reaction as a paradigm for cardiovascular control. In Brooks, C. McC., Koizumi, K. and Sato, A. (eds.) *Integrative Functions of the Autonomic Nervous System*, pp. 443–449 (Tokyo: University Press)

Hilton, S. M., Spyer, K. M. and Timms, R. J. (1979). The origin of the hind limb vasodilatation evoked by stimulation of the motor cortex in the cat. *J. Physiol.*, **287**, 545

Hilton, S. M. and Zbrożyna, A. W. (1963). Amygdaloid region for defence reactions and its efferent pathway to the brainstem. *J. Physiol.*, **165**, 160

Hodges, J. R., Jones, M. T. and Stockham, M. A. (1962). Effect of emotion on blood corticotrophin and cortisol concentrations in man. *Nature*, **193**, 1187

Kelly, D. H. W. and Walter, C. J. S. (1968). The relationship between clinical diagnosis and anxiety, assessed by forearm blood flow and other measurements. *Br. J. Psychiatry*, **114**, 611

Leshner, A. I. (1977). In Candland, D. K., Fell, J. P., Keen, E., Leshner, A. I., Tarpy, R. M. and Plucheck, R. (eds.) *Emotion*, pp. 443–449. (Monterey: Brooks Cole)

Martin, J., Sutherland, C. J. and Zbrożyna, A. W. (1976). Habituation and conditioning of the defence reactions and their cardiovascular components in cats and dogs. *Pflügers Arch.*, **365**, 37

Mason, J. W. (1959). Psychological influences on the pituitary adrenal cortical system. *Recent Prog. Hormone Res.*, **15**, 345

Schramm, L. P., Honig, C. R. and Bignall, K. E. (1971). Active muscle vasodilatation in primates homologous with sympathetic vasodilation in carnivores. *Am. J. Physiol.*, **221**, 768

Sem-Jacobsen, C. W. and Torkildsen, A. (1969). In Ramev, E. R. and O'Doherty, D. S. (eds.) *Electrical Studies on the Unanaesthetized Brain*, p. 275. (New York: Paul B. Hoeber)

Timms, R. J. (1977). Cortical inhibition and facilitation of the defence reaction. *J. Physiol.*, **266**, 98

Section 7:
MORBIDITY AND MORTALITY

21
Schizophrenia and physical disease: a preliminary analysis of the data from the Oxford Record Linkage Study

J. A. BALDWIN

The study reported in this paper originated from a request by the World Health Organisation to participate in the Study of Determinants of Outcome of Severe Mental Disorders which it is co-ordinating as a multinational study in succession to the International Pilot Study of Schizophrenia. One sub-study is of the General Morbidity of Psychiatric Patients and their Families and is based on psychiatric case registers in Denmark, Hawaii, Monro County, N.Y., Moscow, Nagasaki and Oxford. The Oxford study described here was a preliminary analysis of available data as a guide to design of specific studies in the other centres. The results are therefore tentative and subject to revision upon further examination of the data.

BACKGROUND

A review of literature on the relation between physical disease and schizophrenia showed that a large number of disorders have been postulated to be associated either positively or negatively (antagonistically) with schizophrenia at various times throughout the last two millenia, yet there are very few firmly established conclusions (Baldwin, 1979). Most sound observational studies have been of mortality while the adequacy of design and scale of many studies of both mortality and morbidity are questionable. There is therefore a need for a systematic statistical evaluation of the range of illness found in association with schizophrenia in order to concentrate attention on relationships likely to be of aetiological relevance. The requirement is for valid estimates of the *relative risk* of diseases in schizophrenics in comparison with other psychiatric disorders and with the general population from which the patients come. The collection of cumulative personal medical records in the Oxford Record Linkage Study is a convenient source of information for this purpose.

MATERIAL AND METHOD

The Oxford Record Linkage Study is a collection of abstracts of clinical records of all types of hospitalisation together with records of all births, stillbirths and deaths occurring in a defined population at risk. The abstract records contain identifying, demographic, social and clinical data and are arranged so that all the hospitalisation and vital events relating to an individual are linked together in temporal order to form cumulative personal medical records. This medical information system was started in 1963 and continues to the present day. The techniques of collecting and linking the data have been described elsewhere (Acheson, 1967; Baldwin, 1973). Data used for the study reported in this paper were those for the nominal 8 year period from 1963 to 1970 in respect of the County of Oxfordshire and part of the County of Berkshire, representing a mixed urban and rural community of between 750 000 and 800 000. The whole of this geographical area was not covered throughout the 8 year period and the mean period at risk was approximately 3.25 years. The total number of hospitalisation, birth and death records was 559 266 and when linked together formed 366 862 cumulative personal medical records. The diagnostic information consisted of up to 2 diagnoses for each hospitalisation or vital event, which were coded according to the International Classification of Diseases (Seventh and Eighth Revisions). There were 2314 persons diagnosed schizophrenic. Classification to fourth digit level was used wherever numbers permitted (Table 1).

The objective of the study was to estimate whether schizophrenia was preceded or followed by another disease more often than would be expected by chance, making use of all the available diagnostic information from the cumulative personal medical records. Observed numbers of individuals having each disease studied prior to and following schizophrenia were obtained, omitting only repeated diagnostic information. Expected numbers were derived from the sex and age-specific incidence rates for the calendar period at risk of probands using the linked data as numerators and community population at risk as denominators, adjusted for period at risk, variation of risk with time (secular, seasonal and epidemic trends), sex differences in risk, the cohort effect on age, population migration out of the area, and mortality. The statistical

Table 1 Oxford Record Linkage Study. Sub-types among 2314 persons diagnosed as having schizophrenia during the period 1963–1970

Simple	154
Hebephrenia	82
Catatonia	42
Paranoid	375
Acute	83
Latent/residual	18
Schizo-affective	72
Other/not otherwise stated	1720

Note: The total is greater than 2314 because some individuals were diagnosed as in different sub-types at different times

method has been described in detail in Baldwin *et al.* (1979).

Results were expressed as relative risks (ratio of observed to expected numbers) tested for statistically significant deviations from unity. Expectations were considered to be distributed as Poisson variables and exact probabilities of differences from observed values calculated. Except where differences in relative risks for each temporal order of associated diseases appeared likely to be both important and reliable, results for both temporal orders were combined. Simultaneously occurring diagnoses are difficult to handle statistically and were omitted from the main analyses (Baldwin *et al.*, 1979). Where numbers of such cases altered the result significantly the effect is reported and discussed in the text.

Similar calculations were obtained in respect of individuals with the diagnosis of affective psychosis (1489 persons) to ascertain the degree of association of each disease with another functional psychosis, and non-psychotic depression (3915 persons) to ascertain the degree of association with a non-psychotic psychiatric disorder. Using the same method of calculating relative risks for all three psychiatric conditions ensured strict comparability between the findings for schizophrenia and the controls, permitting an estimate of the degree of specificity of any given association with schizophrenia.

The study was intended only as a preliminary analysis to guide further work and the limitations of the data and of the method must be stated at the outset. Relatively small numbers of cases of schizophrenia and controls as well as of many uncommon diseases were available so that the material was not adequate to assess a number of potentially important associations. Where small numbers are involved, even infrequent errors in the clinical data or in the coding and processing of it may cause unreliable results. Results based on small numbers should be verified by reference to original records but this was not practicable with the time and resources allocated for the study. The nominal period of 8 years with a mean period at risk of only 3.25 years was too short to enable conclusions

Table 2 Oxford Record Linkage Study. Relative risk of specified cancers in schizophrenia cases and controls

Disease	No. Cases	Schizophrenia		Affective Psychosis		Depression	
		Observed No.	Relative Risk	Observed No.	Relative Risk	Observed No.	Relative Risk
Breast	2438	7	0.96+	6	0.70	17	1.02
Colon/Rectum	2443	5	0.77	7	1.08	11	0.90
Haematopoetic	1177	1	0.33	1	0.42	2	0.39
Lung/Bronchus	3052	5	0.64	6	1.07	17	1.38
Oesophagus	302	2	2.93	1	1.53	0	–
Pancreas	533	2	1.65	1	0.88	5	2.28
Stomach	1312	5	1.73++	4	1.46	6	1.16

+Marginally significant excess in hebephrenics
++Marginally significant excess in non-specific schizophrenia

Table 3 Oxford Record Linkage Study. Relative risk of diseases of heart and circulatory system in cases of schizophrenia and controls

Disease	No. Cases	Schizophrenia		Affective Psychosis		Depression	
		Observed No.	Relative Risk	Observed No.	Relative Risk	Observed No.	Relative Risk
Arterio-sclerotic Heart Disease	18,404	70	1.71***	60	1.55***	143	1.98***
Hypertensive Heart Disease	1,418	1	0.29	3	0.81	16	2.38**
Other Hypertensive Disease	2,895	9	0.96	12	1.36	41	2.31***
Arteriosclerosis	1,646	5	1.46	7	2.00	17	2.79***
Vascular Lesions of C.N.S.	11,550	31	1.26	45	1.64**	116	2.44***

$p < 0.01 = **$ $p < 0.001 = ***$

to be drawn about relationships between diseases which are likely to occur at widely different ages in individuals.

Deficient ascertainment of morbidity is likely to have distorted some results in various ways. The fact that the collection of data did not commence until 1963 entails that diseases occurring in individuals before this year were incompletely ascertained. Only morbidity leading to admission to a hospital in-patient service or death (in hospital or community) was included so that physical disease treated wholly in mental hospitals or by means of out-patient or primary care was not recorded. A total of 328 schizophrenics were resident in hospital at the end of the follow-up period and had not been transferred to another facility for treatment of a physical disease.

The diagnostic information was in all cases obtained from clinical records. Thus there was likely to have been variation in diagnostic standards over the 8 year period, particularly in respect of psychiatric diagnoses. There are strong associations between the diagnoses of schizophrenia, affective psychosis and depression, many individuals exhibiting features of more than one of these conditions in the course of successive hospital admissions.

The estimation of periods at risk is in some respects imprecise. For example, information on migration out of the population at risk was sparse, the weights given to this factor having been obtained from a single study covering a year following the end of the follow-up period.

These limitations are likely to have had conflicting and varied effects on the results obtained. Deficient ascertainment will have caused underestimation of associations in most instances and for this reason low relative risks should be interpreted with caution. In contrast, high relative risks are likely to be more reliable. Since both the schizophrenia group and the control diagnoses were, in the main, subject to the same constraints, greater confidence may be had in comparative results between these groups than in the absolute values of each group in isolation.

RESULTS

Results are given for conditions claimed or hypothesized to be positively or negatively associated with schizophrenia in previous literature (Baldwin, 1979), or found *de novo* in the course of the analysis.

Cancer

Summary results for some common cancers and for certain cancers noted in previous literature to be positively or negatively associated with schizophrenia are set out in Table 2. There were no robustly significant

Table 4 Oxford Record Linkage Study. Relative risk of pneumonia and bronchitis in schizophrenia and controls

Disease	No. Cases	Schizophrenia		Affective Psychosis		Depression	
		Observed No.	Relative Risk	Observed No.	Relative Risk	Observed No.	Relative Risk
Pneumonia	10770	34	1.63**	37	1.80***	100	2.64***
Bronchitis	9068	23	1.05	33	1.78**	88	2.41***

$p < 0.01 = **$ $p < 0.001 = ***$

Table 5 Oxford Record Linkage Study. Relative risk of pulmonary tuberculosis in cases of schizophrenia and controls

Disease	No. Cases	Schizophrenia		Affective Psychosis		Depression	
		Observed No.	Relative Risk	Observed No.	Relative Risk	Observed No.	Relative Risk
Before Mental illness							
Pulmonary TB	1885	8	2.93**	1	0.47	11	2.28*
Excl. Pleural Effusion	1484	7	3.14**	1	0.59	10	2.52**
After Mental Illness							
Pulmonary TB	1885	4	1.15	4	2.18	13	2.48**
Excl. Pleural Effusion	1484	4	1.47	3	2.35	8	2.01

$p < 0.05 = *$ $p < 0.01 = **$

increases or decreases of relative risk for any cancer or all cancers in relation to either schizophrenia as a whole or the affective psychoses and non-psychotic depressions. There was a marginally significant excess of cancer of the stomach in non-specific schizophrenics and of cancer of the breast in hebephrenic women. A just significant increase in relative risk of cancer of the oesophagus was found in schizophrenics as a whole when simultaneously diagnosed cases were taken into account (relative risk = 4.39, p = 0.03). Although the period at risk was too short for confident evaluation, these results are in general accord with most comparable estimates. Nevertheless, the study did not take account of duration of hospitalisation so that low relative risks for long-stay mental patients reported previously by Katz et al. (1967) may have been masked.

Heart and vascular disease

Table 3 gives summary results for the commonest groups of circulatory and cardiovascular diseases. There was a highly significant excess of arteriosclerotic heart disease in both schizophrenics and control groups but in distinction from the controls there was no significant elevation of relative risk for any other group of circulatory diseases among schizophrenics.

Respiratory disease

There was a significant excess of pneumonia in relation to both schizophrenia and the controls, but in contrast to the control groups there was no excess of bronchitis among schizophrenics (Table 4). Pulmonary tuberculosis occurred more often than expected by chance prior to the diagnosis of schizophrenia and this was evident after exclusion of diagnoses of pleural effusion of presumed but unconfirmed tuberculous origin (Table 5). Non-psychotic depression was also more common than expected after pulmonary tuberculosis.

Epilepsy

Results for the main types of epilepsy are set out in Table 6. Significantly raised relative risks for major epilepsy, epileptic psychosis and unspecified epilepsy were found among both schizophrenics and the control groups. For schizophrenics all these excesses were limited to paranoid and non-specific schizophrenia. When simultaneously occurring diagnoses were included the relative risk of non-specific epilepsy in non-specific schizophrenia was increased to 5.65 and of major epilepsy in paranoid schizophrenia to 24.69 though the validity of these ratios is somewhat uncertain (Baldwin et al., 1979).

Table 6 Oxford Record Linkage Study. Relative risk of specified epilepsies in cases of schizophrenia and controls

Disease	No. Cases	Schizophrenia		Affective Psychosis		Depression	
		Observed No.	Relative Risk	Observed No.	Relative Risk	Observed No.	Relative Risk
Major Epilepsy	201	3	5.32*§	3	10.75**	3	3.82*
Minor Epilepsy	57	0	–	1	12.66	1	4.90
Focal Epilepsy	73	0	–	1	8.62	1	3.28
Epileptic Psychosis	46	5	32.68***§	0	–	4	17.78***
Epilepsy N.O.S.	1888	14	2.76***§	10	3.17**	38	4.45***

$p < 0.05 =$* $p < 0.01 =$** $p < 0.001 =$***

§ Significant excesses among Paranoid Schizophrenics and Non-specific Schizophrenics

Table 7 Oxford Record Linkage Study. Relative risk of Parkinson's disease in cases of schizophrenia and controls

Disease	No. Cases	Schizophrenia		Affective Psychosis		Depression	
		Observed No.	Relative Risk	Observed No.	Relative Risk	Observed No.	Relative Risk
Before Mental Illness	1235	2	2.32	3	2.80	6	3.78**
After Mental Illness	1235	5	2.57*	6	2.60*	9	2.19*

$p < 0.05 =$* $p < 0.01 =$**

Parkinson's disease

There were increases in the relative risks of schizophrenia, affective psychoses and non-psychotic depression in the course of Parkinson's disease, but the excess was significant only in the last of these (Table 7). Parkinsonism was marginally significantly more frequent than expected by chance following all three groups of psychiatric disorder.

Asthma and hay fever

The incidence of allergic conditions was low although within chance limits in schizophrenia but was significantly raised in both control groups.

Peptic ulcer

The relative risk of peptic ulcer, including both gastric and duodenal types, was non-significantly low in schizophrenia, almost unity in affective psychosis and marginally significantly raised in non-psychotic depression, this increase being limited to depression following the occurrence of ulcer (Table 8).

Diabetes mellitus

A marginally reduced relative risk was found among schizophrenics and there was a marginally raised risk of depression following diabetes mellitus (Table 8). Simultaneous diagnoses of schizophrenia and diabetes numbered seven increasing the relative risk to 1.00. The chronicity of diabetes mellitus increases confidence in the validity of the combined figures and the initial reduced relative risk is almost certainly artefactual.

Malabsorption

Though the relative risk of malabsorption in schizophrenics was nearly threefold, this was within the limits of chance (Table 8). There was one additional case in which malabsorption and schizophrenia were diagnosed simultaneously increasing the relative risk to 4.28 ($p = 0.034$). There was one case of hebephrenia following malabsorption which was significantly more than expected. Depression in malabsorption was also three times as common as expected and this was a just significant excess. There were no cases of confirmed coeliac disease in this group of diagnoses.

Table 8 Oxford Record Linkage Study. Relative risk of certain diseases in cases of schizophrenia and controls

Disease	No. Cases	Schizophrenia		Affective Psychosis		Depression	
		Observed No.	Relative Risk	Observed No.	Relative Risk	Observed No.	Relative Risk
Asthma/Hay Fever	3252	6	0.74	11	1.99*	34	2.46***
Peptic Ulcer	3973	11	0.76	10	1.01	31	1.40*
Diabetes Mellitus	4422	6	0.47*	14	1.09	37	1.52*
Malabsorption	266	2	2.85	1	1.81	4	3.06*
Rheumatoid Arthritis	2122	1	0.15**	10	1.38	13	0.94
Osteo-arthritis	3331	5	0.46*	12	1.02	23	1.09
Thyrotoxicosis	1498	5	0.94	10	2.06*	25	2.18***
Myxoedema/Cretinism	339	4	4.47*	4	3.95*	12	5.73***

$p < 0.05 = *$ $p < 0.01 = **$ $p < 0.001 = ***$

Table 9 Oxford Record Linkage Study. Relative risks of diseases of gallbladder and bone in cases of schizophrenia and controls

Disease	No. Cases	Schizophrenia		Affective Psychosis		Depression	
		Observed No.	Relative Risk	Observed No.	Relative Risk	Observed No.	Relative Risk
Gallbladder Disease	1771	5	0.37**	7	0.57	31	1.13
Osteomyelitis and other bone diseases	6454	6	0.30***	7	0.60	37	1.17

$p < 0.01 = **$ $p < 0.001 = ***$

Arthritis

There was a significant deficit of rheumatoid arthritis among schizophrenics as a whole (Table 8). A second unconfirmed case was found in whom the two conditions were diagnosed simultaneously increasing the relative risk to 0.30 ($p = 0.037$). The relative risk of osteo-arthritis was also marginally significantly low in schizophrenia. The relative risk of both conditions was close to unity in both control groups.

Thyroid disorders

While the number of schizophrenics with thyrotoxicosis was similar to that expected, there was a fourfold increase in relative risk of myxoedema which was just significant for schizophrenia as a whole. The excess was restricted to catatonics and non-specific schizophrenics and was significant in both groups (Table 8). One further case had both diagnoses simultaneously raising the overall relative risk to 5.59 ($p = 0.002$). The risk of both conditions was significantly raised among both affective psychoses and non-psychotic depressions, highly significant in respect of the latter.

Gallbladder disease

There was a highly significantly reduced relative risk of gallbladder disease among schizophrenics (Table 9). The risk was also low among affective psychotics but within chance limits, while among the non-psychotic depressions the observed and expected numbers were nearly equal.

Diseases of bone

Osteomyelitis and certain other diseases of bone were very significantly reduced in the group of schizophrenias (Table 9). There was a non-significantly low risk in the affective psychoses but not in the depressions.

Urinary diseases

A very significantly low relative risk of a group of urinary diseases, mainly calculi, was found among male schizophrenics only but not among males with affective psychoses or non-psychotic depressions (Table 10).

Head injury

There was a marginally significant increase in the relative risk of head

Table 10 Oxford Record Linkage Study. Relative risks of certain urinary diseases and head injury in male schizophrenics and controls

Disease	No. Cases	Schizophrenia		Affective Psychosis		Depression	
		Observed No.	Relative Risk	Observed No.	Relative Risk	Observed No.	Relative Risk
Urinary calculus and other urinary diseases	7521	1	0.11***	8	1.62	14	1.21
Head injury	13711	31	1.44*	15	2.00*	61	2.61***

$p < 0.05 =$* $p < 0.001 =$***

Table 11 Oxford Record Linkage Study. Relative risk of certain diseases in female schizophrenics and controls

Disease	No. Cases	Schizophrenia		Affective Psychosis		Depression	
		Observed No.	Relative Risk	Observed No.	Relative Risk	Observed No.	Relative Risk
Appendicitis	7586	1	0.14**	3	0.58	19	1.07
Varicose veins	3884	2	0.18***	6	0.64	20	0.78
Menstrual disorders	7416	11	0.40***	28	1.37	140	2.19***
Utero-vaginal prolapse	3518	7	0.50*	13	0.89	35	1.10
Benign uterine fibroma	3020	3	0.24**	13	1.27	29	1.00

$p < 0.05 =$* $p < 0.01 =$** $p < 0.001 =$***

injury in both male schizophrenics and male affective psychotics and a highly significant increase in association with depression (Table 10).

Appendicitis

Appendicitis was significantly uncommon in the female schizophrenics but not in the control groups (Table 11).

Varicose veins

There was a very significant deficit of varicose veins among female schizophrenics (Table 11), though the deficit was reduced by the addition of two silmultaneously diagnosed cases (relative risk = 0.36, p = 0.014). The relative risk was also low though within chance limits in both control groups.

Menstrual and uterine disorders

There were low relative risks of menstrual disorders, benign uterine fibromas and utero–vaginal prolapse in the group of female schizophrenics (Table 11). The deficit of menstrual disorders was particularly statistically significant. These conditions occurred as frequently as expected in females with affective psychoses. Depression was significantly associated with menstrual disorders.

Certain uncommon diseases

A number of relatively rare diseases have been postulated to be positively or negatively associated with schizophrenia, mainly in relation to the various biochemical aetiologies currently under consideration. The degree of statistical association was ascertained for several of these from the Oxford Record Linkage Study data (Table 12). In most instances the number of cases was very small and no significant associations were found.

DISCUSSION

Results from the preliminary study of Oxford Record Linkage Study data, though subject to certain limitations, may help to clarify and focus attention on diseases apparently associated with schizophrenia which require more definitive study, and indicate the conditions which will have to be fulfilled for confident conclusions to be drawn. Three groups of disease associations can be considered: (1) common diseases previously said to

Table 12 Oxford Record Linkage Study. Observed and expected numbers of certain uncommon diseases in cases of schizophrenia

Disease	No. cases	Observed	Expected	Relative Risk
Adrenal insufficiency	69	0	0.2	–
Ankylosing spondylitis	118	0	.43	–
Blindness	162	1	0.4	2.36
Chronic hepatitis	343	2	.95	2.11
Hepato-lenticular degeneration	1090	2	2.5	0.81
Hypopituitarism	119	0	0.4	–
Multiple sclerosis	492	1	1.8	0.57
Myasthenia gravis	39	0	1.1	–
Pernicious anaemia	591	2	1.7	1.15
Porphyria	94	1	0.3	3.55
Psoriasis	362	1	1.2	0.86
Systemic lupus erythematosus	516	1	1.6	0.64
Ulcerative colitis	382	0	1.4	–

be positively or negatively associated with schizophrenia but which have no generally accepted bearing on current aetiological theories. This group includes cancer, heart and vascular diseases, respiratory diseases and peptic ulcer; (2) diseases predicted from current aetiological hypotheses to be associated with schizophrenia including epilepsy, Parkinson's disease, allergic conditions, diabetes mellitus, malabsorption and coeliac disease, rheumatoid arthritis, thyroid diseases, and a group of rare conditions; and (3) a group of disorders found to be associated with schizophrenia but not previously reported and including gallbladder disease, osteomyelitis and other bone disease, certain urinary diseases, head injury, benign neoplasms, appendicitis, varicose veins, menstrual and uterine disorders.

Common diseases with no current aetiological implication

Cancer

The short period at risk covered by the data precludes definite conclusions about this important group of diseases. Although no reduction of relative risks for common cancers could be demonstrated, since duration of hospitalisation was not taken into account, any effect comparable with that found by Katz *et al.* (1967) may have been masked. The small but significant excess of cancer of stomach is of interest in view of the similar finding of Opsahl (1933). The small excess of cancer of the breast in hebephrenic women may be a consequence of phenothiazine treatment (Ettigi *et al.*, 1973). There is no doubt that much larger numbers of cases followed for a considerably longer time period are necessary to elucidate the relationship between schizophrenia and its sub-types with specific cancers. Duration of hospitalization must be taken into account in order to clarify any effects of the hospital environment and if data relating to the period over which antipsychotic drug therapy has been common practice are used, it may be impossible to control for its effects.

Heart and vascular disease

The highly significant excess of arteriosclerotic heart disease in both schizophrenics and controls is in accord with previous work by such authors as Alström (1942) and Ødegaard (1967), though the absence of excesses of other groups of vascular disorders in schizophrenics is of interest. Recently Born (1979) has suggested that chlorpromazine may reduce the incidence of myocardial infarction, citing the observation of Ødegaard (1967) that the incidence of cardiac disease had not increased over community rates in schizophrenics to the same extent as in other mental patients. Hussar (1962) found no increase in mortality from acute myocardial infarction since tranquilizers had been introduced though there had been an increase in arteriosclerotic heart disease.

Respiratory disease

Increased mortality and morbidity from pneumonia and other respiratory and infectious diseases among mental hospital patients has been widely reported though the excess seems to have been less in more recent times. It is likely that the environmental conditions in mental hospitals coupled with relatively poor hygiene and behavioural anomalies associated with some mental illness are conducive to the spread of such infectious diseases, especially among the aged and infirm. Schizophrenics were formerly subject to marked excess mortality from pulmonary tuberculosis though this has virtually disappeared following introduction of specific treatment and improvement in the physical condition of the patients. It is therefore of some interest that there was an increased relative risk of pulmonary tuberculosis prior to the diagnosis of schizophrenia in the Oxford data.

Peptic ulcer

No association between gastric and duodenal ulceration and schizophrenia was found in the Oxford data, though increased incidence has been reported previously (Ehrentheil, 1957) and excess mortality from this cause was found among Filipino males in Hawaii (Weiner and Marvit, 1977).

Diseases predicted from current aetiological hypotheses

Epilepsy

It is surprising that the Oxford data showed no relation between schizophrenia and minor or focal epilepsy in view of the work of Slater and Beard (1963) and the more recent finding of excess schizophrenia in temporal lobe epilepsy by Taylor (1975). Deficient ascertainment of minor and focal epilepsy in the Oxford data seems likely. The high relative risks of major epilepsy, epileptic psychosis and unspecified epilepsy among paranoid and non-specific schizophrenias are of interest but do not appear to lend support to the biochemical explanation of a negative association offered by Reynolds (1968) and later elaborated by Levi and Waxman (1975). Results from the Oxford data indicate a complex relationship between schizophrenia and epilepsy which requires detailed study.

Parkinson's disease

Parkinsonism is a common side-effect of phenothiazine therapy so that an increased relative risk following the diagnosis of schizophrenia is not surprising. The occurrence of a schizophrenia-like episode of psychosis in the course of long standing Parkinsonism has been described by Crow *et al.* (1976) who suggested it might be relevant to the 'dopamine hypothesis' of the aetiology of schizophrenia.

Allergic conditions

Reduced incidences of asthma, hay fever and other allergic conditions have been reported, as have alternating psychotic and allergic states. Despite a number of studies the role of histamine in schizophrenia is still unclear (Matthysse and Lipinski, 1975). Although the low relative risk obtained in the Oxford data was not significant, there was a contrast with the high relative risks found in the control groups. It seems possible that there may be a low incidence, at least in one or more of the sub-types of schizophrenia, and further detailed study is indicated.

Diabetes mellitus

'Antagonism' between schizophrenia and diabetes mellitus has been postulated by Rassidakis *et al.* (1974). There was no support for this hypothesis in the Oxford data.

Malabsorption

The marginally significant increase in relative risk of malabsorption in schizophrenics obtained when one simultaneously diagnosed case was added to the original analysis must be interpreted with caution since the group may include several forms of malabsorption and confirmation of the diagnoses would be necessary to validate the result. The single case of hebephrenia compared with 0.014 expected may have been a chance occurrence and little weight can be attached to this finding. Apart from the therapeutic studies of Dohan and his colleagues (Dohan *et al.*, 1969) and the gluten challenge test of Singh and Kay (1976), several studies of various kinds have not confirmed the suspected association with coeliac disease (Dean *et al.*, 1975; Stevens *et al.*, 1977). Though the Oxford results do not rule out the possibility, it seems doubtful that the hypothesis of gluten sensitivity can be sustained.

Arthritis

The reduction in relative risk of rheumatoid arthritis in schizophrenia is in accord with a number of earlier studies and no study has contradicted this negative association (Baldwin, 1979). Nevertheless, the possibility of low ascertainment cannot be dismissed since this condition may be treated without transferring patients from psychiatric hospitals to other units and in these instances there would be no record of the arthritic condition in the Oxford Record Linkage Study. Against this must be set the finding of normal risks for this disease in both control groups, suggesting that under-reporting may not be an important factor in the estimated relative risk in schizophrenia.

The recent extensive Swedish study by Österberg (1978) considered the aetiological implications of a reduced risk of rheumatoid arthritis in schizophrenia and other psychiatric disorders. If the risk was reduced in psychiatric illness generally, a genetic or biochemical explanation would be unlikely and personality characteristics would be more likely to account for the relationship. The Oxford data indicate that rheumatoid arthritis is not unusually uncommon in affective psychosis and non-psychotic depression, the evidence being that the reduced risk in schizophrenia is specific. Thus it is reasonable to seek explanations in genetic and biochemical terms.

The only current biochemical hypothesis which predicts a low relative risk of rheumatoid arthritis in schizophrenia is that of prostaglandin deficiency (Horrobin *et al.*, 1978). This postulates that rheumatoid arthritis should be uncommon except in association with schizo-affective and catatonic states. Several of Österberg's (1978) cases were said to be schizo-affective, but the majority, like both the cases in the Oxford study, were non-specific schizophrenia.

Österberg (1978) also discussed the aetiological consequences of relationships between schizophrenia and various other joint diseases, particularly those known to be associated with human leucocyte antigens (HLA). Her data seemed to indicate that ankylosing spondylitis might be over-represented in schizophrenics in comparison with rheumatoid arthritis. The data in the present Oxford study were insufficient to test this suggestion with no cases found and none expected. This was also the position with respect to other possibly relevant diseases including systematic lupus erthematosus and psoriasis. The only other result of interest in this group of conditions was a marginally significant reduction of relative risk of osteoarthritis in schizophrenics especially in males, which did not occur in the control groups.

The reduced relative risk of rheumatoid arthritis in schizophrenia, though not indisputably confirmed, seems likely to be real and specific. This negative association presents one of the most promising leads for further aetiological research and clearly requires further study both in itself and in relation to other joint diseases and their HLA associations. Although some studies of HLA associations with schizophrenia have been carried out, the results so far are inconclusive (McGuffin *et al.*, 1978). The D locus particularly, which is thought to be associated with rheumatoid arthritis (Stastny, 1976), has not been studied in schizophrenics. Nevertheless, the contrast between the low relative risk of rheumatoid arthritis and the purported raised relative risk of coeliac disease which is also associated with the D antigen, perhaps suggests that HLA associations with schizophrenia, if they exist, are not straightforward. Indeed, it may be argued that the search for a genetic marker through the HLA system is premature and that a wide ranging search among as many known markers as possible would be a more logical preliminary step (Böök *et al.*, 1978).

In the light of these observations the Oxford data were analysed to estimate the degree of association between rheumatoid arthritis and malabsorption and yielded a relative risk of 4.68 ($p = 0.01$). Coeliac disease has been shown to be associated with focal epilepsy (Chapman *et al.*, 1978) and this relationship was also found in the Oxford data (observed = 1; expected = 0.2; $p = 0.02$). The interrelationship between these diseases was further demonstrated by the finding of a highly significant association between focal epilepsy and rheumatoid arthritis (relative risk = 20.13; $p = 0.0005$). Though the number of cases in each of these associations was small, the strength of the statistical relationship is such as to suggest a possibly useful lead for further study.

Thyroid disorders

Both thyrotoxicosis and myxoedema were predicted to be associated with schizophrenia by Gilka (1975) in an extensive review of biochemical studies. Horrobin (1979) noted that thyroid deficiency may reduce prostaglandin secretion. If this were the case myxoedema should be more common than expected in schizophrenia. There was no evidence of an increased risk of hyperthyroidism in the Oxford data, but there were significant excesses of myxoedema in catatonics and non-specific schizophrenics, and in both control groups.

Rare diseases

Both the hypothesis advanced by Gilka (1975) of one or more metabolic defects in the tryptophan-niacin pathway, and the prostaglandin deficiency hypothesis of Horrobin (1979), predict associations between schizophrenia and a number of relatively uncommon diseases. The difficulty with virtually all of these is their rarity, since to obtain a robust estimate of relative risks, a very large sample of schizophrenics would have to be obtained and related to a defined population at risk. The observed and expected numbers shown in Table 12 can be used to infer the size of sample which might be required. Much more extensive data should be available from the Oxford Record Linkage Study in the near future and may enable estimation of some of these associations.

Previously unreported associations

Significant reductions of relative risk were obtained for a number of diseases for which no previous reports have been found. Some of these were sex specific, and comparable reductions of risk were not found among the control groups. Although some of these results might be presumed to stem from known characteristics of schizophrenics such as the reduced fertility of schizophrenic women which might account for the low incidence of utero–vaginal prolapse, and the reputed high tolerance of pain and discomfort which might reduce the likelihood of discovery of some disorders, it seems preferable to presume more prosaic explanations until further research can be undertaken. Deficient ascertainment due to the limited span of the available data, or caused by treatment of some conditions within the psychiatric hospital are at least as likely as failure of clinical detection through infrequent or inadequate physical examination or lack of patient reports. Yet not all this group of negative associations can be accounted for in these ways. For example, appendicitis is virtually certain to be detected and could not have been treated in the psychiatric hospitals concerned. Thus there is reason to suppose that some at least of these reduced risks are real rather than artefactual, so that further study should be contemplated.

The only condition in this group with a high relative risk was head injury in male schizophrenics, which was more common than expected after discharge with schizophrenia.

CONCLUSIONS

This preliminary study of data from the Oxford Record Linkage Study on physical morbidity in schizophrenia has been useful in clarifying some of the large number of previously reported positive and negative disease associations. By using epidemiological methods to obtain comparable relative risks in both schizophrenia and control groups, it has focussed attention on a group of diseases which warrant further study and has indicated directions for future research likely to be relevant to aetiological understanding of schizophrenia.

With a few exceptions, most of the diseases predicted to be associated with schizophrenia from current aetiological hypotheses are so uncommon that valid estimates of relative risk cannot be obtained until much larger collections of data become available. The exceptions which are most likely to repay further study are epilepsy, Parkinson's disease, and rheumatoid arthritis. It is fairly well established that there is a reduced incidence of rheumatoid arthritis in schizophrenia but not in some other psychiatric disorders and this negative association perhaps holds the most promise of illuminating schizophrenia aetiology.

References

Acheson, E. D. (1967). *Medical Record Linkage.* (Oxford University Press)

Alström, C. H. (1942). Mortality in mental hospitals with special regard to tuberculosis. *Acta Psychiatr. Neurol.*, **24** (Suppl.)

Baldwin, J. A. (1973). Linked record medical information systems. *Proc. R. Soc. (Lond.)*, **184**, 403

Baldwin, J. A. (1979). Schizophrenia and physical disease: a review. *Psychol. Med.*, **9**, 611

Baldwin, J. A., Fedrick, J., Gill, L. E. and Simmons, H. (1980). Linked diseases in individuals. (In preparation)

Böök, J. A., Wetterberg, L. and Modrzewska, K. (1978). Schizophrenia in a North Swedish geographical isolate, 1900–1977; epidemiology, genetics and biochemistry. *Clin. Genet.*, **14**, 373

Born, G. (1979). Lancet, **1**, 882

Chapman, R. W. G., Laidlow, J. M., Colin-Jones, D., Eade, O. E. and Smith, C. L. (1978). Increased prevalence of epilepsy in coeliac disease. *Lancet*, **2**, 250

Crow, T., Johnstone, E. C. and McClelland, H. A. (1976). The coincidence of schizophrenia and Parkinsonism: some neurochemical implications. *Psychol. Med.*, **6**, 227

Dean, G., Hanniffy, L., Stevens, F. M., Temperley, L., O'Broin, J. D., Scott, J. and Cahalane, S. F. (1975). Schizophrenia and coeliac disease. *J. Ir. Med. Assoc.*, **68**, 545

Dohan, F. C., Grasberger, F. M., Lowell, H. T., Johnston, A., and Arbegast, W. (1969). Relapsed schizophrenics: more rapid improvement on a milk- and cereal-free diet. *Br. J. Psychiatry*, **115**, 595

Ehrentheil, O. F. (1957). Common medical disorders rarely found in psychotic patients. *Arch. Neurol. Psychiatr.*, **77**, 178

Ettigi, P., Lal, S. and Friesen, H. G. (1973). Prolactin, phenothiozines, admission to mental hospital and carcinoma of the breast. *Lancet*, **2**, 266

Gilka, L. (1975). Schizophrenia: a disorder of tryptophan metabolism. *Acta Psychiatrica Scand.* **258**, (Suppl.)

Horrobin, D. F. (1979). Schizophrenia: reconciliation of the dopamine, prostaglandin and opioid concepts and the role of the pineal. *Lancet*, **1**, 529

Horrobin, D. F., Ally, A. I., Karmali, M., Karmazyn, M., Manku, M. S. and Morgan, R. O. (1978). Prostaglandins and schizophrenia: further discussion of the evidence. *Psychol. Med.*, **8**, 43

Hussar, A. E. (1962). Effect of tranquilizers on medical morbidity and mortality in a mental hospital. *J. Am. Med. Assoc.*, **179**, 682

Katz, J., Kunoesky, S., Patten, R. E. and Allaway, N. C. (1967). Cancer mortality among patients in New York mental hospitals. *Cancer*, **20**, 2194

Levi, R. N. and Waxman, S. (1975). Schizophrenia, epilepsy, cancer, methionine and folate metabolism. *Lancet*, **2**, 11

Matthysse, S. and Lipinski, J. (1975). Biochemical aspects of schizophrenia. *Annu. Rev. Med.*, **26**, 551

McGuffin, P., Farmer, A. E. and Rajah, S. M. (1978). Histocompatibility antigens and schizophrenia. *Br. J. Psychiatry*, **132**, 149

Ødegaard, Ø. (1967). Mortality in Norwegian psychiatric hospitals, 1950–1962. *Acta Genetica*, **17**, 137

Opsahl, R., (1933). *Norsk. Mag. f. Laegevidensk*, **94**, 771

Österberg, E. (1978). Schizophrenia and rheumatic disease. *Acta Psychiatr. Scand.*, **58**, 339

Rassidakis, N. C., Erokocritou, Athitakis, Karayannis and Karaiossephides, K. (1974). Schizophrenia, psychosomatic illnesses, diabetes mellitus and malignant neoplasms. *Int. Ment. Health Res. Newsletter*, **21**, 12

Reynolds, E. H. (1968). Epilepsy and schizophrenia: relationship and biochemistry. *Lancet*, **1**, 398

Singh, M. M. and Kay, S. R. (1976). Wheat gluten as a pathogenic factor in schizophrenia. *Science*, **191**, 401

Slater, E. and Beard, A. W. (1963). The schizophrenia-like psychoses of epilepsy (i) psychiatric aspects. *Br. J. Psychiatry*, **109**, 95

Stastny, P. (1976). Mixed lymphocyte cultures in rheumatoid arthritis. *J. Clin. Invest.*, **57**, 1148

Stevens, F. M., Lloyd, R.S., Geraghty, S. M. J., Reynolds, M. T. G., Sarsfield, M. J., McNicholl, B., Fottrell, P. F., Wright, R. and McCarthy, C. F. (1977). Schizophrenia and coeliac disease – the nature of the relationship. *Psychol. Med.*, **7**, 259

Taylor, D. C. (1975). Factors influencing the occurrence of schizophrenia-like psychosis in patients with temporal lobe epilepsy. *Psychol. Med.*, **5**, 249

Weiner, B. P. and Marvit, R. C. (1977). Schizophrenia in Hawaii: analysis of cohort mortality risk in a multi-ethnic population. *Br. J. Psychiatry*, **131**, 497

Section 8:
DRUG TREATMENTS

22
Depot neuroleptics and tardive dyskinesia: a prospective study

A. C. GIBSON

The development over a period of three years of tardive dyskinesia in 90 of a group of 374 schizophrenic outpatients receiving depot neuroleptic injections is described; in the two subsequent years eight more cases appeared, concomitant with dose reduction or change of medication. 375 replies to a questionnaire asking the incidence of generalised chorea in patients taking neuroleptics suggest those receiving depot drugs are more vulnerable, though the data is insufficient for this conclusion to be certain. This may mean that non-compliance of patients receiving oral medication protects them against dyskinesia, and that therefore intermittent pharmacotherapy is desirable: the result of one such 'drug holiday' is described.

CLINICAL OBSERVATIONS

In describing a prospective study of the development of tardive dyskinesia (TD) in a group of 374 outpatient schizophrenics, treated with depot injections, the author (1978) observed that after three years the number of patients suffering from the bucco-linguo-masticatory (BLM) syndrome had risen from 31 to 84. Figure 1 indicates how the incidence of the condition progressed, and its severity. Of these patients, 18 also developed chorea of other parts of the body than the mouth and tongue.

The observations reported covered the three year period to the end of 1976. Since then, those cases without TD have been treated with lower doses (fluphenazine 12.5 mg monthly and flupenthixol three weekly, although two out of five patients have had to revert to higher doses for

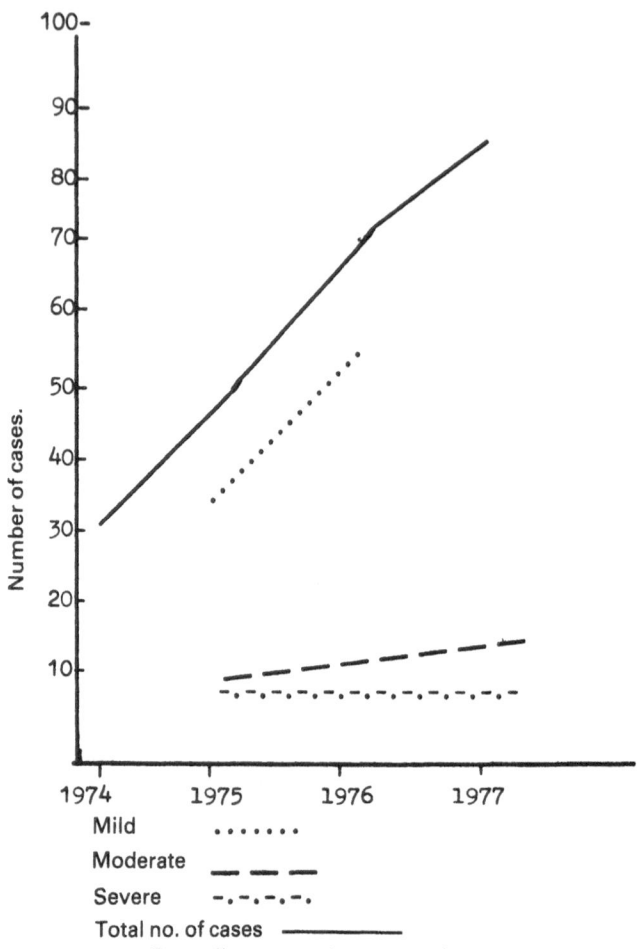

Figure 1   Development of tardive dyskinesia during treatment with depot injections

periods of three to six months) by a change to pimozide (4 mg daily) and by monthly periods of drug abstinence. Pimozide appears to have special properties in opposing dopamine induced dyskinesia in experimental animals (Costall and Naylor 1977). During this time only eight additional cases of TD have appeared, all with the BLM syndrome. Of those who developed TD, and all were treated at the onset of the condition, 41 out of 50 responded to a change of medication to pimozide or fluspirilene, only to relapse within three years; halving the dose of the depot neuroleptic produced remission in all nineteen patients so treated, but after five years fifteen have relapsed. Of the various 'antidotes' recommended, sodium valproate, lithium, clonazepam, amantadine, deanol and bromocryptine were tried with disappointing results.

QUESTIONNAIRE: METHOD AND RESULTS

There were also six patients who developed either severe or fairly severe generalised chorea, within a year of starting depot flupenthixol: three males and three females, with a mean age of 46 years. By 1975 the Committee on Safety of Drugs had received reports of only twelve patients treated with neuroleptics who had developed generalised choreoathetosis, so finding six cases out of 167 on flupenthixol seemed remarkable. Dr. Peter Snaith suggested a questionnaire should be sent to consultant psychiatrists asking them if they had seen a similar phenomenon, and 827 consultants were asked:

Do you have any schizophrenic patients receiving antipsychotic medication who have developed generalised body chorea, with or without involvement of the lower face or tongue. If so, could you please indicate the numbers involved, and the drug(s) that they were receiving at the time the abnormal movements were first observed

Number

Fluphenazine	(Modecate)	
Flupenthixol	(Depixol)	
Fluspirilene	(Redeptin)	
Oral neuroleptic of any kind		

As it was not known which consultants had a special interest, questions were sent to people working in all branches of psychiatry, some of whom would have little contact with schizophrenics. 375 replied; 112 doctors reported 279 cases in all, and it was hoped that the condition is sufficiently rare for psychiatrists to remember their cases without searching records. Through the kindness of the DHSS and the Regional Pharmacists, details were obtained of the number of doses of all neuroleptics prescribed in England and Wales in 1976 both by general practitioners and the hospital services, so it was possible to express the number of cases with generalised chorea as a percentage of the total number receiving the preparation, except for fluspirilene which was the drug six reported chorea cases were receiving. It was assumed that all cases receiving fluphenazine and flupenthixol were schizophrenics, and that flupenthixol is more frequently prescribed than fluphenazine. Of the oral drugs, many would go to non-psychotic patients, often for short periods, but if it is assumed that of the 300 000 schizophrenics in the UK half are receiving neuroleptic treatment then the appropriate calculation expresses the questionnaire results as follows: chorea occurs in one in 320 people receiving depot flupenthixol, one in 370 receiving depot fluphenazine and one in 1800 receiving oral neuroleptics (probably one in 850 schizophrenics). These figures differ from those quoted at the May 1979 meeting at Friends House London, which were based on the belief that flupenthixol is given more frequently than fluphenazine, but an investigation has been brought to my notice that suggests that this is not so.

Without knowledge of previous medication and age of the patient, this information can only, at most, reflect a trend, but it does suggest that patients receiving depot injections should be carefully and frequently monitored for abnormal neurological signs.

INTERMITTENT PHARMACOTHERAPY

If people receiving depot injections are really more prone to TD than those on oral therapy, what is the reason? Adamson *et al*. (1973) showed that 39 out of 97 non-responding schizophrenics were absorbing little of their medication, and injections obviously bypass this mechanism, but clinical experience suggests that, given the chance, patients do not comply well with an oral treatment programme and thereby probably protect themselves against TD.

Table 1   Outcome of drug holiday

Number of patients	Mean age in years	Duration of drug holiday	Number of patients relapsing before holiday complete	Number developing tardive dyskinesia	Number who developed TD and became psychotic before neuroleptic restarted
30	56±12.02 SD	8–9 weeks	5	6	3

Although it is now thirteen years since Ayd (1966) suggested the policy of 'drug holidays', this procedure has never been validated. The questionnaire results indicate that intermittent pharmacotherapy is at present our most potent weapon against dyskinesia, so after looking at the records of 24 drug refusers who took a mean time of 6 months to relapse after stopping neuroleptic injections it was thought safe to give 30 well controlled schizophrenic outpatients an 8–9 week period of drug abstinence. Four relapsed to recover with recommencement of treatment, but a fifth required hospitalisation. Six developed the BLM syndrome, as might be anticipated with the removal of dopamine blocking drugs.

While this may be regarded in a positive light in that it is good to identify patients at risk, and if their dyskinesia disappears with continued withdrawal of medication, all is well; however, three of them became psychotic before the TD had disappeared, and what should be done in these circumstances is debatable.

Such observations may do little to encourage others to use periods of drug abstinence, but the patients involved had been ill for a mean time of eighteen years. In the light of present knowledge intermittent pharmacotherapy represents the logical way of preventing TD but such a programme must be started early in the schizophrenic's treatment life.

One should also beware of exaggerating the problem of TD; most cases are mild, and over a five year period of observation most, in the writer's experience, are not progressive. The inadequately treated psychotic, bombarded by abnormal perceptions, is in a far worse situation than the sufferer from dyskinesia, and neuroleptics must be used in adequate quantity to control the psychosis.

Acknowledgements

I would like to thank the Regional Pharmacists and the Officers of the DHSS, in particular Mrs. Roberts, for all their work in relationship to the questionnaire, and the many doctors who replied. I would also like to thank the Schizophrenia Association of Great Britain for meeting secretarial and postal charges incurred in this study.

References

Adamson, L., Curry, S. H., Bridges, P. K., Firestone, A. F., Lavin, N. I., Lewis, D. M., Watson, R. D., Xavier, C. M. and Anderson, J. A. (1973). Fluphenazine deconate trial in chronic in-patient schizophrenics failing to absorb oral chlorpromazine. *Dis. Nerv. Syst.*, **34**, 181

Ayd, F. J. (1966). Drug Holidays. Intermittent pharmacotherapy for psychiatric patients (continued). *Int. Drug Ther.*, **1**, 1

Costall, B. and Naylor, R. J. (1977). Behavioural characterization of neuroleptic properties. Presented at *Symposium on Schizophrenia and Dopamine*, October 21, Royal Society of Medicine, London

Gibson, A. C. (1978). Depot injections and tardive dyskinesia. *Br. J. Psychiatry*, **133**, 361

23
Recent developments in the drug treatment of schizophrenia

B. COSTALL and R. J. NAYLOR

The development of antischizophrenic drugs via psychopharmacological testing procedures is historically connected with the chance observation that the drug chlorpromazine had antischizophrenic activity in the clinic. The question was raised, what effect did chlorpromazine have, as distinct from other psychoactive agents, in animals and as a result the classical tests for neuroleptic activity evolved; these included the induction of catalepsy, the antagonism of drug induced stereotyped behaviour, the antagonism of conditioned avoidance responses and brain self-stimulation behaviour, the inhibition of locomotor activity, and the inhibition of apomorphine induced emesis (Fielding and Lal, 1974). An effect in all of these behavioural tests has been associated with ability to inhibit cerebral dopamine function and, most important, there would appear to be a close correlation between activity in these animal tests and antischizophrenic activity in the clinic (see review by Costall and Naylor, 1979). Such evidence has been forwarded in support of 'the dopamine hypothesis of schizophrenia'.

Essentially, the classical tests for neuroleptic activity detected drugs having very similar effects on central dopamine mechanisms to chlorpromazine, but this does not negate significant advances in the development of antischizophrenic drugs by use of these tests, since some agents which were developed had decidedly better 'patient acceptability', for example, reduced autonomic and sedative effects, such as with pimozide, or a significantly increased half life, such as with clopimozide or fluspirilene.

At this stage, it becomes essential to recognise that 'central dopamine mechanisms' can be differentiated into well defined systems: the meso-cortical, mesolimbic, extrapyramidal and tubero-infundibular systems, and the mechanisms of the area postrema (Ungerstedt, 1971; Berger *et al.*, 1976). As an oversimplified, but working hypothesis, it is suggested that drug effects on the mesocortical and/or mesolimbic systems may alleviate the mental symptoms of schizophrenia whilst the inhibition of dopamine function in the extrapyramidal system leads to extrapyramidal side effects of the neuroleptics – pseudoparkinsonism, akathisia, dystonic and dyskinetic or antidyskinetic phenomena; blockade in the tubero-infundibular system leads to hormonal changes, particularly the rise in serum prolactin, whilst dopamine blockade in the area postrema relates to the antiemetic action of the neuroleptics. The vast majority of neuroleptic agents will influence all dopamine systems, and it has proved difficult to differentiate antischizophrenic effects from an ability to affect the other dopamine systems which basically give rise to side effects. However, possibly pimozide is one agent which was forwarded from the classical tests as having good antischizophrenic activity with reduced ability to cause extrapyramidal disturbance in man (Pinder *et al.*, 1976).

The major question which has been raised against the usefulness of the classical tests is their failure to detect reliably agents such as thioridazine which shows a very weak and inconsistent effect throughout the battery of tests (Costall and Naylor, 1979), albeit efficacious in the clinic (although not without undesirable effects such as sedation, and autonomic changes). It has since become apparent that effects in the classical tests depend on drug induced changes not only in the mesolimbic and mesocortical systems but also in the extrapyramidal system and, as such, these tests cannot clearly differentiate antischizophrenic ability from potential to cause extrapyramidal side effects. It is therefore possible that the low efficacy of thioridazine in tests such as catalepsy induction may more reflect the low incidence of extrapyramidal side effects caused by this drug in the clinic. It has been shown that thioridazine has low affinity for the striatal neuroleptic (dopamine?) receptor (Leysen *et al.*, 1978) and, in addition, that this agent has powerful anticholinergic properties against striatal cholinergic receptors (see Laduron and Leysen, 1978); both effects could explain the low ability of thioridazine to cause extrapyramidal effects. Most interesting, however, is the development of the concept that a neuroleptic drug may have differential abilities to affect the different cerebral dopamine systems (Blackburn *et al.*, 1978).

The definition of neuroleptic action has classically implied marked ability to inhibit cerebral dopamine mechanisms in experimental animals. However, at the same time as the pharmacologist was attempting to elucidate the differential effects of thioridazine, a further novel agent, sulpiride, was introduced into the clinic in Europe (Justin-Besançon *et al.*, 1967). The properties of sulpiride, which was antischizophrenic (Borenstein *et al.*, 1969), reinforced the concept that the different cerebral dopamine systems could be differentially affected by drugs. The spectrum of activity of sulpiride proved even more remarkable than that of thioridazine. Sulpiride was virtually inactive in all the classical tests for neuroleptics, with the exception of an ability to inhibit emesis (see Costall and Naylor, 1979). Further, far from depressing the locomotor activity of animals, sulpiride appeared to increase vigilance. In the clinic, the antischizophrenic action of sulpiride could be observed in the absence of pseudo-Parkinsonism and, most interestingly, this agent was shown to be valuable in the withdrawn, anergic schizophrenic.

The definition of neuroleptic action must therefore be re-examined. Firstly, it is clear that neuroleptic agents do inhibit cerebral dopamine function in the clinic, the classical neuroleptics apparently affecting all systems with an agent such as sulpiride having a more limited action in those systems which primarily dysfunction in schizophrenia and those which modulate endocrine activity. Therefore, one must question whether the use of animals having 'normal brains' is justified for the assessment of the actions of drugs which are to be used in 'diseased brain'. Should the dopamine mechanisms of an animal's brain be rendered 'abnormal' in a manner most resembling our knowledge of dopamine dysfunction in schizophrenia before the assessment of the potential antischizophrenic activity of a drug? Attempts were made to answer this question by injecting dopamine discretely and directly into mesolimbic or extrapyramidal areas, gaining a change in motor behaviour and then assessing the actions of typical and atypical neuroleptic agents. Very simply, classical neuroleptic agents are able to inhibit a raised dopamine function in both the mesolimbic and extrapyramidal systems; sulpiride is most active against a response caused by raised mesolimbic dopamine function (remembering that this drug is *inactive* in the classical tests for neuroleptics) and, a chemical relative of sulpiride, metoclopramide, is only effective against a raised extrapyramidal dopamine function. The latter observation had far reaching implications since metoclopramide had consistently been forwarded as a false positive in the animal tests, being typically neuroleptic-like in its activity spectrum (Costall and Naylor, 1979) whilst lacking significant antischizophrenic activity in the clinic (Borenstein and Bles, 1965), although clearly able to alter extrapyramidal function as shown by the reports that metoclopramide could elicit dystonic reactions (Robinson, 1973). Two important points emerge, (a) that antischizophrenic agents are more reliably detected by an animal model based on the effects of raised mesolimbic function and (b) that neuroleptic agents may differentially affect mesolimbic and extrapyramidal dopamine mechanisms (see also Costall and Naylor, 1979).

The groups of drugs which have emerged as offering a more specific action in diseases involving cerebral dopamine dysfunction are the benzamide derivatives which include sulpiride and tiapride. These agents not only differ from the neuroleptics in behavioural tests but also biochemically. At the most fundamental level, the benzamides have little or no activity to displace ^{3}H-haloperidol or ^{3}H-spiroperidol from neuroleptic binding sites (Leysen et al., 1978; Jenner et al., 1978), and, unlike classical neuroleptics, fail to block dopamine stimulated adenylate cyclase (Peringer et al., 1976; Roufogalis et al., 1976; Elliott et al., 1977). Both of these biochemical effects are used as precise indices of drug action on neuroleptic/dopamine receptors. Further, if ^{3}H-sulpiride is used to label receptors then this is not subject to displacement by haloperidol (Theodorou et al., 1979). Together, these data indicate obvious differences between what may be termed 'sulpiride receptors' and 'neuroleptic receptors'.

A major problem in the design of drugs for the treatment of schizophrenia is the elimination of side effects. As already outlined, it would appear possible to develop drugs with reduced potential to cause extrapyramidal side effects of pseudoparkinsonism, but a far more serious extrapyramidal effect is that encountered on long term neuroleptic therapy, tardive dyskinesia. Although sulpiride may not cause tardive dyskinesia, this irreversible side effect is probably characteristic of long term therapy with other neuroleptics in present clinical use. It is paradoxical that the only agents which can effectively relieve tardive dyskinesias are larger doses of the neuroleptics which actually cause the dyskinesias. The present situation is, therefore, far from acceptable. Possible advances have been suggested by the analysis of drug action following the stimulation of striatal dopamine function by the intrastriatal injection of dopamine in the guinea pig. The treatment causes a wide range of abnormal involuntary movements in the guinea pig which, at least in appearance, are analogous to components of tardive dyskinesias in man. As in man, the dyskinesias in the animal are remarkably resistant to blockade, even by the neuroleptics themselves and, indeed, from several hundreds of neuroleptic-like compounds assessed in the animal model, only two have shown potent antagonistic ability, oxiperomide and tiapride (Costall and Naylor, 1978a). These drugs have both been forwarded to the clinic, and both have been shown to have antidyskinetic action in man (Bédard et al., 1978; Price et al., 1978). Oxiperomide can depress the normal locomotor activity of animals, and such an effect may limit its clinical usefulness, but tiapride, although clearly effective to antagonize dyskinesias, is generally inactive in other animal tests which may indicate ability to inhibit mesolimbic or extrapyramidal dopamine function (see Costall and Naylor, 1980). Again, it must be emphasized that (a) although tests for antidyskinetic activity have been forwarded which use 'normal animals', only when striatal function is rendered abnormal do the tests specifically detect antidyskinetic agents, and (b) whilst tiapride may have only a limited usefulness in treating schizophrenia per se it may prove useful in combined treatment with antischizophrenic agents to reduce abnormal movements.

Another interesting advance in the treatment of schizophrenia has been the introduction of a benzimidazol derivative, halopemide. This drug shares some properties of the classical neuroleptics in animal tests, but not all. Thus, halopemide is antistereotypic and antiemetic (Niemegeers unpublished data; Costall and Naylor, unpublished data), but fails to cause a dose-dependent catalepsy (Costall and Naylor, unpublished data). Most unexpected, halopemide can antagonize the effects of a raised dopamine function in the striatal area of the extrapyramidal system, but fails to inhibit the effects of enhancing dopamine function in the mesolimbic nucleus accumbens (Costall and Naylor, unpublished data). To add to the complexity of the activity spectrum of this drug, it is reported that it does not show any preferential accumulation in dopamine rich areas of the brain such as the striatum or nucleus accumbens, which do selectively accumulate other neuroleptics, but is accumulated in septal and thalamic areas (Loonen et al., 1978). Clinically, halopemide is reported to be an agent which lacks extrapyramidal side effects and which may be effective for the treatment of psychoses characterised by autism, emotional withdrawal or apathy (Rombaut et al., 1978). It is difficult to reconcile the activity spectrum of this drug with our present understanding of the aetiology of schizophrenia. We would suggest that halopemide may prove more valuable as a tool for investigating the pharmacologically unknown area of autistic behaviour.

Many of the developments in the treatment of schizophrenia have been derived from chance observations in the clinic. Certainly, the clinical activity of halopemide may not have been predicted from the pharmacological experiments, and possibly one should be considering other unexpected observations from the clinic which may forward drugs as tools to further elucidate the aetiology of schizophrenia. The findings with propranolol are a good example. Propranolol can apparently alleviate schizophrenic symptoms (see Yorkston et al., 1978; Elizur et al., 1979) and, at high doses, can modify central dopamine metabolism (Peters and Mazurkiewicz-Kwilecki, 1975; Fuxe et al., 1976; Wiesel, 1976) and, in very high concentrations, can displace ^{3}H-haloperidol in receptor labelling assays (Bremner et al., 1978). In an attempt to characterize the nature of the inhibitory action of dl-propranolol on a raised mesolimbic dopamine function, d- and l-propranolol were assessed in the accumbens dopamine hyperactivity model. It was intriguing that d-propranolol was the most active in causing inhibition of the hyperactivity. This would strongly suggest that β-adrenergic receptor blockade (a property of the l-isomer) is not essentially involved in the behavioural effect. Marked autonomic responses are observed in psychiatric patients taking dl-propranolol, and it would be interesting to assess the importance of these changes to the therapeutic outcome by using the d-isomer. Knowledge

Table 1 Developments in drug therapy in schizophrenia: Activities of antischizophrenic/potential antischizophrenic drugs in man and in animals

Antischizophrenic/ potential antischizophrenic drug	Antipsychotic activity		Induction of pseudoparkinsonism		Increased serum prolactin		Anti-emetic action	
	man	Rodent Inhibition mesolimbic DA	Man	Rodent Catalepsy induction	Man	Animals	Man	Animals
Haloperidol	+	+	+	+	+	+	+	+
Pimozide	+	+	(+)	+	+	+	+	+
Halopemide	+⁻	+	0	0	?	?	+	+
Sulpiride	+	+	0	0	+	+	+	+
Propranolol	+	+	0	0	0	0	0	0
Apomorphine	+	+	0	0	(−)	(−)	(−)	(−)

+ active (in animal tests, this indicates a definite, dose-dependent activity), (+) inconsistent activity, 0 no activity, (−) opposite action to column heading (*decreased* serum prolactin, *induction* of emesis), ? unknown activity here would also be valuable in assessing the real value of the mesolimbic hyperactivity test in rodents for the detection of antischizophrenic agents. However, it must finally be added that it remains an open question as to whether we should be solely considering dopamine systems as a site of drug action for propranolol or whether we should be considering drug action on serotoninergic or other neurotransmitter mechanisms.

Another 'drug action' which would appear unusual is that of apomorphine. Apomorphine has long been accepted as a reference dopamine agonist, and yet, at low doses, this drug has been reported to reduce the symptoms of schizophrenia (see Di Chiara et al., 1978). An explanation for this paradoxical finding could be that apomorphine can activate both presynaptic and postsynaptic dopamine receptors, dependent on the dose. At low doses apomorphine is considered to inhibit presynaptic receptor mechanisms, which are frequently termed autoreceptors and which may be located on the dopamine neurone, to prevent the synthesis and/or release of dopamine (see Di Chiara et al., 1978). Low doses of apomorphine in animals can cause sedation, as do many neuroleptics and, even more indicative of a neuroleptic action, can inhibit the effects of a raised mesolimbic dopamine function (Costall et al., 1979). A drug having specific presynaptic dopamine agonist properties could, therefore, prove to be valuable for the treatment of schizophrenia, and a useful investigative tool (Table 1).

In considering developments or potential developments in the drug therapy of schizophrenia, a mention must be made of the possibility that opiate and other brain peptides may normally be involved in cerebral homeostasis and may dysfunction in schizophrenia. We would take a cautious approach here and refer the reader to Chapters 1–6.

For many years 'new' neuroleptics remained essentially similar to chlorpromazine and the interchangeability of the terms 'neuroleptic' and 'antischizophrenic' was as accepted as the hypothesis that an antischizophrenic agent was essentially one which blocked cerebral postsynaptic dopamine receptors. Now, with the use of agents such as propranolol and halopemide, it may be questioned whether the term neuroleptic can be so widely applied to agents which are antipsychotic. Indeed, it is particularly interesting that Rombaut and colleagues (1978) actually entitled their clinical paper 'Halopemide, a new potent non-neuroleptic dopamine-blocker with psychotropic properties'. Further, drug mechanisms must now encompass the knowledge that there are different dopamine systems in the brain and that the nature of the dopamine mechanisms may differ between the systems (for example, metoclopramide may affect those dopamine receptor mechanisms in the striatum, but not those in the nucleus accumbens) and within the areas (for example, one group of receptor mechanisms in the nucleus accumbens appear to modulate stereotyped behaviour whilst another group, requiring different structural characteristics for stimulation, appear to modulate locomotor activity). Further, an important addition is the concept of dopamine agonist action on autoreceptors to inhibit dopamine function. Finally, in addition to considering that neuroleptic agents may have differing affinities for the different cerebral dopamine mechanisms, it must be appreciated that neuroleptic agents may also have different effects on systems which modulate dopamine. Although, so far, we have considered neuroleptic drug action in terms of influence on cerebral dopamine systems, neuroleptic agents clearly interact either directly or indirectly with, at least, serotonin, GABA, noradrenaline and acetylcholine. For example, an enhanced serotonin effect within the mesolimbic system is important for neuroleptic action (Costall *et al.*, 1977; Costall and Naylor, 1978b). An interaction with GABA may facilitate a selective action on the mesolimbic system (Fuxe *et al.*, 1976). Therefore, the future development of drugs for the treatment of schizophrenia may require not only a differentiation of complex interactions with different dopamine mechanisms, but also the development of agents to specifically modulate GABA and serotonin systems.

References

Bédard, P., Parkes, J. D. and Marsden, C. D. (1978). Effect of new dopamine-blocking agent (oxiperomide) on drug induced dyskinesias in Parkinson's disease and spontaneous dyskinesias. *Br. Med. J.*, **1**, 954

Berger, B., Thierry, A. M., Tassin, J. P. and Moyne, M. A. (1976). Dopaminergic innervation of the rat prefrontal cortex: a fluorescence histochemical study. *Brain Res.*, **106**, 133

Blackburn, K. J., Bremner, R. M., Greengrass, P. and Morville, M. (1978). Selective affinities of bromocriptine and lergotrile for rat limbic dopamine binding sites. *Br. J. Pharmacol.*, **64**, 413

Borenstein, P. and Bles, B. (1965). Effects cliniques et électroencephalographiques du métoclopramide en psychiatrie. *Therapie*, **20**, 975

Borenstein, P., Champion, C., Cujo, Ph., Gekiers, P., Olivenstein, C. and Kramarz, P. (1969). An original psychotropic drug: sulpiride. *La Semaine des Hopitaux*, **19**, 1301

Bremner, R. M., Greengrass, P. M., Morville, M. and Blackburn, K. J. (1978). Effect of tolamolol and other β-ardenoceptor blocking drugs on (^{5}H)-haloperidol binding to rat striatal membrane preparations. *J. Pharm. Pharmacol.*, **30**, 388

Costall, B., Fortune, D. H. and Naylor, R. J. (1977). 5HT-antagonists inhibit neuroleptic and morphine antagonism of the hyperactivity induced by dopamine from the nucleus accumbens. *Br. J. Pharmacol.*, **60**, 206

Costall, B., Hui, S.-C. G. and Naylor, R. J. (1979). A demonstration of the ability of apomorphine to act on dopamine receptors on nerve terminals in the nucleus accumbens to reduce locomotor hyperactivity. *Br. J. Pharmacol.*, **67**, 475P

Costall, B. and Naylor, R. J. (1978a). Experimental studies of dopamine function in movement disorders. In Legg, N. J. (ed.) *Neurotransmitter Systems and their Clinical Disorders*, pp. 129–142. (London: Academic Press)

Costall, B. and Naylor, R. J. (1978b). Neuroleptic interaction with the serotonergic-dopaminergic mechanisms in the nucleus accumbens. *J. Pharm. Pharmacol*, **30**, 257

Costall, B. and Naylor, R. J. (1980). Assessment of the test procedures used to analyse neuroleptic action. *Rev. Res. Pharm. Sci.* (In press)

Di Chiara, G., Corsini, G. U., Moreu, G. P., Tissari, A. and Gessa, G. L. (1978). Self-inhibitory dopamine receptors: their role in the biochemical and behavioural effects of low doses of apomorphine. In Roberts, P. J., Woodruff, G. N. and Iversen, L. L. (eds.) *Advances in Biochemical Psychopharmacology, Vol. 19 Dopamine,* pp. 275–292. (New York: Raven Press)

Elizur, A., Segal, Z., Yeret, A., Davidson, S. and Atsmon, A. (1979). Antipsychotic effect of propranolol on chronic schizophrenics: a study of gradual treatment regimen. *Psychopharmacology,* **60,** 189

Elliott, P. N. C., Jenner, P., Huizing, G., Marsden, C. D. and Miller, R. (1977). Substituted benzamides as cerebral dopamine antagonists in rodents. *Neuropharmacology,* **16,** 333

Fielding, S. and Lal, H. (1974). *Neuroleptics, Vol. 1 Industrial Pharmacology,* (New York: Futura Publishing Company)

Fuxe, K., Bolme, P., Agnati, L. and Everitt, B. J. (1976). The effect of DL-, L- and D-propranolol on central monoamine neurones. I. Studies on dopamine mechanisms. *Neurosci. Lett.,* **3,** 45

Fuxe, K., Hökfelt, T., Ljungdahl, A., Agnati, L., Johnasson, O. and Perez de la Mora, M. (1976). Evidence for an inhibitory gabergic control of the mesolimbic dopamine neurones: possibility of improving treatment of schizophrenia by combined treatment with neuroleptics and gabergic drugs. *Med. Biol.,* **58,** 177

Jenner, P., Clow, A., Reavill, C., Theodorou, A. and Marsden, C. D. (1978). A behavioural and biochemical comparison of dopamine receptor blockade produced by haloperidol with that produced by substituted benzamide drugs. *Life Sci.,* **23,** 545

Justin-Besançon, L., Thominet, M., Laville, Cl. and Margarit, J. (1967). Constitution chimique et proprietes du sulpiride. *C.R. Acad. Sci. (Paris),* **265,** 1253

Laduron, P. M. and Leysen, J. E. (1978). Is the low incidence of extrapyramidal side-effects of antipsychotics associated with antimuscarinic properties? *J. Pharm. Pharmacol.,* **30,** 120

Leysen, J. E., Niemegeers, C. J. E., Tollenaere, J. P. and Laduron, P. M. (1978). Serotonergic component of neuroleptic receptors. *Nature,* **272,** 168

Loonen, A. J. M., Van Wijngaardan, L., Janssen, P. A. J. and Soudijn, W. (1978). Regional localisation of halopemide, a new psychotropic agent, in the rat brain. *Eur. J. Pharmacol.,* **50,** 403

Peringer, E., Jenner, P., Donaldson, I. M. and Marsden, C. D. (1976). Metoclopramide and dopamine receptor blockade. *Neuropharmacology,* **15,** 463

Peters, D. A. V. and Mazurkiewicz-Kwilecki, I. M. (1975). Tyrosine hydroxylase activity in rat brain regions after chronic treatment with ±-propranolol. *J. Pharm. Pharmacol.,* **27,** 671

Pinder, R. M., Brogden, R. N., Sawyer, P. R., Speight, T. M., Spencer, R. and Avery, G. S. (1976). Pimozide: a review of its pharmacological properties and therapeutic uses in psychiatry. *Drugs,* **12,** 1

Price, P., Parkes, J. D. and Marsden, C. D. (1978). Tiapride in Parkinson's disease. *Lancet,* **2,** 1106

Robinson, O. P. W. (1973). Metoclopramide – side effects and safety. *Postgrad. Med. J.,* **49,** 77

Rombaut, N., Depoorter, H. and Brugmans, J. (1978). Halopemide, a new potent non-neuroleptic dopamine-blocker with psychotropic properties. Presented at the *XIth C.I.N.P. Congress,* July 9–16, Vienna

Roufogalis, B. D., Thornton, M. and Wade, D. N. (1976). Specificity of the dopamine sensitive adenylate cyclase for antipsychotic antagonists. *Life Sci.,* **19,** 927

Theodorou, A., Crockett, M., Jenner, P. and Marsden, C. D. (1980). Specific binding of ^{3}H-sulpiride to rat striatal preparations. *J. Pharm. Pharmacol.* (In press)

Ungerstedt, U. (1971). Stereotaxic mapping of the monoamine pathways in the rat brain. *Acta Physiol. Scand. (Suppl.),* **367,** 1

Wiesel, F. A. (1976). Effects of high dose propranolol treatment on dopamine and norepin-ephrine metabolism in regions of rat brain. *Neurosci. Lett.*, **2**, 85

Yorkston, N. J., Zaki, S. A. and Havard, C. W. H. (1978). Propranolol in the treatment of schizophrenia: an uncontrolled study with 55 adults. Roberts, I. E. and Amacher, P. (eds.) *Propranolol and Schizophrenia* pp. 39–68 (New York: Alan R Liss Inc.)

Index